FREE Study Skills Videos/DVD Offer

Dear Customer,

Thank you for your purchase from Mometrix! We consider it an honor and a privilege that you have purchased our product and we want to ensure your satisfaction.

As part of our ongoing effort to meet the needs of test takers, we have developed a set of Study Skills Videos that we would like to give you for FREE. These videos cover our *best practices* for getting ready for your exam, from how to use our study materials to how to best prepare for the day of the test.

All that we ask is that you email us with feedback that would describe your experience so far with our product. Good, bad, or indifferent, we want to know what you think!

To get your FREE Study Skills Videos, you can use the **QR code** below, or send us an **email** at studyvideos@mometrix.com with *FREE VIDEOS* in the subject line and the following information in the body of the email:

- The name of the product you purchased.
- Your product rating on a scale of 1-5, with 5 being the highest rating.
- Your feedback. It can be long, short, or anything in between. We just want to know your impressions and experience so far with our product. (Good feedback might include how our study material met your needs and ways we might be able to make it even better. You could highlight features that you found helpful or features that you think we should add.)

If you have any questions or concerns, please don't hesitate to contact me directly.

Thanks again!

Sincerely,

Jay Willis
Vice President
jay.willis@mometrix.com
1-800-673-8175

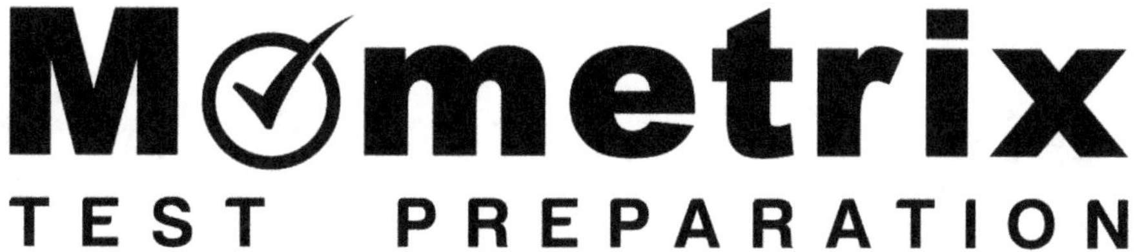

50% OFF
Online CNOR Prep Course!

By Mometrix

Dear Customer,

We consider it an honor and a privilege that you chose our CNOR Study Guide. As a way of showing our appreciation and to help us better serve you, we are offering **50% off our online CNOR Prep Course**. Many Certified Perioperative Nurse courses are needlessly expensive and don't deliver enough value. With our course, you get access to the best CNOR prep material, and **you only pay half price**.

We have structured our online course to perfectly complement your printed study guide. The CNOR Prep Course contains **in-depth lessons** that cover all the most important topics, **20+ video reviews** that explain difficult concepts, over **1,000+ practice questions** to ensure you feel prepared, and more than **500 digital flashcards**, so you can study while you're on the go.

Online CNOR Prep Course

Topics Included:

- Pre/Postoperative Patient Assessment and Diagnosis
- Individualized Plan of Care Development and Expected Outcome Identification
- Intraoperative Activities
- Communication and Documentation
- Infection Prevention and Control
- Emergency Situations
- Professional Accountabilities

Course Features:

- CNOR Study Guide
    - Get content that complements our best-selling study guide.
- Full-Length Practice Tests
    - With over 1,000 practice questions, you can test yourself again and again.
- Mobile Friendly
    - If you need to study on the go, the course is easily accessible from your mobile device.
- CNOR Flashcards
    - Our course includes a flashcard mode with over 500 content cards to help you study.

To receive this discount, visit us at mometrix.com/university/cnor or simply scan this QR code with your smartphone. At the checkout page, enter the discount code: **cnor50off**

If you have any questions or concerns, please contact us at support@mometrix.com.

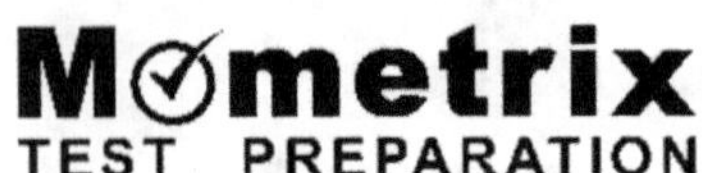

CNOR®

Exam Secrets

Study Guide

Your Key to Exam Success

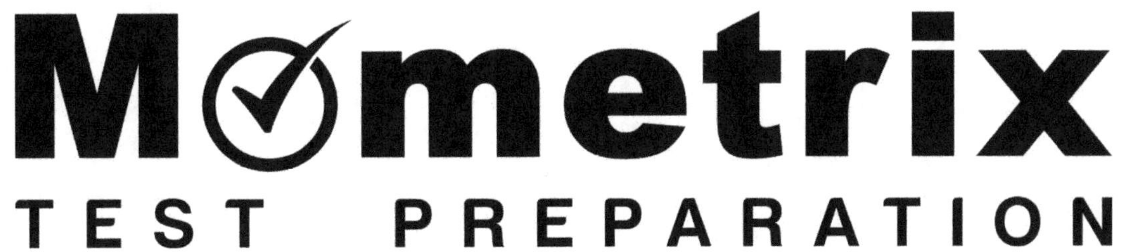

Written and edited by the Mometrix Nursing Certification Test Team

Paperback
ISBN 13: 978-1-60971-000-2
ISBN 10: 1-60971-000-2

Ebook
ISBN 13: 978-1-62120-292-9
ISBN 10: 1-62120-292-5

Hardback
ISBN 13: 978-1-5167-1363-9
ISBN 10: 1-5167-1363-X

DEAR FUTURE EXAM SUCCESS STORY

First of all, **THANK YOU** for purchasing Mometrix study materials!

Second, congratulations! You are one of the few determined test-takers who are committed to doing whatever it takes to excel on your exam. **You have come to the right place.** We developed these study materials with one goal in mind: to deliver you the information you need in a format that's concise and easy to use.

In addition to optimizing your guide for the content of the test, we've outlined our recommended steps for breaking down the preparation process into small, attainable goals so you can make sure you stay on track.

We've also analyzed the entire test-taking process, identifying the most common pitfalls and showing how you can overcome them and be ready for any curveball the test throws you.

Standardized testing is one of the biggest obstacles on your road to success, which only increases the importance of doing well in the high-pressure, high-stakes environment of test day. Your results on this test could have a significant impact on your future, and this guide provides the information and practical advice to help you achieve your full potential on test day.

Your success is our success

We would love to hear from you! If you would like to share the story of your exam success or if you have any questions or comments in regard to our products, please contact us at **800-673-8175** or **support@mometrix.com**.

Thanks again for your business and we wish you continued success!

Sincerely,
The Mometrix Test Preparation Team

Need more help? Check out our flashcards at:
http://mometrixflashcards.com/CNOR

Table of Contents

Introduction

Thank you for purchasing this resource! You have made the choice to prepare yourself for a test that could have a huge impact on your future, and this guide is designed to help you be fully ready for test day. Obviously, it's important to have a solid understanding of the test material, but you also need to be prepared for the unique environment and stressors of the test, so that you can perform to the best of your abilities.

For this purpose, the first section that appears in this guide is the **Secret Keys**. We've devoted countless hours to meticulously researching what works and what doesn't, and we've boiled down our findings to the five most impactful steps you can take to improve your performance on the test. We start at the beginning with study planning and move through the preparation process, all the way to the testing strategies that will help you get the most out of what you know when you're finally sitting in front of the test.

We recommend that you start preparing for your test as far in advance as possible. However, if you've bought this guide as a last-minute study resource and only have a few days before your test, we recommend that you skip over the first two Secret Keys since they address a long-term study plan.

If you struggle with **test anxiety**, we strongly encourage you to check out our recommendations for how you can overcome it. Test anxiety is a formidable foe, but it can be beaten, and we want to make sure you have the tools you need to defeat it.

Review Video Directory

As you work your way through this guide, you will see numerous review video links interspersed with the written content. If you would like to access all of these review videos in one place, click on the video directory link found on the bonus page: **mometrix.com/bonus948/cnor**

Secret Key #1 – Plan Big, Study Small

There's a lot riding on your performance. If you want to ace this test, you're going to need to keep your skills sharp and the material fresh in your mind. You need a plan that lets you review everything you need to know while still fitting in your schedule. We'll break this strategy down into three categories.

Information Organization

Start with the information you already have: the official test outline. From this, you can make a complete list of all the concepts you need to cover before the test. Organize these concepts into groups that can be studied together, and create a list of any related vocabulary you need to learn so you can brush up on any difficult terms. You'll want to keep this vocabulary list handy once you actually start studying since you may need to add to it along the way.

Time Management

Once you have your set of study concepts, decide how to spread them out over the time you have left before the test. Break your study plan into small, clear goals so you have a manageable task for each day and know exactly what you're doing. Then just focus on one small step at a time. When you manage your time this way, you don't need to spend hours at a time studying. Studying a small block of content for a short period each day helps you retain information better and avoid stressing over how much you have left to do. You can relax knowing that you have a plan to cover everything in time. In order for this strategy to be effective though, you have to start studying early and stick to your schedule. Avoid the exhaustion and futility that comes from last-minute cramming!

Study Environment

The environment you study in has a big impact on your learning. Studying in a coffee shop, while probably more enjoyable, is not likely to be as fruitful as studying in a quiet room. It's important to keep distractions to a minimum. You're only planning to study for a short block of time, so make the most of it. Don't pause to check your phone or get up to find a snack. It's also important to **avoid multitasking**. Research has consistently shown that multitasking will make your studying dramatically less effective. Your study area should also be comfortable and well-lit so you don't have the distraction of straining your eyes or sitting on an uncomfortable chair.

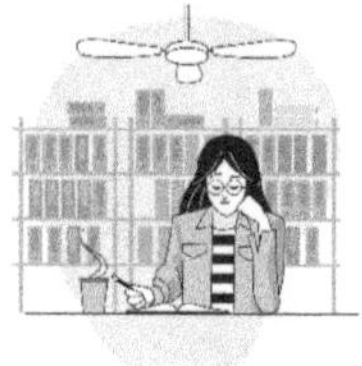

The time of day you study is also important. You want to be rested and alert. Don't wait until just before bedtime. Study when you'll be most likely to comprehend and remember. Even better, if you know what time of day your test will be, set that time aside for study. That way your brain will be used to working on that subject at that specific time and you'll have a better chance of recalling information.

Finally, it can be helpful to team up with others who are studying for the same test. Your actual studying should be done in as isolated an environment as possible, but the work of organizing the information and setting up the study plan can be divided up. In between study sessions, you can discuss with your teammates the concepts that you're all studying and quiz each other on the details. Just be sure that your teammates are as serious about the test as you are. If you find that your study time is being replaced with social time, you might need to find a new team.

Secret Key #2 – Make Your Studying Count

You're devoting a lot of time and effort to preparing for this test, so you want to be absolutely certain it will pay off. This means doing more than just reading the content and hoping you can remember it on test day. It's important to make every minute of study count. There are two main areas you can focus on to make your studying count.

Retention

It doesn't matter how much time you study if you can't remember the material. You need to make sure you are retaining the concepts. To check your retention of the information you're learning, try recalling it at later times with minimal prompting. Try carrying around flashcards and glance at one or two from time to time or ask a friend who's also studying for the test to quiz you.

To enhance your retention, look for ways to put the information into practice so that you can apply it rather than simply recalling it. If you're using the information in practical ways, it will be much easier to remember. Similarly, it helps to solidify a concept in your mind if you're not only reading it to yourself but also explaining it to someone else. Ask a friend to let you teach them about a concept you're a little shaky on (or speak aloud to an imaginary audience if necessary). As you try to summarize, define, give examples, and answer your friend's questions, you'll understand the concepts better and they will stay with you longer. Finally, step back for a big picture view and ask yourself how each piece of information fits with the whole subject. When you link the different concepts together and see them working together as a whole, it's easier to remember the individual components.

Finally, practice showing your work on any multi-step problems, even if you're just studying. Writing out each step you take to solve a problem will help solidify the process in your mind, and you'll be more likely to remember it during the test.

Modality

Modality simply refers to the means or method by which you study. Choosing a study modality that fits your own individual learning style is crucial. No two people learn best in exactly the same way, so it's important to know your strengths and use them to your advantage.

For example, if you learn best by visualization, focus on visualizing a concept in your mind and draw an image or a diagram. Try color-coding your notes, illustrating them, or creating symbols that will trigger your mind to recall a learned concept. If you learn best by hearing or discussing information, find a study partner who learns the same way or read aloud to yourself. Think about how to put the information in your own words. Imagine that you are giving a lecture on the topic and record yourself so you can listen to it later.

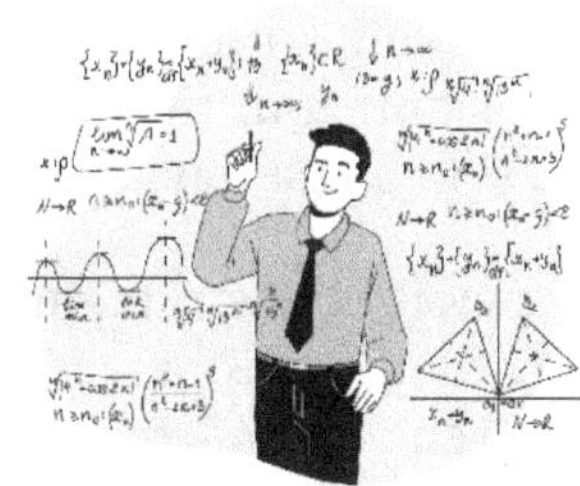

For any learning style, flashcards can be helpful. Organize the information so you can take advantage of spare moments to review. Underline key words or phrases. Use different colors for different categories. Mnemonic devices (such as creating a short list in which every item starts with the same letter) can also help with retention. Find what works best for you and use it to store the information in your mind most effectively and easily.

Secret Key #3 – Practice the Right Way

Your success on test day depends not only on how many hours you put into preparing, but also on whether you prepared the right way. It's good to check along the way to see if your studying is paying off. One of the most effective ways to do this is by taking practice tests to evaluate your progress. Practice tests are useful because they show exactly where you need to improve. Every time you take a practice test, pay special attention to these three groups of questions:

- The questions you got wrong
- The questions you had to guess on, even if you guessed right
- The questions you found difficult or slow to work through

This will show you exactly what your weak areas are, and where you need to devote more study time. Ask yourself why each of these questions gave you trouble. Was it because you didn't understand the material? Was it because you didn't remember the vocabulary? Do you need more repetitions on this type of question to build speed and confidence? Dig into those questions and figure out how you can strengthen your weak areas as you go back to review the material.

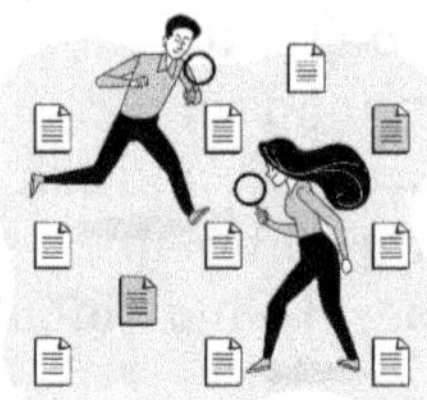

Additionally, many practice tests have a section explaining the answer choices. It can be tempting to read the explanation and think that you now have a good understanding of the concept. However, an explanation likely only covers part of the question's broader context. Even if the explanation makes perfect sense, **go back and investigate** every concept related to the question until you're positive you have a thorough understanding.

As you go along, keep in mind that the practice test is just that: practice. Memorizing these questions and answers will not be very helpful on the actual test because it is unlikely to have any of the same exact questions. If you only know the right answers to the sample questions, you won't be prepared for the real thing. **Study the concepts** until you understand them fully, and then you'll be able to answer any question that shows up on the test.

It's important to wait on the practice tests until you're ready. If you take a test on your first day of study, you may be overwhelmed by the amount of material covered and how much you need to learn. Work up to it gradually.

On test day, you'll need to be prepared for answering questions, managing your time, and using the test-taking strategies you've learned. It's a lot to balance, like a mental marathon that will have a big impact on your future. Like training for a marathon, you'll need to start slowly and work your way up. When test day arrives, you'll be ready.

Start with the strategies you've read in the first two Secret Keys—plan your course and study in the way that works best for you. If you have time, consider using multiple study resources to get different approaches to the same concepts. It can be helpful to see difficult concepts from more than one angle. Then find a good source for practice tests. Many times, the test website will suggest potential study resources or provide sample tests.

Practice Test Strategy

If you're able to find at least three practice tests, we recommend this strategy:

Untimed and Open-Book Practice

Take the first test with no time constraints and with your notes and study guide handy. Take your time and focus on applying the strategies you've learned.

Timed and Open-Book Practice

Take the second practice test open-book as well, but set a timer and practice pacing yourself to finish in time.

Timed and Closed-Book Practice

Take any other practice tests as if it were test day. Set a timer and put away your study materials. Sit at a table or desk in a quiet room, imagine yourself at the testing center, and answer questions as quickly and accurately as possible.

Keep repeating timed and closed-book tests on a regular basis until you run out of practice tests or it's time for the actual test. Your mind will be ready for the schedule and stress of test day, and you'll be able to focus on recalling the material you've learned.

Secret Key #4 – Pace Yourself

Once you're fully prepared for the material on the test, your biggest challenge on test day will be managing your time. Just knowing that the clock is ticking can make you panic even if you have plenty of time left. Work on pacing yourself so you can build confidence against the time constraints of the exam. Pacing is a difficult skill to master, especially in a high-pressure environment, so **practice is vital**.

Set time expectations for your pace based on how much time is available. For example, if a section has 60 questions and the time limit is 30 minutes, you know you have to average 30 seconds or less per question in order to answer them all. Although 30 seconds is the hard limit, set 25 seconds per question as your goal, so you reserve extra time to spend on harder questions. When you budget extra time for the harder questions, you no longer have any reason to stress when those questions take longer to answer.

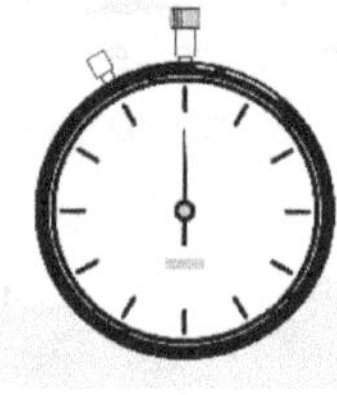

Don't let this time expectation distract you from working through the test at a calm, steady pace, but keep it in mind so you don't spend too much time on any one question. Recognize that taking extra time on one question you don't understand may keep you from answering two that you do understand later in the test. If your time limit for a question is up and you're still not sure of the answer, mark it and move on, and come back to it later if the time and the test format allow. If the testing format doesn't allow you to return to earlier questions, just make an educated guess; then put it out of your mind and move on.

On the easier questions, be careful not to rush. It may seem wise to hurry through them so you have more time for the challenging ones, but it's not worth missing one if you know the concept and just didn't take the time to read the question fully. Work efficiently but make sure you understand the question and have looked at all of the answer choices, since more than one may seem right at first.

Even if you're paying attention to the time, you may find yourself a little behind at some point. You should speed up to get back on track, but do so wisely. Don't panic; just take a few seconds less on each question until you're caught up. Don't guess without thinking, but do look through the answer choices and eliminate any you know are wrong. If you can get down to two choices, it is often worthwhile to guess from those. Once you've chosen an answer, move on and don't dwell on any that you skipped or had to hurry through. If a question was taking too long, chances are it was one of the harder ones, so you weren't as likely to get it right anyway.

On the other hand, if you find yourself getting ahead of schedule, it may be beneficial to slow down a little. The more quickly you work, the more likely you are to make a careless mistake that will affect your score. You've budgeted time for each question, so don't be afraid to spend that time. Practice an efficient but careful pace to get the most out of the time you have.

Secret Key #5 – Have a Plan for Guessing

When you're taking the test, you may find yourself stuck on a question. Some of the answer choices seem better than others, but you don't see the one answer choice that is obviously correct. What do you do?

The scenario described above is very common, yet most test takers have not effectively prepared for it. Developing and practicing a plan for guessing may be one of the single most effective uses of your time as you get ready for the exam.

In developing your plan for guessing, there are three questions to address:

- When should you start the guessing process?
- How should you narrow down the choices?
- Which answer should you choose?

When to Start the Guessing Process

Unless your plan for guessing is to select C every time (which, despite its merits, is not what we recommend), you need to leave yourself enough time to apply your answer elimination strategies. Since you have a limited amount of time for each question, that means that if you're going to give yourself the best shot at guessing correctly, you have to decide quickly whether or not you will guess.

Of course, the best-case scenario is that you don't have to guess at all, so first, see if you can answer the question based on your knowledge of the subject and basic reasoning skills. Focus on the key words in the question and try to jog your memory of related topics. Give yourself a chance to bring the knowledge to mind, but once you realize that you don't have (or you can't access) the knowledge you need to answer the question, it's time to start the guessing process.

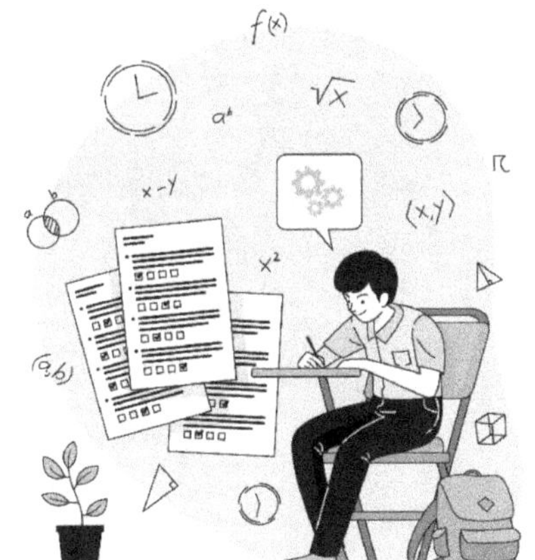

It's almost always better to start the guessing process too early than too late. It only takes a few seconds to remember something and answer the question from knowledge. Carefully eliminating wrong answer choices takes longer. Plus, going through the process of eliminating answer choices can actually help jog your memory.

Summary: Start the guessing process as soon as you decide that you can't answer the question based on your knowledge.

How to Narrow Down the Choices

The next chapter in this book (**Test-Taking Strategies**) includes a wide range of strategies for how to approach questions and how to look for answer choices to eliminate. You will definitely want to read those carefully, practice them, and figure out which ones work best for you. Here though, we're going to address a mindset rather than a particular strategy.

Your odds of guessing an answer correctly depend on how many options you are choosing from.

Number of options left	5	4	3	2	1
Odds of guessing correctly	20%	25%	33%	50%	100%

You can see from this chart just how valuable it is to be able to eliminate incorrect answers and make an educated guess, but there are two things that many test takers do that cause them to miss out on the benefits of guessing:

- Accidentally eliminating the correct answer
- Selecting an answer based on an impression

We'll look at the first one here, and the second one in the next section.

To avoid accidentally eliminating the correct answer, we recommend a thought exercise called **the $5 challenge**. In this challenge, you only eliminate an answer choice from contention if you are willing to bet $5 on it being wrong. Why $5? Five dollars is a small but not insignificant amount of money. It's an amount you could afford to lose but wouldn't want to throw away. And while losing $5 once might not hurt too much, doing it twenty times will set you back $100. In the same way, each small decision you make—eliminating a choice here, guessing on a question there—won't by itself impact your score very much, but when you put them all together, they can make a big difference. By holding each answer choice elimination decision to a higher standard, you can reduce the risk of accidentally eliminating the correct answer.

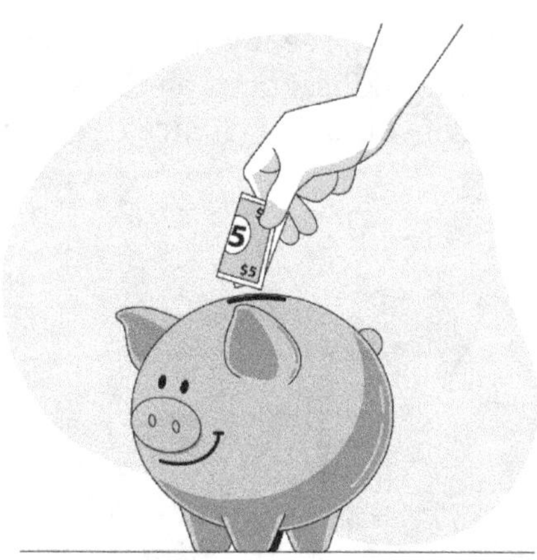

The $5 challenge can also be applied in a positive sense: If you are willing to bet $5 that an answer choice *is* correct, go ahead and mark it as correct.

Summary: Only eliminate an answer choice if you are willing to bet $5 that it is wrong.

Which Answer to Choose

You're taking the test. You've run into a hard question and decided you'll have to guess. You've eliminated all the answer choices you're willing to bet $5 on. Now you have to pick an answer. Why do we even need to talk about this? Why can't you just pick whichever one you feel like when the time comes?

The answer to these questions is that if you don't come into the test with a plan, you'll rely on your impression to select an answer choice, and if you do that, you risk falling into a trap. The test writers know that everyone who takes their test will be guessing on some of the questions, so they intentionally write wrong answer choices to seem plausible. You still have to pick an answer though, and if the wrong answer choices are designed to look right, how can you ever be sure that you're not falling for their trap? The best solution we've found to this dilemma is to take the decision out of your hands entirely. Here is the process we recommend:

Once you've eliminated any choices that you are confident (willing to bet $5) are wrong, select the first remaining choice as your answer.

Whether you choose to select the first remaining choice, the second, or the last, the important thing is that you use some preselected standard. Using this approach guarantees that you will not be enticed into selecting an answer choice that looks right, because you are not basing your decision on how the answer choices look.

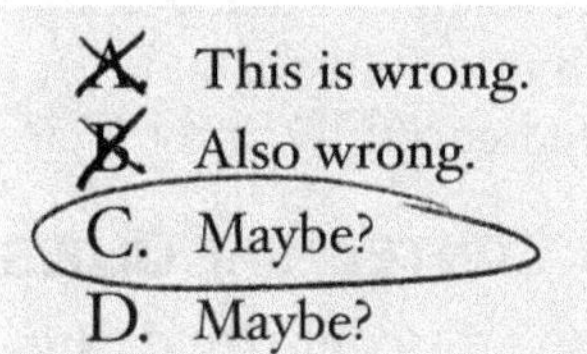

This is not meant to make you question your knowledge. Instead, it is to help you recognize the difference between your knowledge and your impressions. There's a huge difference between thinking an answer is right because of what you know, and thinking an answer is right because it looks or sounds like it should be right.

Summary: To ensure that your selection is appropriately random, make a predetermined selection from among all answer choices you have not eliminated.

Test-Taking Strategies

This section contains a list of test-taking strategies that you may find helpful as you work through the test. By taking what you know and applying logical thought, you can maximize your chances of answering any question correctly!

It is very important to realize that every question is different and every person is different: no single strategy will work on every question, and no single strategy will work for every person. That's why we've included all of them here, so you can try them out and determine which ones work best for different types of questions and which ones work best for you.

Question Strategies

☑ Read Carefully

Read the question and the answer choices carefully. Don't miss the question because you misread the terms. You have plenty of time to read each question thoroughly and make sure you understand what is being asked. Yet a happy medium must be attained, so don't waste too much time. You must read carefully and efficiently.

☑ Contextual Clues

Look for contextual clues. If the question includes a word you are not familiar with, look at the immediate context for some indication of what the word might mean. Contextual clues can often give you all the information you need to decipher the meaning of an unfamiliar word. Even if you can't determine the meaning, you may be able to narrow down the possibilities enough to make a solid guess at the answer to the question.

☑ Prefixes

If you're having trouble with a word in the question or answer choices, try dissecting it. Take advantage of every clue that the word might include. Prefixes can be a huge help. Usually, they allow you to determine a basic meaning. *Pre-* means before, *post-* means after, *pro-* is positive, *de-* is negative. From prefixes, you can get an idea of the general meaning of the word and try to put it into context.

☑ Hedge Words

Watch out for critical hedge words, such as *likely*, *may*, *can*, *sometimes*, *often*, *almost*, *mostly*, *usually*, *generally*, *rarely*, and *sometimes.* Question writers insert these hedge phrases to cover every possibility. Often an answer choice will be wrong simply because it leaves no room for exception. Be on guard for answer choices that have definitive words such as *exactly* and *always.*

☑ Switchback Words

Stay alert for *switchbacks*. These are the words and phrases frequently used to alert you to shifts in thought. The most common switchback words are *but*, *although*, and *however*. Others include *nevertheless*, *on the other hand*, *even though*, *while*, *in spite of*, *despite*, and *regardless of.* Switchback words are important to catch because they can change the direction of the question or an answer choice.

☑ FACE VALUE

When in doubt, use common sense. Accept the situation in the problem at face value. Don't read too much into it. These problems will not require you to make wild assumptions. If you have to go beyond creativity and warp time or space in order to have an answer choice fit the question, then you should move on and consider the other answer choices. These are normal problems rooted in reality. The applicable relationship or explanation may not be readily apparent, but it is there for you to figure out. Use your common sense to interpret anything that isn't clear.

Answer Choice Strategies

☑ ANSWER SELECTION

The most thorough way to pick an answer choice is to identify and eliminate wrong answers until only one is left, then confirm it is the correct answer. Sometimes an answer choice may immediately seem right, but be careful. The test writers will usually put more than one reasonable answer choice on each question, so take a second to read all of them and make sure that the other choices are not equally obvious. As long as you have time left, it is better to read every answer choice than to pick the first one that looks right without checking the others.

☑ ANSWER CHOICE FAMILIES

An answer choice family consists of two (in rare cases, three) answer choices that are very similar in construction and cannot all be true at the same time. If you see two answer choices that are direct opposites or parallels, one of them is usually the correct answer. For instance, if one answer choice says that quantity x increases and another either says that quantity x decreases (opposite) or says that quantity y increases (parallel), then those answer choices would fall into the same family. An answer choice that doesn't match the construction of the answer choice family is more likely to be incorrect. Most questions will not have answer choice families, but when they do appear, you should be prepared to recognize them.

☑ ELIMINATE ANSWERS

Eliminate answer choices as soon as you realize they are wrong, but make sure you consider all possibilities. If you are eliminating answer choices and realize that the last one you are left with is also wrong, don't panic. Start over and consider each choice again. There may be something you missed the first time that you will realize on the second pass.

☑ AVOID FACT TRAPS

Don't be distracted by an answer choice that is factually true but doesn't answer the question. You are looking for the choice that answers the question. Stay focused on what the question is asking for so you don't accidentally pick an answer that is true but incorrect. Always go back to the question and make sure the answer choice you've selected actually answers the question and is not merely a true statement.

☑ EXTREME STATEMENTS

In general, you should avoid answers that put forth extreme actions as standard practice or proclaim controversial ideas as established fact. An answer choice that states the "process should be used in certain situations, if..." is much more likely to be correct than one that states the "process should be discontinued completely." The first is a calm rational statement and doesn't even make a definitive, uncompromising stance, using a hedge word *if* to provide wiggle room, whereas the second choice is far more extreme.

⊘ Benchmark

As you read through the answer choices and you come across one that seems to answer the question well, mentally select that answer choice. This is not your final answer, but it's the one that will help you evaluate the other answer choices. The one that you selected is your benchmark or standard for judging each of the other answer choices. Every other answer choice must be compared to your benchmark. That choice is correct until proven otherwise by another answer choice beating it. If you find a better answer, then that one becomes your new benchmark. Once you've decided that no other choice answers the question as well as your benchmark, you have your final answer.

⊘ Predict the Answer

Before you even start looking at the answer choices, it is often best to try to predict the answer. When you come up with the answer on your own, it is easier to avoid distractions and traps because you will know exactly what to look for. The right answer choice is unlikely to be word-for-word what you came up with, but it should be a close match. Even if you are confident that you have the right answer, you should still take the time to read each option before moving on.

General Strategies

⊘ Tough Questions

If you are stumped on a problem or it appears too hard or too difficult, don't waste time. Move on! Remember though, if you can quickly check for obviously incorrect answer choices, your chances of guessing correctly are greatly improved. Before you completely give up, at least try to knock out a couple of possible answers. Eliminate what you can and then guess at the remaining answer choices before moving on.

⊘ Check Your Work

Since you will probably not know every term listed and the answer to every question, it is important that you get credit for the ones that you do know. Don't miss any questions through careless mistakes. If at all possible, try to take a second to look back over your answer selection and make sure you've selected the correct answer choice and haven't made a costly careless mistake (such as marking an answer choice that you didn't mean to mark). This quick double check should more than pay for itself in caught mistakes for the time it costs.

⊘ Pace Yourself

It's easy to be overwhelmed when you're looking at a page full of questions; your mind is confused and full of random thoughts, and the clock is ticking down faster than you would like. Calm down and maintain the pace that you have set for yourself. Especially as you get down to the last few minutes of the test, don't let the small numbers on the clock make you panic. As long as you are on track by monitoring your pace, you are guaranteed to have time for each question.

⊘ Don't Rush

It is very easy to make errors when you are in a hurry. Maintaining a fast pace in answering questions is pointless if it makes you miss questions that you would have gotten right otherwise. Test writers like to include distracting information and wrong answers that seem right. Taking a little extra time to avoid careless mistakes can make all the difference in your test score. Find a pace that allows you to be confident in the answers that you select.

✓ KEEP MOVING

Panicking will not help you pass the test, so do your best to stay calm and keep moving. Taking deep breaths and going through the answer elimination steps you practiced can help to break through a stress barrier and keep your pace.

Final Notes

The combination of a solid foundation of content knowledge and the confidence that comes from practicing your plan for applying that knowledge is the key to maximizing your performance on test day. As your foundation of content knowledge is built up and strengthened, you'll find that the strategies included in this chapter become more and more effective in helping you quickly sift through the distractions and traps of the test to isolate the correct answer.

Now that you're preparing to move forward into the test content chapters of this book, be sure to keep your goal in mind. As you read, think about how you will be able to apply this information on the test. If you've already seen sample questions for the test and you have an idea of the question format and style, try to come up with questions of your own that you can answer based on what you're reading. This will give you valuable practice applying your knowledge in the same ways you can expect to on test day.

Good luck and good studying!

Pre/Postoperative Patient Assessment and Diagnosis

Anatomy and Physiology

Anatomical Body Planes and Directional Terms

Body planes include the following:

- **Sagittal/Lateral**: The vertical plane that separates the body into right and left.
- **Median/Midsagittal**: The sagittal plane at midline (middle) that separates the body into equal halves.
- **Coronal/Frontal**: The vertical plane that separates the body into anterior (front) and posterior (back).
- **Axial/Transverse**: The horizontal plane that separates the body into superior (upper) and inferior (lower) parts.
- A **cross-section** is an axial/transverse (horizontal) cut through a tissue specimen or body structure while a **longitudinal section** is a sagittal or coronal (vertical) cut.

Body planes and anatomic terms

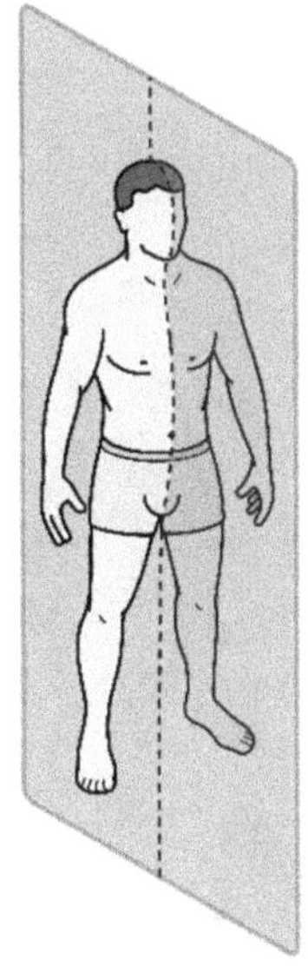

Sagittal/Lateral

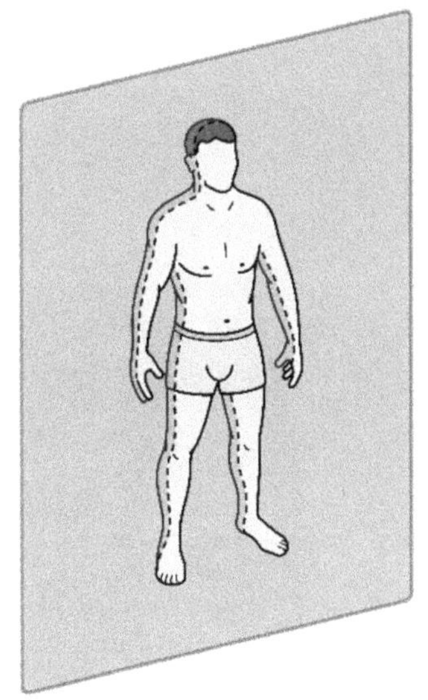

Coronal/Frontal

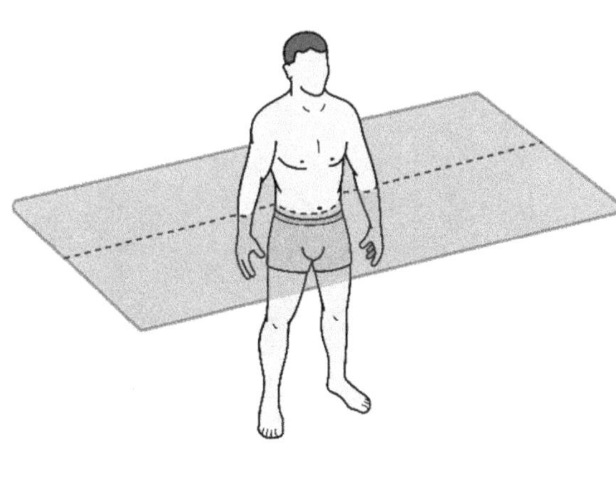

Axial/Transverse

Directional terms used when describing the body include the following:

- **Medial** is toward the midline while **lateral** is away from the midline and to the side.
- **Distal** is farthest from the point of reference and **proximal** is closest.
- **Superior** is above, **inferior** is below, **anterior** is toward the front, and **posterior** is toward the back.
- **Superficial** is close to the surface, and **deep** is away from the surface.
- When describing an area of the patient's body, the description should be patient-oriented, using phrases such as "the patient's left" and "the patient's right" to ensure accurate interpretation.

Abdominal Regions of the Body and Underlying Organs

Abdominal regions include the following:

- **A: Right hypochondriac**—right kidney, liver, gallbladder, and small intestine
- **B: Epigastric** (Epi = on, above)—stomach, liver, adrenal glands, pancreas, spleen, small intestine
- **C: Left hypochondriac**—left kidney, spleen, pancreas, and colon
- **D: Right lumbar**—ascending colon, liver, gallbladder
- **E: Umbilical**—small intestine, duodenum, umbilicus
- **F: Left lumbar**—descending colon, left kidney
- **G: Right iliac**—cecum, appendix
- **H: Hypogastric** (Hypo = below, beneath, less than normal)—bladder, female internal reproductive organs, sigmoid colon
- **I: Left iliac**—descending and sigmoid colon

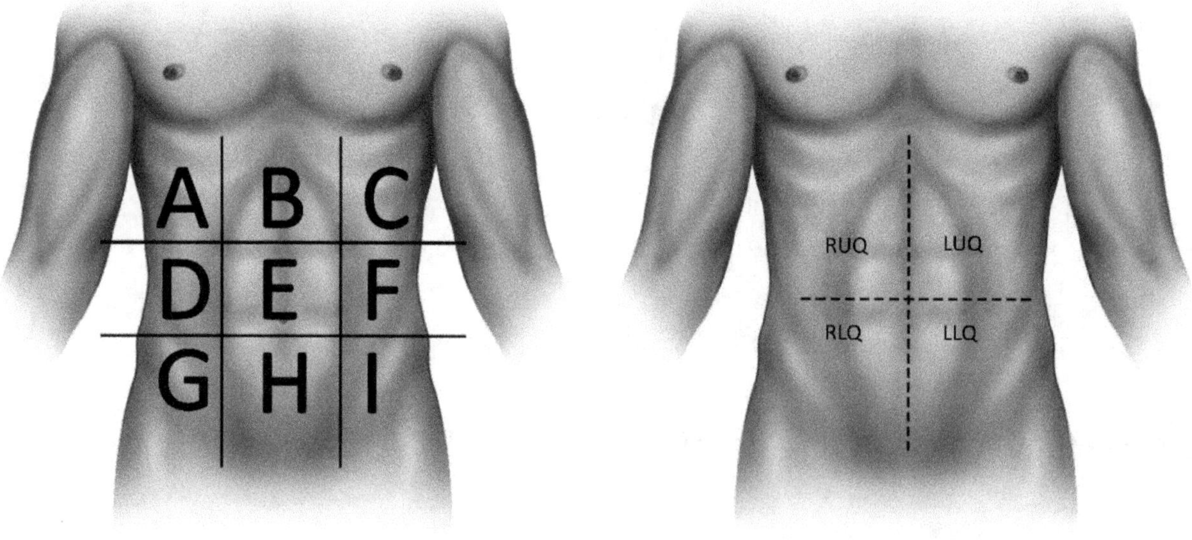

ABDOMINAL QUADRANTS

The abdomen may also be divided into four **quadrants** (sections) with the umbilicus (navel) at the center, helping to identify the position of organs:

- **Right upper quadrant** (RUQ): Duodenum, part of the ascending and transverse colon, hepatic flexure, liver, gallbladder, pancreas (head), right kidney, and right adrenal gland
- **Right lower quadrant** (RLQ): Cecum, appendix, right ureter, right fallopian tube, and right ovary
- **Left upper quadrant** (LUQ): Stomach, liver (left lobe), pancreas (body), left kidney, left adrenal gland, splenic flexure, spleen, part of transverse and descending colon
- **Left lower quadrant** (LLQ): Left ureter, left fallopian tube, left ovary, part of descending colon, and sigmoid colon

VENTRAL CAVITY

The ventral cavity, located on the anterior aspect of the trunk, comprises the thoracic and the abdominopelvic cavities, separated by the diaphragm. The walls of both cavities are comprised of skin, skeletal muscles, and bone. The organs within the cavities are the viscera.

- **Thoracic cavity**: The thoracic cavity is above the diaphragm and contains the lungs and the mediastinum, which separates the cavity into a right and left compartment. The heart, trachea, esophagus, and thymus gland lie within the mediastinum.
- **Abdominopelvic cavity**: The abdominopelvic cavity extends below the diaphragm to the pelvic floor, contains the upper abdominal cavity and the lower pelvic cavity (not physically separated). The organs within the abdominal cavity include the stomach, liver, gallbladder, spleen, kidneys, pancreas, large and small intestines. The pelvic cavity, encased in the pelvic bones, contains the internal reproductive organs, the bladder, and the distal part of the colon.

The cavities are lined with thin serous membranes, which secrete serous fluid that separates the parietal layer (lining the cavity walls) from the visceral layer (lining the organs). The membrane lining the thoracic cavities is referred to as the parietal pleura. The pericardial membrane lines the heart and the peritoneal membrane lines the abdominopelvic cavity.

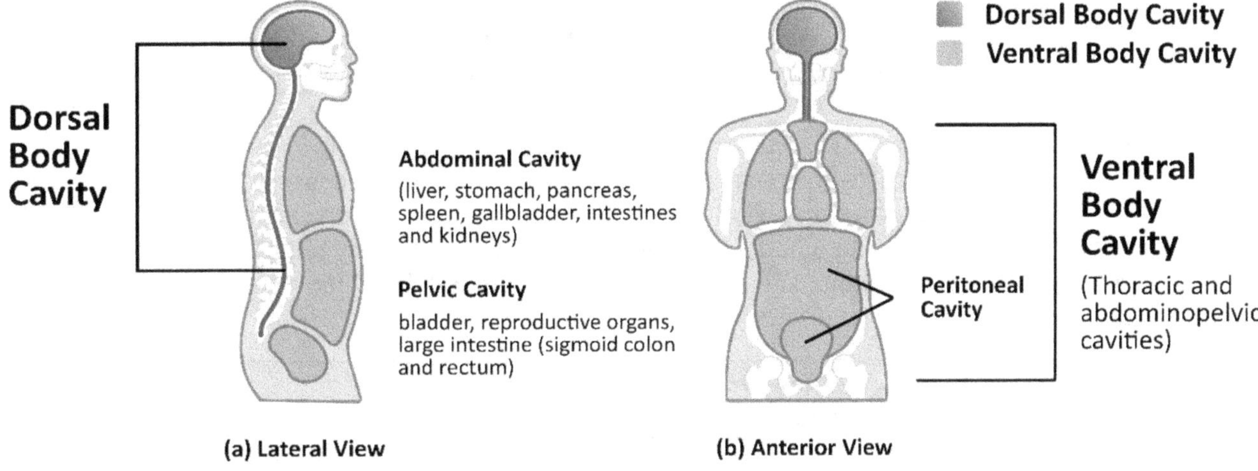

Dorsal Cavity

The dorsal cavity is located on the posterior (dorsal) aspect of the body and contains the brain and the spinal cord.

Cranial cavity: Encased in cranial bones at the bottom and the skull cap the top, this cavity contains the brain, the 12 cranial nerves, and the pituitary gland. The meninges (comprised of the dura mater, arachnoid mater, and pia mater) line the cavity and surround the brain and the spinal cord and contain cerebrospinal fluid between the arachnoid mater and pia mater in the subarachnoid space. The meninges and cerebrospinal fluid protect and cushion the dorsal cavity. The vascularized pia mater is adhered to the surface of the brain and the spinal cord. The middle layer, the arachnoid mater, contains connective tissue but not nerves or blood vessels. The enervated, vascularized dura mater is the outer layer that lies next to the bones and folds inward in places in the cavity and separates the brain into different compartments. The dura mater has two layers: The endosteal layer lines the cranial bones. The meningeal layer, which lines the endosteal layer within the cranium, lines the vertebral cavity.

Vertebral cavity: The vertebral cavity contains the vertebrae and the spinal cord. The meninges extend from the cranial cavity to enclose the vertebral cavity.

Body Systems

Each body system plays an important role in maintaining the life and function of the body.

Circulatory/Cardiovascular System

The circulatory system comprises the heart, arteries, and veins and pumps about 7000 liters of blood throughout the body each day to oxygenate and provide nutrients to the organs and tissues and to remove waste products. The circulatory system helps to maintain a stable body temperature and to maintain blood pressure.

Review Video: Functions of the Circulatory System
Visit mometrix.com/academy and enter code: 376581

Review Video: Heart Anatomy and Physiology
Visit mometrix.com/academy and enter code: 569724

Review Video: Heart Blood Flow
Visit mometrix.com/academy and enter code: 783139

Respiratory System

The respiratory system comprises the nasal passages, oral cavity, pharynx, larynx, trachea, bronchi, bronchioles, and lungs, which contain alveoli where oxygen/carbon dioxide exchange occurs. The respiratory system oxygenates the blood and removes carbon dioxide. Oxygenated blood returns to the heart and the circulatory system, and carbon dioxide is exhaled. Lung movements facilitate blood circulation.

Review Video: Respiratory System
Visit mometrix.com/academy and enter code: 783075

Digestive/Gastrointestinal System

The digestive system comprises the 8-meter alimentary canal that is continuous from the mouth to the anus and includes the mouth, pharynx, esophagus, small intestine, large intestine (colon), rectum, and anus. Mechanical digestion breaks down large food particles, and chemical digestion breaks down nutrients into a form that can be absorbed into the circulatory system in the small intestine. Fluid is reabsorbed into the circulatory system in the large intestine. Accessory organs that aid in digestion include the salivary glands, liver, gallbladder, and pancreas.

> **Review Video: Gastrointestinal System**
> Visit mometrix.com/academy and enter code: 378740

Endocrine System

The endocrine system produces the hormones that help to regulate the functioning of many organs.

Hypothalamus

The hypothalamus links the endocrine and nervous systems. It produces hormones that are stored in the posterior lobe of the pituitary gland and stimulates the pituitary to release hormones.

Pineal Gland

The pineal gland secretes melatonin and dimethyltryptamine, which control sleep cycles and dreaming.

Pituitary Gland

The posterior lobe of the pituitary gland secretes oxytocin (uterine contractions/lactation) and vasopressin (i.e., antidiuretic hormone, which raises blood pressure and promotes water reabsorption). The anterior lobe secretes hormones that control cell growth (somatotropin) and body growth (growth hormone), controls thyroid release of hormones (thyrotropin), controls release of steroids from the adrenal glands (corticotropin), and controls reproductive functions (follicle stimulating hormone and luteinizing hormone).

Thyroid Gland

The thyroid secretes hormones that control protein production, basal metabolic rate, and oxygen consumption (T3, T4, and calcitonin).

Parathyroid Glands

The parathyroid glands secrete parathyroid hormone, which controls the use of calcium.

Adrenal glands

The adrenal glands produce cortisol (roles in metabolism), aldosterone (water and sodium levels), and androgens (male hormones).

Ovaries

The ovaries secrete female hormones (estrogen and progesterone).

Testes

The testes secrete androgens (testosterone).

> **Review Video: Endocrine System**
> Visit mometrix.com/academy and enter code: 678939

INTEGUMENTARY SYSTEM

The integumentary system consists of the skin. The epidermis is the outer layer, and the dermis is the thicker inner layer. The two are separated by the basement membrane. The skin adheres to the underlying tissue by a subcutaneous layer (hypodermis) of connective and adipose tissue that is not part of the skin but insulates the internal organs and helps to conserve body heat. The skin provides barrier protection, prevents water loss, helps to control body temperature, contains sensory receptors, synthesizes chemicals (vitamin D), and excretes waste products.

Review Video: Integumentary System
Visit mometrix.com/academy and enter code: 655980

LYMPHATIC SYSTEM

The lymphatic system comprises lymphatic vessels, lymph nodes, tonsils, adenoids, and spleen and thymus. It is part of the body's immune system. Lymph circulates through the system and is filtered in the lymph nodes to remove harmful particles before fluid is returned to the blood. Hundreds of lymph nodes produce and store cells that fight infection. T-cells mature in the thymus, and the spleen filters blood produces and stores antibody-producing lymphocytes.

Review Video: Immune System
Visit mometrix.com/academy and enter code: 622899

MUSCULAR SYSTEM

The muscular system comprises about 700 muscles. Skeletal muscles attach to the skeletal system to allow movement; smooth muscles are contained inside organs such as the stomach and vessels to help propel substances, such chyme and blood. Cardiac muscle is found only in the heart and facilitates the circulation of blood. Muscle contractions also generate body heat and promote venous return.

Review Video: Muscular System
Visit mometrix.com/academy and enter code: 967216

SKELETAL SYSTEM

The skeletal system comprises 206 bones (adult), cartilage, and ligaments. Its functions include facilitating movement and support, storing minerals and controlling levels of calcium and other minerals in the plasma, storing fat in yellow bone marrow, and producing red blood cells in red bone marrow.

Review Video: Skeletal System
Visit mometrix.com/academy and enter code: 256447

EXCRETORY SYSTEM

The urinary system comprises the kidney, ureters, bladder, and urethra. The kidneys are responsible for the fluid and acid-base balance in the body. Kidneys filter out waste products from the blood, help to control blood pressure, and maintain fluid balance. The nephron is the functional unit responsible for filtering the blood (known as the glomerular filtration rate which ranges from 90-120 mL/min) and removing waste products.

Review Video: Urinary System
Visit mometrix.com/academy and enter code: 601053

Reproductive System

The female reproductive system includes the ovaries (which produce eggs and estrogen), fallopian tubes, uterus, cervix, vagina, vulva, labia minora, labia majora, and the clitoris, as well as the breasts. Functions include ovulation, fertilization, menstruation, pregnancy, and lactation. The male reproductive system includes the scrotum, testes (which produce sperm, androgens, and estrogen), epididymis, vas deferens, seminal vesicle, prostate, urethra, and penis. Functions include fertilization.

Review Video: Reproductive Systems
Visit mometrix.com/academy and enter code: 505450

Nervous System

The nervous system comprises the central nervous system (brain and spinal cord) and peripheral nervous system (cranial and spinal nerves), which contains sensory receptors. The somatic nervous system controls voluntary activities (such as muscle movement), and the autonomic nervous system controls involuntary activities (such as the function of organs). The functional unit is the neuron. The primary function of the nervous system is to receive sensory input, interpret it, and respond to it, as well as maintain homeostasis and control muscles and glands.

Review Video: What is the Function of the Nervous System
Visit mometrix.com/academy and enter code: 708428

Preoperative Preparation

Elements of Preoperative Preparation

Elements of preoperative preparation include the following:

- **IV placement**: An intravenous catheter is typically placed in a distal vein in the right or left arm. In some cases, a central line or a second IV catheter is placed (such as when blood transfusions are needed or anticipated).
- **Jewelry removal**: Jewelry removal is dependent upon the procedure being performed. Jewelry that may be a cause of trauma during surgery, that presents a risk of infection, and that may cause possible burns from metal during electrosurgical procedures should be removed prior to surgery.
- **Hair removal**: Hair does not need to be removed in most cases, but if hair at a procedural site is thick, it should be clipped rather than shaved if possible because shaving may cause micro skin abrasions that increase the risk of infection. However, antiseptic agents require a longer drying time on hairy skin surfaces. If hair removal is absolutely necessary, then clippers or chemical depilatories are generally preferred to razors.

Transporting Patients from Preoperative Area to Operating Room

The following are various considerations to be mindful of when transporting a patient from the preoperative area to the operating room:

- Confirm the patient's **identity** with two patient identifiers and check the **chart** to verify the correct site, the correct operation, and that the correct patient is being transported to the correct area. This can also be done verbally if the patient is able to respond.
- If the patient is able, they should confirm the **procedure** to be done, including which side if applicable, or the site.
- At this time the RN can check to make sure that the following are present on the **chart**: current history and physical, surgical consent, preanesthesia assessment and anesthesia consent, and labs or x-rays indicated. Also check that blood products ordered are crossmatched and ready and check for any devices or implants.
- Whether or not and how the patient is allowed to **ambulate** to the operating room is determined by patient condition.
- If a **stretcher** is used, it must have side rails, a safety belt, locking wheels, and be able to position the patient in various configurations.
- In transport with a stretcher, **side rails** should always be up and the **safety belt** in place. The comfort and dignity of the patient are maintained via the use of appropriate coverings.
- If **special equipment** (ventilators, EKG monitoring, etc.) or **additional personnel** are needed for transport, the nurse must secure these before transport begins.

Pre- and Post-Operative Assessment

CHART REVIEW

A chart review is a critical aspect of the preoperative health assessment. The entire record should be reviewed to look for information that may impact surgical outcomes, including the following:

- **Advance directives**, including DNR, which provide guidance regarding emergency situations.
- **Family history** that indicates a problem with surgery, such as sudden death after anesthesia.
- **Health history** that indicates bleeding, immunosuppression, antibiotic resistance, or negative response to anesthesia.
- **Allergy lists**, noting especially allergies to latex, foods, and medications. This should trigger the application of an allergy band to any patient with an allergy.
- **Surgical history**, including any operations that may include metal implants in order to ensure safe placement of grounding pads.
- **Laboratory findings**, including CBC, clotting times, and any other preoperative tests.
- **Imaging** results important to the surgical procedure.
- **Baseline vital signs**—BP, pulse, respirations—and oxygen saturation level if noted.
- **Medication list**, including medications that have been withheld (such as anticoagulants) and any medications taken the morning of the surgical procedure.
- **NPO** status.

PHYSIOLOGIC ASSESSMENT

The preoperative physiologic assessment may include the following:

- **Name, age, diagnosis, and surgical site**: To confirm the correct patient and the correct procedure, and identify whether the patient is very young or very old
- **Height and weight**: To identify alterations from normal that may pose potential risk to the patient and alter positioning in the surgical area
- **Allergies**: To prevent adverse medication reactions intraoperatively
- **Vital signs and diagnostic or laboratory acquisition**: To identify any abnormalities that may require special preoperative or intraoperative precautions or those that may possibly prevent a patient from being able to have the procedure performed before certain parameters are corrected
- **Medications**: To identify any medications that could interfere with physiologic parameters
- **Previous surgeries**: To identify any previous effects or complications from surgery
- **Nothing by mouth**: NPO status (to avoid delay of surgery)
- **Skin condition**: To assess for hydration or the presence of lesions
- **Impairments**: Sensory, mobility, prosthetic devices to identify anything that may alter positioning, postsurgical needs, or intraoperative considerations

VITAL SIGNS

Electronic or mechanical (manual) monitoring of vital signs is done preoperatively to establish baseline readings and done continuously through surgery by the anesthesia provider to monitor condition. The monitor is able to capture these vitals in real time so that the surgical team can track the patient's status throughout the procedure. The heart rate is measured through the electrodes attached to the patient's chest (generally a 3- or 5-lead). Respirations are also tracked through those electrodes, although movements or coughs can skew the reading and the patient generally should be visually assessed for any abnormal reading. When attached to a ventilator, the ventilator will monitor both respirations and ventilation more accurately. The blood pressure is monitored using a cuff that is attached to the patient's arm, and then to the monitor. The monitor can be set to measure the patient's blood pressure at any given time interval, depending on the patient's status and procedure. Any abnormal readings or alarms by the monitor should be followed up by an assessment of the patient and manual measurements.

NORMAL RANGES

Age	Heart rate	Respirations	BP (mmHg)
Neonate (newborn)	100-220 (average 140-160); begins to slow after 3 months	40-60 for a few minutes, then 30-40	Systolic 70-90
Toddler (12-36 mo.)	80-130	20-30	Systolic 70-100
Pre-school (3-5)	80-120	20-30	Systolic 80-110
School-age (6-12)	70-110	20-30	80-120/60-80
Adolescence (13-18)	55-100	12-20	110-131/64-84
Early adulthood (19-40)	60-100 (average 80)	12-20	100-119/60-79 to 140/90 (high)
Mid Adulthood (41-60)	60-100 (average 80)	12-20	100-119/60-79 to 140/90 (high)
Late adulthood (61+)	60-100 (average 70)	12-20	100-119/60-79 to 140/90 (high)

Review Video: Vital Signs and How to Check Them
Visit mometrix.com/academy and enter code: 330799

Additional Considerations

Additional elements of the preoperative physical assessment include the following:

- **Mobility**: Any physical limitations (paresis, paralysis, contractures, inability to walk, back pain, nerve damage) must be noted, as they may affect assessment during and after surgical procedures and may affect decisions about positioning in order to avoid causing further damage.
- **Body piercing**: Jewelry in and around the mouth should be removed prior to surgical procedures because those on the tongue, lip, or nose may interfere with visualization of the airway and may become dislodged and aspirated. In the case of electrosurgery, body piercings may conduct electricity, causing burns, if electrocautery is utilized. Therefore, the site of piercings should be evaluated as they relate to the location of the electrosurgery. Piercings may also interfere with imaging, causing artifacts, and cause burns or punctures if left in place during an MRI. All metal jewelry must be removed prior to MRI. Jewelry removal procedures vary, and some patients will want the tract maintained. In such cases, sutures or small catheters may be fed through the tract or non-metallic retainers placed if they do not interfere with the procedure or increase risk to the patient.
- **Implants or foreign objects**: Any implants or shrapnel must be noted as placing grounding pads over metal must be avoided. Breast implants may dictate a change in incision.

Preoperative Assessment Tools

Scott triggers are four items that are assessed. If 2 out of the 4 qualifications are met, this indicates increased risk of perioperative pressure injury.

- Age 62 or older
- Serum albumin <3.5 g/L or BMI <19 or >40
- ASA 3 or greater
- Estimated surgery time over 3 hours/180 minutes

The **Munro scale** is used to assess the risk of pressure injuries in each phase of surgery. Pre-procedural assessment includes weight and calculation of BMI, baseline temperature, and blood pressure.

Parameter	1	2	3
Weight loss in 30-180 days	No change or up to 7.4% weight loss	7.5-9.9% weight loss	≥10% weight loss
Intraoperative temperature	27.8-36.1 °C Temperature maintained	<36.1 °C or >37.8 °C Fluctuation of up to 2 °C	<36.1 °C or >37.8 °C Fluctuation of >2 °C
Intraoperative hypotension	Absent or ≤10% BP change	Fluctuating or 11-20% BP change	Persistent or 21-50% BP change

BRADEN SCALE

The Braden scale is a risk assessment tool that has been validated clinically as predictive of the risk of patient's developing pressure sores. It was developed in 1988 by Barbara Braden and Nancy Bergstrom and is in wide use. The scale scores six different areas with five areas scored 1-4 points, and one area 1-3 points. The lower the score, the greater the risk.

Area	Score of 1	Score of 2	Score of 3	Score of 4
Sensory perception	Completely limited	Very limited	Slightly limited	No impairment
Moisture	Constantly moist	Very moist	Occasionally moist	Rarely moist
Activity	Bed	Chair	Occasional walk	Frequent walk
Mobility	Immobile	Limited	Slightly limited	No limitations
Nutritional pattern	Very poor	Inadequate	Adequate	Excellent
Friction and shear	Problem	Potential problem	No apparent problem	

AMERICAN SOCIETY OF ANESTHESIOLOGISTS PHYSICAL STATUS CLASSIFICATION SYSTEM

ASA I	Normal, healthy, non-smoking, no or minimal alcohol use
ASA II	Mild systemic disease without substantive functional limitations. Includes current smoker, social drinker, pregnancy, obesity (BMI 30-40), mild lung disease, controlled diabetes mellitus/hypertension
ASA III	Severe systemic disease with substantive functional limitations, poorly controlled diabetes mellitus or hypertension, COPD, morbid obesity (BMI ≥40). May include active hepatitis, substance abuse, pacemaker, moderately decreased ejection fraction, ESRD with dialysis, history (>3 months) of MI, CVA, TIA, CAD/stents
ASA IV	Life-threatening severe systemic disease with history of recent (<3 months) MI, CVA, TIA, CAD/stents, ongoing cardiovascular disease (ischemia, severe valve dysfunction, decreased ejection fraction), shock, sepsis, DIC, ARD or ESRD but not having regular dialysis
ASA V	Moribund and likely to die without surgery: ruptured abdominal/thoracic aortic aneurysm, massive trauma, intracranial bleeding, ischemic bowel, multiple system dysfunction
ASA VI	Brain dead organ donor

Assessing for Surgery Positioning

The following are factors to assess for when considering positioning for surgery:

- **Skin integrity**: The intactness of the skin; the presence or absence of edema, lesions, erythema, and ecchymosis; adequate capillary refill
- **Cardiovascular integrity**: Blood pressure and heart rate, whether or not peripheral pulses are present, temperature of the skin, presence or absence of mottling
- **Neuromuscular integrity**: Intactness of reflexes, joint flexibility, presence or absence of numbness or tingling, ability to flex or extend limbs, strength
- **Pulmonary integrity**: Ability of lungs to ventilate, whether pulmonary disease might prevent proper ventilation in surgery
- **Surgical procedure to be performed**: Including positioning required, time of surgery, potential pressure points
- **Patient characteristics**: Age, height, weight, amount of muscle and fat deposition on body and location of deposition, nutritional status

Psychological Assessment

Psychological assessment elements include the following:

- **Understanding** of the procedure being performed, the site of surgery, expected outcomes of the procedure, and other perioperative activities to take place. The patient should have a basic knowledge of what will happen when the surgery is completed and what will be in the patient's potential discharge plan.
- Assessment of the patient's **ability** to understand information about the surgery and ability to comprehend information provided in patient teaching.
- Assessment of the patient's **readiness** to learn.
- Ability of the patient to **cope** with the situation or the procedure to be performed. This includes the assessment of anxieties about the procedure or outcomes of the procedure.
- Assessment of any **personal beliefs**, cultural aspects, or spiritual beliefs related to surgery.

Assessment of Nutritional Status

Assessment data a nurse may obtain regarding the nutritional status of a patient include the following:

- **Vital signs** may indicate problems with nutritional status (increased blood pressure may indicate too much sodium in the diet).
- Assessment of the patient's **diet** may indicate potential concern for proper nutrition (vegan diets, alcohol consumption and potential vitamin deficiency, high-fat or high-cholesterol diets).
- **Laboratory values** may indicate the presence or absence of anemia, hypoalbuminemia, or electrolyte imbalances.
- **Skin assessment** may indicate hydration status (dryness of skin or mucous membranes), ability to heal (presence of nonhealing wounds), and fragility of skin (skin tears).
- **Height and weight** may help to indicate whether the patient is over- or under-eating.
- **Increased weight** can also indicate fluid retention, which may also be indicated by the presence of ankle or leg edema and jugular venous distention. The urine can also be tested for specific gravity, which can indicate hydration status.
- **Urine and blood** can be tested for quality of diabetic control by looking for blood sugar values.

Assessment for Pain Control

Some assessment data a nurse may obtain regarding pain control for a patient include the following:

- Assess the patient for ability to **communicate pain** and for **developmental level**. If the patient is unable to communicate, variations in vital signs can be one indicator for pain control. For very young patients who cannot indicate number values of pain, facial expressions may help to indicate the presence of pain. Verbal patients who are able to communicate number values may be asked to use a 1-10 value system on rating pain.
- Assess a patient on **regular intervals** regarding the presence or absence of pain.
- When a patient indicates pain, assess methods available for **pain control** and any potential **side effects**.
- When various forms of pain control are used, assess the **effectiveness of the analgesia** at appropriate intervals after administration. Patients who have frequent pain may need alternative forms of pain management including the use of patient-controlled analgesia pumps to effectively manage their pain.

Postoperative Electrolyte Imbalances

Postoperative electrolyte imbalances may include:

- **Hypocalcemia** (<8.2 mg/dL) is associated with parathyroidectomy because of postoperative end-organ parathyroid hormone resistance and possible operative trauma. Other possible causes include impaired calcium absorption following pancreatectomy because of the loss of pancreatic enzymes needed in the duodenum and jejunum. Additionally, bowel resection may result in less available surface area for calcium absorption.
- **Hypokalemia** (<3.5 mEq/L) is a common finding after major abdominal surgery, such as gastric bypass or other bariatric procedures.
- **Hyperkalemia** (>5.5 mEq/L) may also occur and is associated with rhabdomyolysis, hypovolemia, massive transfusions, tissue ischemia, and trauma. Some medications, such as beta blockers and succinylcholine, increase risk of hyperkalemia.
- **Hyponatremia** (<135 mEq/L) is the most common electrolyte imbalance postoperatively and may be attributed to hypovolemia from vomiting or hypotonic fluid overload as well as SIADH and the administration of diuretics or excessive desmopressin to control diabetes insipidus. Hyponatremia is associated with hysteroscopy and a wide variety of surgical procedures.
- **Hypernatremia** (>145 mEq/L) is common after surgery involving the pituitary or hypothalamus because of increased incidence of diabetes insipidus.

Assessments in Patients with High Risks

Injuries Related to Wound Closure and Healing

The following are some things the perioperative nurse can assess for in the patient with a nursing diagnosis of high risk for injury related to wound closure and healing:

- Assess **wound edges** for good approximation including absence of dehiscence (separation) or evisceration (protrusion through wound).
- Assess for potential for **infection** or delayed healing secondary to class of wound, and whether wound is being allowed to close via primary, secondary, or delayed primary closure.
- Assess site for quality and amount of **drainage** from site, presence of erythema, pain, or cellulitis.
- Assess site for type of **closure** performed and whether sutures are absorbable, nonabsorbable, mono- or multifilament, and potential complications related to each type.
- Assess for **scar formation**, spitting of suture material at the wound site (although not done until sometime after surgery, perhaps on return of patient to surgery due to complications).
- Assess **drains** for proper use and functioning.
- Assess patient for **nutritional status and skin integrity** regarding ability to heal after surgery.

Injuries Related to Wound Infection

The following are some things the perioperative nurse can assess for in the patient with a nursing diagnosis of high risk for injury related to wound infection:

- Assessment can be made of the patient's **vital signs** to look for indications of infection (increased blood pressure, heart rate, or temperature).
- Assess **wound site** for evidence of purulent drainage, abscess formation, cellulitis, edema, and erythema.
- Assess **potential for infection** related to type of surgery performed, type of closure of wound and materials used, and potential for retained fragments in surgery.
- Assess the **process of asepsis** during surgical procedure to help prevent contamination of the wound site.
- Assess the patient for **nutritional status and skin integrity** before surgery for indications regarding ability to heal after surgery. Patients who are on immunosuppressive agents or who have chronic inflammatory conditions may indicate potential difficulty fighting infection and healing post-surgery.
- Check the chart for **prescribed antibiotics** to be given before, during, or after surgery to prevent infection.

Preventing Complications Related to High Risk of Infection

When a patient has a diagnosis of high risk for infection, the nurse can perform assessments of the patient and the environment in order to help prevent infection including:

- Assessment of **materials** to be used including storage, condition of packaging, sterility indicators, ventilation, and traffic through the operating suite. These assessments may reduce risk of infection from contaminated sources that may be presented to the patient during surgery.
- Assessment of the **patient** may include nutritional status, NPO status, skin integrity, hydration status, vital signs, and potential allergies to various forms of disinfectants. Poor nutritional status, potential for aspiration, and potential allergic reactions may contribute to the patient developing an infection during or after surgery.
- The nurse may assess the **type of surgery** to be performed and positioning desired during surgery, as more invasive surgery and certain positions required for surgery may potentiate infection in the surgical patient.

Preventing Complications Related to High Risk for Surgical Site Infection

When a patient has a diagnosis of high risk for surgical site infection, the nurse can perform assessments of the patient and the environment in order to help prevent infection including:

- Assess all materials used **prior to surgery** for sterility and proper functioning. Instruments that do not function properly can cause further injury and damage to surrounding tissues, allowing for potentially more areas for surgical site infection.
- Assess self and other members of the healthcare team for maintenance of **aseptic techniques.**
- Assess what surgery is to take place that day and the degree of **risk** or potential complications regarding the extensiveness or invasiveness of the surgery.
- Assess patient for **fever, erythema, induration, cellulitis, edema, drainage, abscess formation, dehiscence** post-surgery. Some of these factors will not present directly postoperatively, but any evidence of their formation should be assessed and indicated if present.

Injuries Related to Electrosurgery

The following are some things the perioperative nurse can assess for in the patient with a nursing diagnosis of high risk for injury related to electrosurgery:

- Before the procedure begins, an assessment can be made of the chart to ensure the proper type of **electrosurgical device** is being used.
- Assessment should be made that all proper parts of the electrosurgery device are **present,** that it has been adequately **inspected** by the biosurgical team according to hospital protocol, and that they found it to be in good working order.
- The nurse can assess that a **dispersing electrode** is being placed on the patient accurately. If there are weight limits, they should be taken into consideration.
- Assess whether the patient is in contact with **metallic surfaces** during the surgery, and that proper action is being taken to prevent such contact.
- Assessment and documentation of the **skin** before, during, and after the procedure will help to delineate if injury to the skin has occurred during surgery.

Injuries Related to Anesthesia

The following are some things the perioperative nurse can assess for in the patient with a nursing diagnosis of high risk for injury related to anesthesia:

- Assess the patient **prior** to administration of anesthesia for information necessary to have during the procedure in case of need, risk for injury during anesthesia, and if any premedications are to be administered.
- Assess the patient for **adverse reactions** to anesthetics in the past or potential reactions in the future.
- Assess for difficult airway, aspiration risks, and patient allergies.
- Assess **type of anesthesia** to be provided and any potential complications related to that particular agent or mode of delivery. Local anesthetics and moderate sedative procedures are of lower risk than general anesthesia.
- Assess the patient for proper **ventilation, perfusion, and vital signs** during and after anesthesia.
- **During** anesthesia administration, observe the amount of anesthesia the patient receives, and note the relaxation of the musculature in response to anesthesia.
- **After** anesthesia, assess the amount of sedation, ability to ventilate, cognition, circulation, and speed of emergence.

Injuries Related to Instrument Use in Surgery

The following are some things the perioperative nurse can assess for in the patient with a nursing diagnosis of high risk for injury related to instrument use in surgery:

- All instruments should be **assessed** for quality, sharpness, lubrication, that moving parts do so smoothly, that edges align appropriately, etc. All instruments should be assessed for integrity of packaging and sterility.
- **During** the surgery, assessment should include checking to see if an instrument is broken; **after** the surgery, instruments should be assessed for missing parts that were present before surgery (for potential retained fragments).
- Assessment should be made of the patient's **skin** before, during, and after surgery to detect edema, ecchymosis, or discoloration that may indicate injury to the surgical site. This also includes assessing the patient's vital signs frequently to assess for potential infection or injury related to poor instrumentation use.
- If an instrument is needed during surgery, and the nurse needs to sterilize it for use, assess whether or not the instrument is properly handled, cleaned, sterilized, and handed back off to the sterile environment without **contamination**.

Injuries Secondary to Bleeding and Hemostasis

The following are some things the perioperative nurse can assess for in the patient with a nursing diagnosis of high risk for injury secondary to bleeding and hemostasis:

- Assessment can be made of the patient's chart regarding **medication usage and doses** being taken, and whether or not all medications that may potentiate bleeding were stopped appropriately before surgery. Also check the chart for any allergies to any potential hemostatic devices to be used.
- Assess the patient for signs or symptoms of **adverse bleeding** (excessive ecchymosis, hematoma, low blood pressure, increased heart rate, signs of external bleeding, etc.) before, during, and after surgery.
- Assessment should be made of the type of device to be used for obtaining **hemostasis** in surgery and that the device is in good working order, with all appropriate equipment, and that all equipment is being used appropriately.
- Assess the patient's **blood type**, and whether or not the patient has any banked blood available for use during the surgery if indicated.

Assessment in Patients with Retained Surgical Fragments

The following are some things the perioperative nurse can assess for in the patient with a retained surgical fragment:

- The nurse can assess the patient's vital signs for **fever** and **increased heart rate or blood pressure** (which are difficult to differentiate between normal postoperative elevations and those due to retained fragments).
- **Cramping, pain, or abscess** of the site are also things the nurse may assess for that might indicate a potential retained fragment, although again, immediately postoperatively, these symptoms can be secondary to the surgery as well.
- The nurse can look at **x-ray films** of the surgical site (although these are ordered and read by the physician) to potentially view any evidence of retained fragments of the surgical site postoperatively.
- Most often all these symptoms will occur **later** in the healing process and after the patient goes home, indicating that the patient's surgical site needs to be reassessed, as there may be potential retained fragments within the surgical site.

Assessment Data Regarding Patient Safety

The following are some assessment data a nurse may obtain regarding a patient's safety:

- Assess **potential for injury** related to cognitive ability, age, and developmental level. Some populations have higher safety concerns related to their own ability to prevent injury or communicate discomfort or danger. Patients undergoing anesthesia are at high risk for injury related to inability to communicate discomfort.
- Assessment should be made of the **environment** in which a patient is located to prevent potential complications related to environmental hazards. These may include assessments of the presence of fire extinguishers in case of fire and fire exit routes, or potential sources of infection.
- Assessment of **patient positioning** at all times can help to keep a patient safe, including methods for transfer (adequate numbers of personnel for transfer, safety straps intact and holding patient appropriately) and equipment used in transfer (equipment is intact, functioning properly, side rails up, wheels lock properly).

Culturally Appropriate Interview Techniques

Nurses must remain culturally sensitive when conducting patient interviews in order to promote better communication and to avoid some misperceptions. When conducting a culturally appropriate interview, the nurse should keep in mind the ethnic and social background of the patient, including potential beliefs about health and healing, life experiences, language barriers, spiritual beliefs, and physical practices that may vary from Western medicine. When performing an assessment, the nurse should recognize the acceptable form of communication of the patient and practice it, particularly if this means using an interpreter. The nurse should identify spiritual practices that are important to the patient. Each nurse should recognize their own body language and consider how their nonverbal language is perceived by the patient, involve family members in the assessment if possible (if this is acceptable to the patient), and avoid developing biases or criticizing the patient for following practices that may be different from the nurse's beliefs.

Medication Reconciliation

Assessing Medication History

Assessing the patient's medication history is important to ensure **medication reconciliation**, which is the process of reviewing prescriptions when the patient is admitted in order to avoid errors. Assessing the patient's medical history is important to ensure that the patient is not taking any drugs that could interfere with surgical medications. For example, if a patient takes anticoagulants, this information is essential for providers to know so that steps to prevent excessive bleeding can be taken. If the patient must be NPO for surgery, that day's dose of medication may not be administered or may be delayed, depending on the medication and the type of surgery being performed. Medication assessment also includes the patient's use of herbal remedies. All herbal supplements should be brought to the attention of the nurse because there may be interactions between these preparations and the medications used for surgery. Additionally, the patient should clarify if there is a history of drug or alcohol abuse, as this can be damaging to the body and may impact the effectiveness of surgical medications.

Medications to Discontinue Prior to Surgery

Some medications may need to be discontinued for a period of time prior to surgery to prevent complications such as bleeding, dysrhythmias, and drug interactions. This is dependent upon the surgery, the prescribing physician, and the facility/operating surgeon. It is important to communicate this clearly to the patient. Encourage the patient to contact their prescribing physician if there are any discrepancies. Medications that may need to be discontinued prior to surgery and their general timeline for discontinuation include the following:

- **Aspirin or aspirin-containing compounds**: Stop 7 days preoperatively to reduce the risk of bleeding. Some surgeons may permit low-dose aspirin, depending on the operative procedure.
- **NSAIDS**, such as Celebrex, Naprosyn, and ibuprofen: Stop 7 days preoperatively to reduce the risk of bleeding.
- **Anticoagulants**, such as warfarin and Plavix: Time is determined by the physician on an individual basis, but generally stopped about 5 days before the operative procedure.
- **OTC herbs** (such as garlic and ginger tablets, ginkgo, St. John's wort, ginseng, chondroitin, and omega 3 fatty acids): Stop 14 days preoperatively to reduce risk of bleeding.
- **Vitamin E**: Vitamin E is often avoided for 14 days preoperatively because of increased risk of bleeding.
- **MAO inhibitors** (such as phenelzine, rasagiline, and selegiline): Stop 15 days preoperatively as they may interfere with some anesthetics.
- **Dabigatran, rivaroxaban, apixaban**: Hold 24-48 hours before surgery.
- **ACE inhibitors** and **ARBs**: Usually held on the day of surgery.
- **Diuretics** and **bisphosphonates**: Hold on the day of surgery.

MEDICAL MARIJUANA

Marijuana is prepared from the *Cannabis sativa* plant. The psychoactive element of marijuana is *delta-9-tetrahydrocannabinol* (THC). When marijuana is smoked, about 60% of THC is absorbed systemically. If ingested orally, only 6-20% is absorbed systemically, so oral doses must be 3-10 time higher to attain the same effect. Marijuana legalization has become more widespread, currently legal for recreational use in 15 states and the District of Columbia. Regardless of legality, it has been widely used for many recreational and medicinal purposes, such as to relieve anxiety, treat glaucoma, relieve symptoms of MS, reduce pain, and reduce nausea and vomiting. The FDA has approved a small number of drugs derived from marijuana, including:

- **Epidiolex (cannabidiol/CBD)**: The only directly cannabis-derived drug recently FDA-approved to treat severe forms of epilepsy (Dravet and Lennox-Gastaut syndrome).
- **Dronabinol (Marinol and Syndros)**: A synthetically derived drug that is used to treat nausea and vomiting and to stimulate appetite in AIDS patients.
- **Nabilone (Cesamet)**: A synthetically derived drug that is used to treat nausea and vomiting.

Perioperative Nursing Diagnoses

NANDA Nursing Diagnoses

North American Nursing Diagnosis Association (NANDA) (founded in 1982) is an association of professional nurses developed to standardize nursing terminology. In 2002, NANDA became NANDA International. NANDA developed a taxonomy of approved standardized nursing diagnoses that are used throughout nursing practice in the United States and other countries as well. The taxonomy is regularly evaluated and updated and new diagnoses added. For example, in the 11th edition of *NANDA International Nursing Diagnoses: Definitions and Classification, 2018-2020* (one of NANDA's official publications), the new categories of "associated conditions" and "at risk populations" were added. Nursing diagnoses are not the same as medical diagnoses, which identify the cause of a patient's problems. Rather, nursing diagnoses provide information about a patient's problems, such as "Activity intolerance related to weakness and fatigue," in order to guide nursing care. Taxonomy II, currently in use, organizes information in 3 levels: Domains (such as "Health Promotion" and "Perception/Cognition"), classes (class 1-6), and diagnoses.

PNDS

The Perioperative Nursing Data Set (PNDS), produced by AORN, is a standardized nursing language that categorizes perioperative nursing practice and provides terms and definitions for clinical problems (nursing diagnoses), interventions, and patient outcomes in order to reduce risks. PNDS is used to document standards of care. It is not itself a standard of care but is based on the Perioperative Patient Focused Model with its 4 domains:

1. Patient safety
2. Physiological response to surgery
3. Patient/family behavioral response to surgery
4. Health system

The PNDS domains are similar:

1. Safety
2. Physiological response
3. Behavioral responses
    a. Knowledge
    b. Rights and ethics
4. Health system

PNDS provides a common method of communication. The current edition (3rd) of PNDS provides language for 148 interventions, 39 outcomes, and 156 NANDA nursing diagnoses. Each component is coded with unique alphanumeric identifiers (diagnoses codes are consistent with NANDA). For example, E550 indicates evaluation of response to instructions under domain 3A:

Alpha	Numeric
A = assessment	Domain 1 = 0 – 199
IM = implementation	Domain 2 = 200 – 499
E = evaluation	Domain 3A = 500 – 699
O = outcome	Domain 3B = 700 – 899
	Domain 4 = 900 – 1100

Formulating a Nursing Diagnosis

Steps to formulating a nursing diagnosis include:

1. Attending to the patient's immediate concerns and needs, such as control of pain or toileting, so that the patient's needs can be more accurately assessed.
2. Completing and/or reviewing the patient's history and physical examination.
3. Reviewing laboratory and imaging reports.
4. Collecting data, such as vital signs, weight, reports of pain, and mobility limitations.
5. Questioning the patient about any concerns important to the patient.
6. Reviewing all data for commonalities that may suggest a nursing diagnosis.
7. Identifying problems and matching them to the NANDA nursing diagnoses.
8. Prioritizing nursing diagnoses and delineating expected outcomes.
9. Developing long-term and short-term goals based on the nursing diagnoses.
10. Identifying nursing interventions for each nursing diagnoses in order to facilitate expected outcomes.
11. Documenting nursing diagnoses, goals, and interventions, including a timeline when appropriate.

Individualized Plan of Care Development and Expected Outcome Identification

Individualized Plan of Care

PREOPERATIVE BEHAVIORAL RESPONSES OF PATIENTS

Common preoperative behavioral responses of patients include:

- **Anxiety**: Patients may exhibit anxiety in different ways. Some withdraw, children and adolescents may exhibit negative behaviors, and others exhibit self-comforting measures, such as rubbing hands together. In severe cases, a benzodiazepine, such as diazepam, may be indicated; however, keeping the patient informed, providing comfort measures, allowing their favorite toy/blanket, and reassuring the patient may help to reduce anxiety. If possible, patients should be allowed to listen to music as studies have shown doing so reduces anxiety.
- **Fear**: Some patients are fearful of needles, procedures in general, and anticipated pain and discomfort, and others face life-threatening procedures. Patients may appear panicked, so encouraging them to express feelings, listening, keeping the patient informed, and providing reassurance may help to reduce fear.
- **Pain**: Some patients who are experiencing pain may exhibit pain responses, such as moaning, crying, and moving about or lying in the fetal position. The patient should receive pain medication and comfort measures, such as heated blankets.
- **Confusion**: With confusion, patients should be monitored carefully, reassured, distracted (if possible), and given explanations in simple terms.

AGE SPECIFIC OPERATIVE NEEDS

The following are age specific operative needs:

Element	Pediatrics	Geriatrics
Room temperature	Patients have poor thermal insulation so operating room temperature must be increased before the child enters. Infants and toddlers may need overhead radiant heat. Temperature should be monitored continuously.	Thermal regulation may be impaired, increasing risk of hypothermia, so the patient should be kept warm during the operative procedure.
Instrument size	Special pediatric instruments are smaller in size and can be used in small spaces.	Instrument size depends on the patient's body size.
Anesthesia impact/ response	Repeated or prolonged use of anesthetic agents may result in developmental impairments in children under 3 years of age. Sevoflurane is preferred for inhaled induction. General anesthesia is needed for most procedures. Dosages of anesthetic agents must be titrated for age and size.	Patients may have exaggerated response to anesthetic agents, so the dosage may have to be adjusted. Agents on Beers criteria (such as benzodiazepines and meperidine) should be avoided. Chronic disease may impact choice of anesthetic agent. Anesthesia may increase risk of delirium.

Age-Related Needs Related to Surgical Plan of Care

All surgical patients must have a plan of care, in which problems such as comfort, hydration, skin integrity, or mobility are addressed with interventions. The patient's age can alter the plan of care, as age-related changes impact the patient's condition. Very young patients who are having surgery may not have the capacity to understand what is happening and need an adult to remain with them. They may be unable to explain how they are feeling, and the nurse should understand how young age impacts the ability to communicate and make appropriate accommodations. Alternatively, older age can affect the surgical procedure. Changes such as alterations in skin integrity, mobility, circulation, joint health, sensory impairments, and memory are all examples of age-related changes that the nurse may encounter. These changes should be identified as part of the pre-op assessment and the surgical plan of care should be modified to reflect these changes and to make accommodations.

Family Patterns to Consider with Surgical Patients

Family power structures vary widely; however, in many families, power rests with one person who makes ultimate decisions and whose opinions affect other family members, such as those having surgery. In many traditional cultures (Hispanic, Asian, Middle Eastern) power lies with the father, a grandparent, or another family member. However, in American society, this may vary because of diversity. Power may be shared or rest with the mother, the father, or another person.

Family patterns	
Nuclear	In this model, the husband is the provider (and often the decision-maker), and the mother stays home to care for the children, representing about 7% of current American families.
Dual career/ Dual earner	Both parents work, which is the case for about 65% of two-parent families. One parent may work more than another or both may work fulltime. There may be disparities in income that affect family dynamics.
Childless	10-15% have no children because of infertility or choice.
Extended	This may include multigenerational families or shared households with friends, parents, or other relatives.
Stepparent	Stepparent families are common. There may be harmony or jealousy and resentment on the part of siblings and estranged family members.
Extended kin network	Two or more nuclear families live closely together, sharing goods and services and supporting each other, including caring for children. This model is most common in the Hispanic community.
Single parent	The single parent (usually the mother) may be widowed, divorced, or separated, but more commonly never married. Children may have minimal or no contact with one parent, often the father. Single parents often suffer economic hardship.
Binuclear/ Co-parenting	Children share time between two primarily nuclear families because of joint custody agreements. While this may at times result in conflict, the child benefits from having a continued relationship with both parents although parents may hold different opinions about important matters.
Cohabiting	Unmarried heterosexual or homosexual couples live together. The relationships within this model may vary, with some similar to the nuclear family.
LGBTQ	Family structures vary widely; for example, lesbian couples may use sperm donors, and gay couples may adopt or use a surrogate to have children. Relationships may be open or traditional.

Cultural and Religious Considerations

Transcultural Nursing Theory

Madeline Leininger developed the theory of culture care diversity and universality (transcultural nursing theory) in 1974, based on anthropological concepts. Transcultural nursing considers cultural issues as central to providing care and promotes the study of cultural differences in relation to people's beliefs about illness, behavioral patterns, and caring behavior as well as nursing behavior. Leininger recognized that response to illness is often rooted in cultural beliefs and traditions. Based on research, the goal is to identify and provide care that is both culture-specific (fitting the needs of a specific cultural group based on their belief systems and behavior) and universal (based on belief systems and behavior that hold true for all cultures). Nurses are expected to assess and analyze transcultural factors to determine the most appropriate approach to care, considering not only the needs of ethnic or minority populations but also gender issues. The transcultural theory tries to find ways to accommodate traditional belief systems with modern medicine and to prevent cultural conflict.

Conscientious Objection

Conscientious objection is objecting or refusing to participate in an activity or treatment based on religious or moral grounds. In healthcare, conscientious objection most often relates to refusal of different types of treatment. Religious beliefs that may affect medical care include:

- **Christian Scientists**: They believe that prayer is the first treatment for sickness or disease. While the religion leaves participation in regular medical treatments up to the individual, many choose to have no medications or treatments. This can pose real challenges when parents have the power to make decisions regarding a child's care.
- **Jehovah's Witnesses**: They have traditionally shunned transfusions and blood products as part of their religious belief. However, they can receive fractionated blood cells, thus allowing hemoglobin-based blood substitutes.
- **12-step followers**: People with a history of addiction may be very reluctant on moral grounds to accept pain medication because of the fear of addiction.

Practices and Situations That May Impact Surgical Preparation

Practices and situations that may impact surgical preparation include:

- **Language barriers**: While using pictures, demonstrations, and pantomime and having family members translate may help to convey basic meaning, if a patient does not speak English, an official translator with experience in healthcare vocabulary should be used, if possible, to ensure that the patient understands and is able to convey concerns.
- **Rites and Ceremonies**: Before surgery those with different religious beliefs may want specific sacraments; for example, Buddhist patients may want to meditate or chant and Catholics have the Sacrament of the Sick with confession and Holy Communion. Muslim patients may want to pray and may avoid care provided by healthcare providers of the opposite gender. Native Americans may want healing ceremonies or other rituals.
- **Attire**: Members of the LDS (Mormon) church often wear sacred undergarments, but they can be removed for surgical procedures. The garments should never be placed on the floor or thrown away, even if soiled with blood. In that case, they should be sealed in a plastic bag and returned to the patient. Muslim patients may want to maintain modesty and keep their arms and legs covered as much as possible.

PATIENT-CENTERED CARE STAFFING MODEL

Patient-centered care is a staffing model used in acute care. Patients are aggregated not by diagnoses but by a similar need for care and services. Key elements of patient-centered care include the use of protocols or clinical pathways for clinical processes while customizing the nursing care plan according to the patient's needs and wishes. Staffing needs may vary according to the acuity level of the aggregate. Additionally, cross-training of staff is critical to ensure that staff members can assume different roles and have flexibility. While training adds value, it can also be time-consuming and costly, especially initially. All staff members, even housekeeping, are considered caregivers who must consider the needs, goals, and safety of the patient. Therefore, training must extend to all departments. The care plan is centered on the patient's needs, and communication with the patient should be open and honest with the patient having ready access to the health record.

Developing a Plan of Care

Presurgical Setting

Developing a plan of care for the patient in the presurgical setting involves both psychological and physical preparations for the patient. Obtaining an accurate and thorough assessment will lead to the development of appropriate desired outcomes and will assist the nurse in implementing interventions in order to meet those outcomes in the perioperative setting. Knowledge of the procedure being performed and any standards involved in the particular procedure or written preoperative orders will assist the nurse in performing pertinent activities for the patient, including medication administration and/or laboratory acquisition. In addition, knowledge of hospital policies and standards for medication administration and/or laboratory acquisition will assist the nurse in performing these activities at the appropriate time before the surgery takes place.

Review Video: Plan of Care
Visit mometrix.com/academy and enter code: 300570

Knowledge Deficit and Anxiety

Patients can have a deficit of knowledge about many different aspects of surgery. It can be due to a mere a lack of teaching, communication barriers (such as language differences), impairment in ability to learn, or other reasons. The desired outcome for a patient with this diagnosis would be that they will demonstrate knowledge in whatever area is necessary. The nurse can facilitate this by simply reiterating information, initiating a translator, identifying teaching needs, etc. Patients can be anxious at any point in the preoperative period and may or may not be able to delineate the exact reasons for feeling anxious. They may have physiological responses to anxiety (such as tachypnea, tachycardia, etc.). The desired outcome for patients with anxiety is that their anxiety level will decrease. This can be accomplished through the nurse actively listening to the patient's fears, providing information about the procedure, and providing reassurance.

High Risk for Infection

The following are some things the perioperative nurse can do to prevent injury in a patient who has a diagnosis of high risk for infection:

- Decrease **traffic flow** in the operating room area.
- **Dispose** of single-use devices instead of reusing them.
- If a patient is not NPO before surgery, notify the physician for **potential nasogastric tube placement**, gastric gavage.
- Use proper **positioning techniques** to prevent injury and subsequent source for infection.
- Use a proper **scrubbing agent** that the patient is not allergic to.
- Maintain good aseptic technique.
- **Clean instruments** properly during the procedure.
- Remove all contaminated items and nonsterile items from the field and replace with **sterile** ones if necessary.
- Make sure to include a **proper nutrition consult or plan** in the plan of care.
- If **antibiotics** are prescribed for the patient preoperatively, make sure they are given in a timely manner.

High Risk for Surgical Site Infection

Some things the perioperative nurse can do to prevent injury in a patient who has a diagnosis of high risk for surgical site infection include:

- Maintain good **aseptic technique**. Remove all jewelry, watches, artificial nails, etc. before scrubbing for the procedure.
- Remove **contaminated items** from the surgical field and replace if necessary.
- Accurately and effectively **communicate** with other members of the surgical team if contamination or a break in sterility occurs.
- Properly **clean and cover** operating room equipment before surgery to prevent sources of contamination to the surgical site.
- Perform adequate **skin prep**, cleaning the area from the surgical site outward, clean to dirty, etc.
- Wear proper surgical **personal protective equipment** including hats, masks, eye shields, gloves, and gown for prevention of transfer of organisms to patient.
- **Minimize talking** in the operating room to prevent bacterial invasion of the surgical area.

High Risk of Injury Related to Tourniquet Use

The following are some things the perioperative nurse can assess for in the patient with a nursing diagnosis of high risk for injury related to tourniquet use:

- Before the tourniquet is applied, the nurse will assess the **chart** and consult the **physician** for information regarding what type of tourniquet to use, on which extremity, location/type of procedure, length of time of the procedure, and to what pressure the tourniquet is to be applied.
- When applying a tourniquet, the skin should be assessed at the site of tourniquet placement for **skin integrity**.
- After applying the tourniquet, the nurse can assess for adequate **hemostasis** in the extremity by absence of capillary refill and pulselessness in that extremity.
- While prepping the skin for the procedure, assessment must be made to ensure that the **solution** has not been trapped in or around the tourniquet.
- The tourniquet must be assessed for adequate **pressure** throughout the procedure.
- **After** the procedure, the extremity can be assessed for nerve injury, bruise/blister formation, swelling of the extremity, and pain.

High Risk for Injury Related to Retained Surgical Fragments

The following are some things the perioperative nurse can do to prevent injury in a patient with the diagnosis of high risk for injury related to retained surgical fragments:

- Make accurate and appropriate **surgical counts** when setting up the operating area.
- Accurately **document** those counts in the appropriate areas (forms). If any additional materials are added to the field, be sure to document those materials as well.
- During the surgery, methodically keep **materials** that are used counted and together.
- Perform adequate surgical counts **after** the surgery has been completed and before closure of the patient begins.
- If an **inaccurate count** occurs, immediately and effectively communicate that information to the surgical and assisting personnel so the missing instrument/material can be looked for and located before closure begins.
- Do not **remove items** from the room until the procedure is completed and the patient has left the room.
- Once the patient has left the room, all materials are **removed** from the room to prevent miscounting with the next case.

Hemostasis and Increased Risk of Bleeding

A plan of care for a patient in surgery regarding hemostasis and increased risk of bleeding includes the following:

- Assess **medication usage** by the patient preoperatively and intraoperatively, searching for items that may potentiate bleeding. If items are identified, then those items are communicated quickly with the rest of the surgical team to ensure measures are undertaken to prevent injury to the patient.
- Check vital signs and other assessment data frequently for **signs or symptoms of bleeding** (decreased blood pressure, increased heart rate, hematoma formation, obvious external bleeding).
- **Coagulation studies** are monitored for adequate bleeding times.
- If a **tourniquet** is used, adequate pressure is maintained throughout the procedure.
- **Hemostatic agents** will be reconstituted appropriately before use.
- Ensure the **electrocautery device** is functioning properly and that all pieces of equipment are available and set up appropriately.
- The patient's **blood type** is adequately documented on the chart, and any banked autologous blood to be given intraoperatively is on hand.

DECREASING INJURY SECONDARY TO USE OF INSTRUMENTATION IN SURGERY

A plan of care for decreasing injury in a patient secondary to the use of instrumentation in surgery is described below:

- Assessment is performed of all **instrumentation** before use in surgery for adequate sterilization, packaging, storage, sharpness, lubrication, and movement. In addition, instruments that are tested by biological engineering are adequately tagged indicating proper functioning.
- Instruments will be added to the surgical field using **aseptic technique**.
- Instruments will be periodically **inspected for integrity** during the procedure, and all items that show signs of breakage or wear will be identified, removed from the field, and replaced. Any signs of broken instruments will be inspected to ensure that all fragments are removed from the surgical site.
- All instruments will be used in a manner in which they were designed or in a manner that is **appropriate** for use.
- Instruments needed for use during the procedure that have become contaminated or are not readily available will be properly **cleaned, disinfected, and sterilized** before use.

Expected Outcomes

Preoperative Setting

It is desirable that the patient who is being prepared for surgery be fully knowledgeable about the procedure that is being performed, the expected outcomes of the surgery to be performed, and any potential risks that are involved with the procedure. Once the patient demonstrates knowledge of the procedure, the patient should confirm this knowledge by signing consent for the procedure. Even at this point, the patient should have a basic knowledge of the expected length of stay after the procedure in the hospital, the intended amount of participation involved in recovery, and the expected discharge plan. In this setting, the patient should also be allowed to express any feelings of anxiety/fear and should be minimally anxious about the procedure to be performed. Additional outcomes such as freedom of infection or injury can be developed based on information received through the patient assessment.

Conscious Sedation and Regional Anesthesia

The following are expected outcomes for a patient undergoing conscious sedation and regional anesthesia:

- The patient will be as free from **anxiety** and **fear** as possible.
- The patient will be able to respond to **verbal stimulation** during the procedure, and complete anesthesia is not obtained.
- The patient will be able to maintain adequate **ventilation** and **perfusion** throughout the procedure with little or no assistance.
- The patient will not suffer **adverse/allergic reactions** to the anesthetic agents used.
- The patient achieves adequate levels of **sedation** and **analgesia** during and after the procedure.
- The patient's **vital signs** remain stable throughout the procedure.
- The patient will not suffer adverse effects from **spinal anesthesia** including headache, total spinal anesthesia, or intravascular injection.
- The patient will have a successful **recovery** from the sedative/anesthetic agents used and will return rapidly to their psychological and physiological pre-anesthesia state.

Anesthesia

The following are expected outcomes for a patient undergoing anesthesia:

- The patient will be as free from **anxiety** as possible before anesthesia begins.
- The patient will achieve adequate **anesthesia** and **analgesia**.
- The patient will have proper **musculature relaxation** during anesthesia.
- The patient will be free from signs or symptoms of an **adverse/allergic reaction** to the anesthetic agent including malignant hyperthermia.
- The patient will maintain adequate **ventilation** and **perfusion** during anesthesia throughout the post-anesthesia recovery period.
- The patient's **vital signs** will remain stable during anesthesia.
- The patient will not exhibit signs or symptoms of **aspiration** during anesthesia.
- The patient will not suffer **adverse effects** from anesthesia, including pain secondary to tissue disruption secondary to not being able to communicate areas of excessive discomfort or pressure.
- The patient will have a successful **recovery** from anesthesia to their pre-anesthesia state psychologically and physiologically.

Pain Control

The following are expected outcomes for a patient with regard to pain control:

- An accurate method for obtaining the patient's **level of pain control** is indicated (scale of 1-10, facial expression, and vital sign interpretation).
- The patient's pain will be adequately controlled using the least amount of **intervention** possible.
- The patient will not suffer adverse effects from the use of **pain medications**, including allergic reactions or undesirable side effects (nausea and vomiting).
- Patients with **high needs for pain control** will be adequately assessed and their pain managed appropriately with the use of epidural, patient-controlled anesthesia devices, etc.
- The patient's pain will **decline** over time, allowing pain control methods to be periodically decreased.
- The patient will not suffer other **adverse effects** from pain including anxiety, nausea, or vomiting.

Nutrition

The following are expected outcomes for a patient with regard to nutrition:

- The patient's **vital signs** will remain stable.
- Patients with **vegan/vegetarian diets** will consume adequate amounts of proteins and minerals.
- **Electrolyte imbalances** in patients with poor nutrition will be corrected and then maintained.
- The patient with **anemia** will achieve and maintain adequate iron stores and/or receive blood transfusions as indicated.
- The patient will achieve and maintain good **hydration status**.
- The patient will consume adequate amounts of **calories** for their metabolic needs.
- The patient will achieve and maintain adequate control of **blood sugar levels**.
- The patient will exhibit no adverse effects from being **NPO**. During NPO and after NPO status is reversed, adequate nutritional requirements are met.
- The patient will achieve and maintain adequate **protein stores** during hospitalization.

Wound Closure

The following are expected outcomes for a patient secondary to wound closure:

- The patient will have good **wound approximation.**
- **Pocket formation/hematoma** formation will not occur.
- The patient will be free of signs or symptoms of **infection** related to wound closure.
- The patient will be free from **dehiscence or evisceration.**
- The wound will exhibit **adequate healing** related to the age of the wound. Scar formation will be adequate, but not excessive.
- **Suture spitting** will not occur.
- Sutures with an appropriate **tensile strength** will be used to maintain wound closure.
- **Absorbable sutures** used will be properly absorbed by the body.
- The **skin** around the wound closure site will not be adversely affected by wound closure devices.
- **Drainage devices** will adequately drain the site of undesired fluids and maintain good wound approximation internally.
- **Dressings** will remain clean, dry, and intact as appropriate. Wet-to-dry dressings will adequately debride wound to allow for proper granulation tissue formation.

Electrosurgery

The following are some expected outcomes for a patient on whom electrosurgery is used:

- **Hemostasis** will be achieved throughout the procedure.
- The patient's skin will remain free of **burn injury** secondary to electrosurgical unit use postoperatively in areas that do not include the surgical site.
- The patient will not obtain injury related to **insulation failure**, **direct coupling**, or **capacitive coupling**.
- There will not be **excessive coagulation tissue** to cause sloughing and improper wound healing.
- If **fulguration** is being performed, adequate fulguration and removal of tissue is achieved.
- The patient will not be in contact with **metallic surfaces** during the procedure and while electrosurgery is being performed.
- Injury will not be incurred via initiation of fire by the **electrosurgical unit**.
- The patient will not suffer adverse effects from **plume inhalation** during the procedure.

Tourniquet Use

The following are expected outcomes for a patient on whom a tourniquet is used:

- The patient will be free from injury related to **tourniquet use** in surgery.
- The patient will be free from injury to the integumentary system related to use of **prep solutions**. Prep solutions will not be allowed to pool in or around the tourniquet.
- The patient will not suffer **bruise, blister, or other laceration** from use of the tourniquet.
- The patient will not suffer **hematoma** related to inappropriate tourniquet use/inflation.
- The tourniquet will maintain **adequate pressure** throughout the procedure.
- **Hemostasis** will be maintained throughout the procedure.
- Tourniquet **inflation time** will be kept to a minimum as desired by protocol/procedure/surgeon preference.
- The patient will not suffer **nerve or other musculoskeletal injury** related to tourniquet use.
- If two tourniquets are used, the patient will not suffer adverse effects from **excessive metabolite release** into the blood stream upon deflation of the tourniquet.

Instrumentation Use

The following are expected outcomes regarding the use of instrumentation in surgery:

- The patient is free from injury related to **instrumentation use** in surgery.
- The patient is free from signs or symptoms of **infection** systemically or at the surgical site.
- The patient has had no unintended **tissue disruption** secondary to the use of instrumentation.
- The patient will not suffer **adverse effects** from instruments not processed appropriately.
- **Instruments** will be used, packaged, cleaned, and transported in a manner that prevents excessive wear and damage to the instrument, thus maintaining cost containment.
- **Cutting instruments** will be handled by personnel appropriately to prevent injury to themselves or fellow personnel.
- Instruments are kept **moist** during and after surgery, gross contamination is removed, and instruments are kept free from environments that may potentiate **biofilm formation**.

Safety in the Perioperative Area

The following are expected outcomes for a patient with regard to safety and emergency situations in the perioperative area:

- The patient will not incur injury relating to **fire breakout** in the perioperative area.
- The patient will not suffer injury related to **chemical spill**.
- The patient will not suffer injury related to **natural disaster, bomb threat, or terrorist attack.**
- The patient will not suffer injury related to **electrical or radiation exposure**.
- The patient will not exhibit signs or symptoms of **infection**.
- The patient will not suffer injury related to **anesthesia administration**.
- The patient will be free from injury related to **impaired physicians, nurses, or other colleagues or families.**
- The patient will not suffer injury related to **positioning** or **transfer** into or out of the perioperative area.
- All **equipment** used for any of the above safety hazards mentioned will be in good working order at all times during need/use during an emergency situation.

Positioning

The following are expected outcomes for the patient with regard to positioning include:

- The patient's **skin** will remain intact and without evidence of superficial or deep tissue injury.
- **Dignity** and **comfort** will be maintained.
- The patient will not suffer **adverse cardiovascular effects** from positioning. The patient's heart rate, blood pressure, and pulses will remain intact to maintain adequate perfusion. The skin will remain warm and dry with brisk capillary refill.
- The patient will have no evidence of **nerve damage** postoperatively. All range of motion activities preoperatively will be maintained postoperatively, including strength and reflexes. The patient will not have postoperative pain, numbness, or tingling related to nerve compression or damage.
- The patient will maintain adequate **ventilation** during the procedure. Pulse arterial oxygen saturations will be maintained at adequate levels. As a more specific measurement, the patient's arterial blood gases will demonstrate adequate ventilation and oxygenation of the blood.

Intraoperative Activities

Operative Safety

Surgical Care Improvement Project (SCIP) Protocol

The Surgical Care Improvement Project (SCIP) evolved from the National Surgical Infection Preventions (SIP) Project, which was a joint venture of the CDC and the CMS intended to decrease the rates of surgical morbidity and mortality. Multiple national agencies are involved in this project. Hospitals must report rates of compliance with SCIP measures, which affects Medicare payments. These rates are subsequently published on Hospital Compare on the internet. Accrediting agencies, such as the Joint Commission, include the SCIP core measure set as part of evaluation. The SCIP core measure set includes: antibiotic prophylaxis given one hour prior to onset of surgery, appropriate antibiotic selection, antibiotic discontinuation with 24 hours postoperatively, controlled blood glucose level at 6 AM postoperatively, appropriate removal of hair, perioperative temperature management, receipt of beta-blocker when appropriate during perioperative period, and thromboembolism prophylaxis as indicated.

Fire Precautions in the Operating Room

Electrosurgical units (ESUs) cause 68% of fires in the OR and lasers cause 13%. Around 75% of OR fires occur because oxygen pools in drapes about the face and neck or inside the throat. This oxygen-enriched atmosphere (OEA) sparks easily. Oxygen, heat, and fuel combine to create combustion:

- **Oxygen**: Leakage from about connections and pooled oxygen in drapes and body cavities
- **Heat**: ESUs, lasers, and fiberoptic equipment
- **Fuel**: Ointments, solutions, dressing supplies, electrical equipment, and body and facial hair

Precautions include:

- Allow antiseptic solutions to dry for 2-3 minutes before drapes are applied about the head and neck and place drapes carefully to avoid creating pockets for oxygen to pool.
- Apply wet packing and keep it wet.
- Keep sponges and dressings wet to prevent ignition.
- Keep all dressing materials away from heat sources.
- Apply water-soluble jelly to facial hair.
- Use medical air (<30% oxygen) to decrease risk. If the patient requires more oxygen, a laryngeal mask or endotracheal airway should be utilized.
- Ensure the integrity of all anesthesia tubing to prevent leakage of gas.
- Keep sterile water or normal saline on the back table.
- Follow regulations for storing flammable solutions.

Prevention and Interventions for Fire, Chemical Spills, and Toxic Fumes

Preventative measures and interventions for a fire in the operating room include the following:

- Participate in **fire drills**.
- Instill a **fire prevention and management plan** that is built after a **fire prevention assessment** of the unit is conducted and analyzed.
- Be aware of the **fire triad**: Oxygen, fuel, and ignition. Have controls in place for these three contributing elements of fire ignition.
- Train to use firefighting equipment properly using the **PASS** and **RACE** protocols.
- Know where the **gas** panels, **electrical** panels, and **ventilation** systems are, and who is to shut them off, how, and when.
- Know how to set the **fire alarm** off and notify others of fire danger.
- Know how to contact the local **fire department**.

Preventative measures and interventions for **toxic fumes/chemical spills** in the operating room include the following:

- Know where all **SDSs** are kept.
- Be familiar with the **chemicals** used in the area and protocols for cleanup.
- Know who to **call** in case of caustic chemical spills.
- Know hospital policy for potential **removal** of patients and staff from an area for cleanup.

Roles of Healthcare Team Members During a Fire in Operating Room

Interventions in the case of a fire in the operating room are specific to the location of the fire:

- **Airway**: The anesthesiologist/anesthetist removes the tracheal tube and stops the flow of gases into the airway. The surgeon removes burning/flammable materials. The scrub nurse or surgeon pours water/saline into the burning airway and maintains the sterile field. The circulating nurse provides supplies and sounds alarms as needed. When fire is eliminated, the anesthesiologist/anesthetist reestablish ventilation and examines the ETT, and the physician assesses the patient's general condition and extent of injury.
- **Other parts of the body**: The anesthesiologist/anesthetist stops the flow of gases into the airway, the scrub nurse and surgeon remove all flammable or burning materials and use saline or water to put out the flames. The scrub nurse maintains the sterile field. The circulating nurse provides supplies and assistance and sounds alarms as needed. When fire is eliminated, the anesthesiologist/anesthetist assesses non-intubated patients for smoke inhalation, and the surgeon assesses the patient's general status and determines whether the procedure should be continued.

If the fire cannot be immediately extinguished, the circulating nurse should provide a CO_2 extinguisher and activate the fire alarm. The team should evacuate the patient if possible and close the door to the room. The circulating nurse or other designated team member should shut off gas to the room.

Laser Safety

The laser light used in surgical procedures poses a risk of fire. A laser safety officer (LSO) should be designated by the laser safety committee in any facility that utilizes lasers, in addition to a deputy LSO. The LSO should be aware of all laser safety procedures and precautions and should enforce the following:

- **Sterile water** should be available to put out small fires and to keep sponges and dressings moist to prevent ignition.
- **Laser-retardant drapes** should be used and wet dressings placed on the drapes about the surgical site.
- **Flammable solutions**, such as alcohol, should be **avoided**.
- Halon fire extinguishers should be available.
- For surgical procedures in the **mouth or larynx**, flame-resistant ETTs are indicated with the balloon inflated with water.
- For surgical procedures on the **head and neck**, oxygen and nitrous oxide may accumulate under drapes, risking ignition. These gases should be stopped or minimized while the laser is in use near the patient's head.
- The patient should be advised to **avoid hair spray** before surgery and the hair should be covered with wet dressings.
- The **laser foot pedal** must be placed correctly and away from other foot pedals to avoid confusion.
- **Eye protection** must be provided to the patient and surgical team to avoid accidental exposure injury.
- **Fire retardant surgical gowns** should be worn, and the circulating nurse should wear a flame-retardant scrub jacket that covers the arms.
- **Avoid instruments with reflective surfaces** as the laser reflection can damage the field.
- **Laser safety audits** should occur annually and when indicated by the LSO.

Chemical and Radiation Safety

Chemical safety requires facilities to strictly adhere to all local and federal guidelines as they pertain to chemical handling and chemical waste. A safety data sheet (SDS) must detail all chemicals that are used in the facility and should include procedures for safe handling and storage in addition to proper response to spills. Anesthesia machines may vent vapors from anesthetic agents, so gas-scavenging systems are essential as these vapors may lead to disease, such as cancer and liver disorders. Bone cement (methyl methacrylate or MMA) releases harmful vapors when the liquid and powder that makes the cement is combined, causing eye irritation and irritation of mucous membranes. A vapor evacuation system should be utilized during the mixing procedure. Formalin, which is used to preserve specimens, may irritate the respiratory tract and should be used only by those wearing masks and only in areas that are well-ventilated.

Radiation safety should be established and enforced by the radiation safety committee, led by the radiation safety officer, in all facilities where radiation exposure occurs. A radiation time out should occur before all procedures involving radiation to discuss the settings and procedure in addition to patient risk factors (in particular, pregnancy). Surgical procedures utilizing imaging, such as the C-arm or intraoperative CT/x-rays pose a risk of ionizing radiation. Exposure should be of the shortest possible duration, and adequate distance and shielding must be maintained with pregnant team members avoiding exposure. Lead (or lead alternatives such as tungsten, antimony, or bismuth-antimony) aprons should be worn under gowns during procedures that may expose the staff to radiation. Lead thyroid shields should also be used during fluoroscopic procedures and lead gloves for those handling x-ray cassettes. Perioperative team members exposed to radiation use should wear radiation monitors (dosimeters) that monitor their level of exposure.

Electrosurgery Safety

Complications of Electrosurgery

Direct Coupling

Direct coupling occurs when the active electrode from the electrosurgery instrument is charged when there is another instrument close by. This is most likely to occur during laparoscopic procedures when the instruments are in a relatively small space. The second instrument will become energized. This energy, or electric current, will then look for a way to travel back to the return electrode. This means that significant patient injury can occur as the electrical current travels through the tissue or body to follow the path of least resistance back to the return electrode. The main injuries seen with this complication are tissue burns. The spark that is generated when this occurs can result in tremendous heat production. If the spark occurs with metal clips it may result in damage or necrosis of the underlying tissue which could cause the clip to fall off the tissue or organ. The electrocautery instrument should never be activated unless all other instruments can be visualized and are not in close proximity.

Insulation Failure

Insulation failure can occur when there are breaks or holes in the insulation. These are usually caused by reprocessing or damage from use. These breaks in the insulation can serve as an alternative pathway for current to leave the electrode as it completes its circuit to the return electrode. If the generator is activated, the current can exit directly into patient tissue that is lying adjacent to the insulation. This can produce significant tissue damage. This can frequently occur outside of the surgical field of vision so the problem may go undetected until there is extensive tissue damage. To prevent an insulation failure from occurring, the insulation should be carefully inspected before every procedure. It should be examined for small cracks and defects, even on brand new units. The generator should not be activated until it is very close to the target tissue. This will ensure that the circuit can be completed through the target tissue without a deviation of the circuit into healthy tissue.

Preventing Patient Injury During Electrosurgery

When using an electrosurgery instrument, the lowest possible power setting should be used. This prevents accidental burning of tissue. The power setting can be adjusted if it is found that the lowest level is not effective. Before beginning a procedure, the instrument should be examined to assess for any breaks or cracks in the insulation. This should not be done only on older, reusable models, but also on brand new disposable cauterizers. Bipolar electrosurgery is safe because the electrical current is passed through one electrode, through the tissue that is grasped in the instrument, and back into the return electrode. There is no risk of the electrical current traveling through a large portion of tissue without warning. That is if all of the settings on the generator are correct and the patient does not receive a monopolar charge. Be very conscious of where the electrode is placed before activating the charge. This can prevent contact with other metal instruments within the patient's body, especially with laparoscopic procedures.

Before Surgery

The following are some things that can be implemented to prevent injury by electrosurgical burn **before surgery** takes place:

- Assess the patient for metal jewelry on the areas of the body located between the dispersing electrode and the active electrode. This jewelry should be removed. If the jewelry cannot be removed, alternative measures may be required, the patient educated on risks for burns, and the areas monitored.
- Place EKG electrodes away from the surgical site.
- Any electrodes used should be compatible with their subsequent **generators**.
- **Inspection** should take place of the generator and all subsequent parts for intactness and appropriateness for use.
- **Biomedical engineering** should inspect equipment regularly.
- **Alarms** should be set loud enough to hear adequately.
- All **cords** should be free of bending/kinking, and stretching.
- The generator should be kept free from contamination by **liquids**.
- Single-use electrodes should not be **re-used**. Reusable electrodes should not be used past anticipated lifespan of the instrument.
- The active electrode should be **shielded** on the field before surgery to prevent accidental burn injury.
- Dispersive electrodes should not be **altered** beyond their intended use. An appropriate electrode should be used according to patient size.
- If the patient has a metal implant (pacemaker, pump, etc.) the manufacturer should be contacted to confirm safety protocols for the device in the context of electrosurgery. If a pacemaker or ICD has to be turned off for the procedure, a defibrillator should be bedside.

During Surgery

Measures must be taken **during surgery** to prevent electrosurgical burns, including the following:

- Power settings should be **doubly confirmed verbally** with the surgeon prior to implementation.
- **Electrocautery** should only be used in well-ventilated areas away from flammable fumes/agents.
- The active **electrode** should periodically be cleaned with a moist sponge to prevent buildup.
- Placing the **dispersive electrode** on dry skin, close to the surgical site, over a large muscle mass helps to disperse current sufficiency. Scarred, fatty, or bony areas are not good places for placement.
- Keep the dispersive electrode away from **warming devices** to prevent thermal burn.
- Protect the patient from all **metal surfaces.**
- Frequently check adequate **connection** of the patient to the dispersive electrode.
- Any **defective parts** that are identified should be retained and sent to biomedical engineering so as to prevent injury to another patient.

Patient Positioning

Positioning Devices

There are various positioning devices that can be used to safely place the patient in proper positioning, including the following:

- **Foam products, pillows with silicone gel, cotton, sheepskin, and felt** are used on pressure point areas to reduce the amount of pressure on joints, limbs, nerves, etc.
- **Padded dressings** can be placed over bony prominences such as the heels, sacrum, or elbows to prevent pressure injury. They should be applied in a single layer.
- **Pillows** are used for positioning, elevating, and bolstering and can also help to protect certain pressure points.
- **Sandbags** are used to immobilize certain body parts.
- **Beanbags** can be formed to position body parts when air is removed from the bag via suction.
- **Tape** can be used to secure body parts for positioning if the patient is not allergic to adhesives.
- **Body rolls** and a **laminectomy frame** support the body.
- **Eye pads** keep the eyes closed and protect the eyes from injury. The eyes may also be lubricated if risk factors indicate, and/or dressings may be used for eyelid closure.

Of note, **blankets and sheets** are used to keep the patient warm, but AORN guidelines discourage their use for positioning due to increased risk for pressure injuries.

Transferring Patients from Stretcher to Operating Room Table

Considerations to be mindful of when transferring a patient from the stretcher to the operating room table include the following:

- The patient's **identification** is checked to make sure the correct site, operation, and patient are in the correct area.
- If a **stretcher** is used, the side rail closest to the table is lowered, the stretcher is butted against the table, wheels are locked, and the stretcher/table is moved up/down until they are the same height. All **lines and catheters** are identified and moved to prevent extubation in transfer.
- One member stands at the **far side** of the table to receive the patient, one member **behind** the patient, and ideally one member at the **head** and at the **foot** of the patient for transfer. The person at the head of the patient indicates that all members are ready for transfer and that all lines are free to move. The patient should be lifted via a roller or lifting sheet to the table and dragging should be avoided to prevent injury.

Positioning Patients Before Anesthetization

Various techniques can be used when positioning a patient before anesthetization takes place, including the following:

- Proper **body alignment** is taken into account when positioning the patient. Legs and arms are secured with the table strap and draw sheets as appropriate to prevent hanging.
- The patient should never be left on the table **unattended**.
- For patients who are awake, all positioning movements should be **described and explained** to the patient. The patient should be questioned whether they are comfortable and adjustments made accordingly. Warm blankets may be applied for comfort as well as elevating the head (for those patients who have trouble lying flat) until anesthesia ensues. The legs/ankles should be uncrossed before anesthesia begins.
- Care should be undertaken to make sure no body part of the patient contacts the **metal surfaces** of the table to prevent compression injury or potential electrical burn.
- No body parts are to **hang free** off the table. The entire body should be supported by the table.

Supine Position

The supine position (dorsal recumbent position) is the most common position for surgery.

Considerations include the following:

- This position is used for **head, neck, extremity, abdominal, thoracic surgeries**, and for **surgeries that are minimally invasive**.
- When the patient is in the supine position, the patient is on their **back** with the palms facing upward or inward.
- Arms may be positioned **in line with the body** and secured with the sheet (tucked between the back and mattress) or an arm guard, or they are positioned on an arm board extended from the body. The arms on an arm board are not extended more than 90 degrees. Arms can also be **flexed across the body** and secured.
- **Lumbar support** with a pad or pillow may be indicated as back strain may occur when relaxation occurs with anesthesia. Knees should be slightly flexed (5 to 10 degrees) to reduce pressure and DVT risk.
- The **table strap** is placed over the patient's legs, 2 inches above the knees to prevent hyperextension of the knees.
- Legs should be **parallel** and **heels raised**.
- Protective **padding** is placed on pressure points to prevent skin injury.

POTENTIAL COMPLICATIONS

Potential complications to the patient in the supine position include the following:

- Potential areas of **skin injury** due to pressure points in this position include the occiput, scapulae, thoracic vertebrae, styloid processes, olecranon, sacrum, coccyx, and the calcaneus. These areas are often padded, especially when the surgery is anticipated to last longer than 2 hours, with various padding pillows/devices.
- **Nerve groups at risk for injury** in this position include the brachial plexus, radial, ulnar, median, common peroneal, and tibial nerve groups. Care is taken that overextension of these nerves and extensive compression of these nerve groups is avoided.
- Due to decreased expansion of the rib cage in the posterior direction, the patient's **pulmonary vital capacity** is reduced. Care is taken to monitor the patient's ventilation and perfusion throughout the procedure to make sure that adequate oxygenation takes place.

TRENDELENBURG POSITION

The Trendelenburg position is essentially the supine position with the body and head positioned lower than the feet.

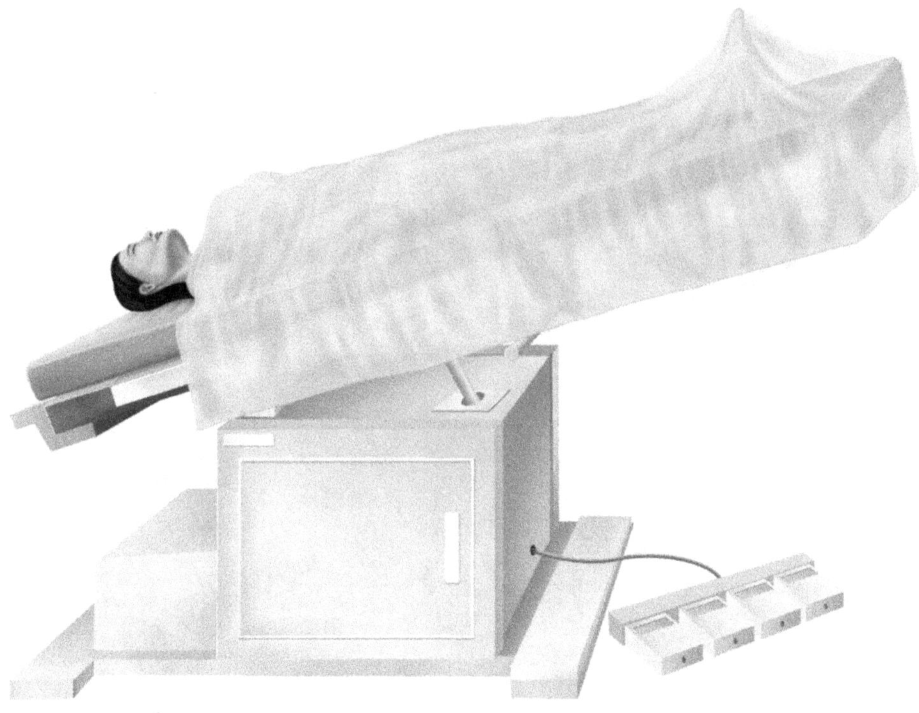

Considerations and precautionary measures include the following:

- **Pelvic surgery** and **lower abdominal surgeries** are commonly performed in this position. Patients who develop hypovolemic shock are also sometimes placed into this position to aid blood return to the vital organs.
- **Positioning devices** are used to help maintain the patient in the proper position and prevent friction injuries resulting from sliding. **Shoulder braces are no longer recommended** due to risk for compression of the brachial plexus.
- **Hands and arms** are properly secured to prevent extension beyond the mattress.
- Major redistribution of **blood volume and abdominal contents** occurs in this position, increasing intrathoracic, intracranial, and intraocular pressure. To reduce complications from this pressure, movement into and out of this position is done slowly at established intervals, and the patient is maintained in this position for as little time as possible.
- This position is **contraindicated in the severely obese** due to issues with oxygenation. If this position must be utilized in this patient, close monitoring of oxygenation and ventilation is required.

Reverse Trendelenburg Position

The reverse Trendelenburg position is achieved when the patient is in the supine position, and the table is left flat and tilted so that the head of the bed is elevated above the feet.

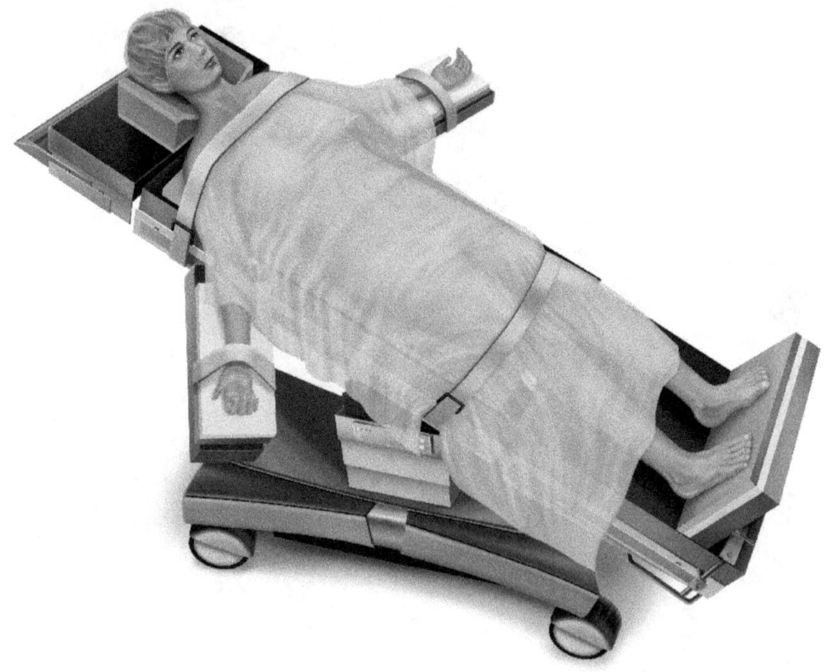

Considerations and precautionary measures include the following:

- **Head and neck surgeries** are often performed in this position.
- **Padding** for the supine position also takes place for the reverse Trendelenburg position, although additional padding is in place under the feet to prevent extensive compression against the soles and to help support the patient's body.
- It is important to maintain **sequential compression devices** and/or antiembolic stockings on the patient in this position, since pooling of blood is likely to occur.
- **Blood volume to the vital organs** is likely to be decreased in this position secondary to pooling of blood in the lower vasculature.

LITHOTOMY

The lithotomy position is a modification of the supine position in which the legs are secured in stirrups, which elevate and abduct them. Buttocks are positioned even with the break or the end of the table.

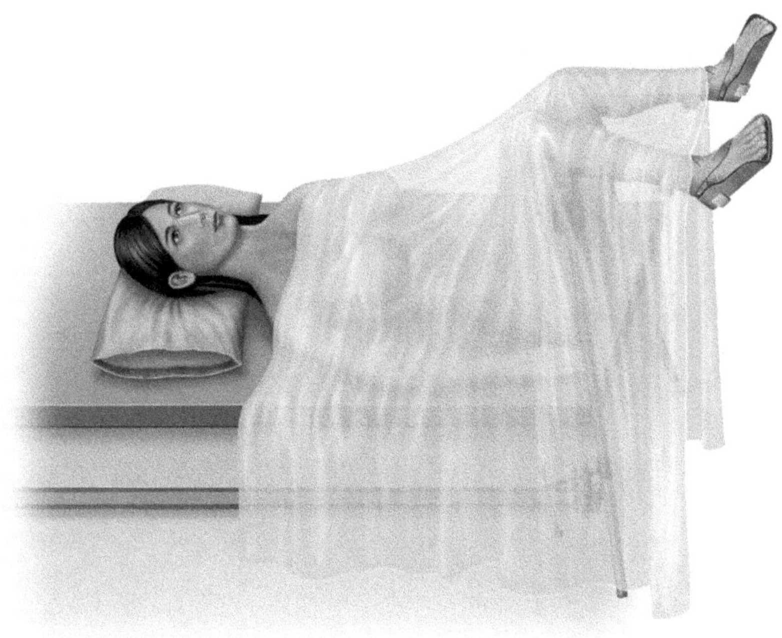

Considerations include the following:

- Surgery involving the **perineum, pelvis, and genitalia** utilizes this position.
- **Arms** are secured on arm boards.
- Padding may be placed under the **lumbar area** to prevent straining of this area, and all other standard padding for the supine position is utilized. The buttocks should rest even with the end of the bed so that the sacrum is secured over the bed.
- The legs are lifted **slowly** to prevent strain on the hip joints. Hips are not excessively flexed, extended, or rotated.
- The legs are secured in **evenly leveled stirrups** with the **heels in the lowest position possible**, then the lower section of the table is removed for the procedure to commence. The lower section of the table is returned before the legs are removed from the stirrups, brought together, and simultaneously lowered again after the procedure has completed.

Potential Complications

Potential complications with the lithotomy position include the following:

- There are many potential areas for **skin and nerve compression/damage** in this position and care is taken to pad all points of the stirrups, that they do not impinge on either side of the leg, and that they are at an appropriate height for the size of the patient's legs (preventing over extension/flexion of the legs). The femoral epicondyle, tibial condyles, and lateral and medial malleolar areas are of potential concern when positioning in stirrups.
- When the legs are lowered from the stirrups back onto the table at the completion of the procedure, blood diverts back from the body to the legs, and **hypovolemia** may occur. Lowering the legs carefully and slowly helps prevent this complication.
- Although blood flow to the lungs is usually good in this position, the patient's **respiratory capacity** is reduced secondary to pressure from the thighs and the abdominal contents on the diaphragm. This position should be avoided in the severely obese.

Prone Position

The prone position is achieved with the patient initially in the supine position on a stretcher. The patient is then transferred to the operating table slowly while turning the patient onto their abdomen.

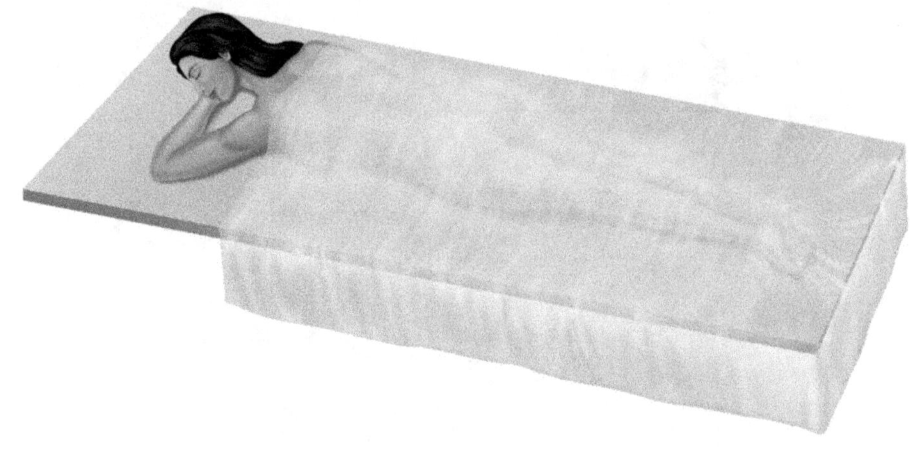

Considerations include the following:

- **Back, spinal, rectal, and posterior extremity surgery** is done in this position.
- The prone position **improves ventilation and perfusion to the lungs**.
- The **arms** may be placed with arm boards by the side or abducted outward no more than 90 degrees with palms facing downward, or they may be secured by the sides with a sheet or arm guards with palms faced inward.
- **Knee, chest, head, and ankle/foot pillows** are in place before the patient is turned onto the table.
- The **head** is positioned to the side to allow for adequate ventilation or can be placed midline with a face positioner.
- The **eyes** are closed and padded to prevent corneal abrasion and excessive eye pressure.
- The **chest** is supported on a laminectomy frame or rolls. Care is taken to prevent injury to breasts, genitalia, etc.
- A **table strap** is placed over the thighs above the knees to secure the body.

Sitting Position

The sitting (semi-sitting, semi-Fowlers, lawn chair) position is achieved by placing the patient on the table supine, lowering the feet, flexing the knees and pelvis, and raising the upper portion of the table.

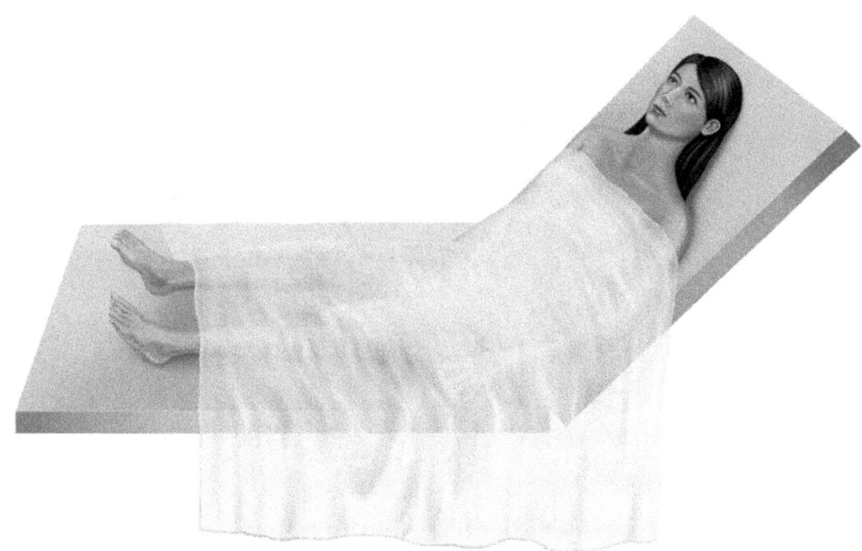

Considerations and precautionary measures include the following:

- Some **cranial procedures** are performed in this position. The semi-sitting position is used for nasopharyngeal, facial, breast, and neck surgery.
- A **body strap** is used to support the body upright across the thighs.
- To avoid hyperextension and dependency, the **arms are often flexed** and supported on a pillow placed on the legs/abdomen.
- **Padding** is done of the scalp, scapulae, olecranon process, popliteal areas, sacrum, ischial tuberosities, calcaneus, and the bottom of the feet.
- **Sequential compression devices** and/or antiembolic stockings are utilized to prevent pooling of blood in the extremities.
- **Negative pressure** occurs in the head in this position and a central venous pressure monitor with Doppler is used to monitor/protect from air embolism.

Lateral Position

The lateral position is a side-lying position in which the patient lies on either the right or left side, depending on the procedure being performed.

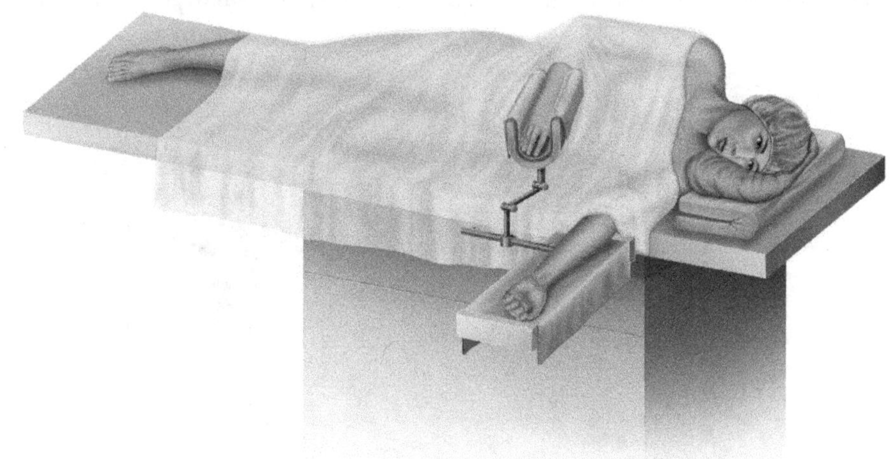

Considerations include the following:

- In the right **lateral position**, the patient lies on the right side with the left side up, and vice versa for the left lateral position.
- **Thoracic, kidney, retroperitoneal, and hip surgeries** are performed in this position.
- For **kidney surgery**, the patient's flank must be positioned over the kidney rest with the iliac crest below the table break. The table is flexed at the center break and the kidney rest portion of the table is raised.
- The **lower leg** is flexed.
- **Padding** is done of the lateral aspects of the legs, the feet/ankles, and the lower rib cage/axilla to prevent injury.
- The **table strap** is applied over the upper hip for support.
- The **arms** are secured on parallel, two-level arm boards, palms toward the center of the body, and allowed to slightly flex (they are not extended more than 90 degrees to prevent brachial plexus injury).

Potential Complications

Potential complications with the lateral position include the following

- **Peroneal damage, malleolar damage, and brachial plexus injury** can occur without proper padding of the lateral legs, feet/ankles, and dependent axilla, respectively.
- The ankles, knees, greater trochanter, iliac crest, shoulders, elbows, and wrists are prone to **pressure point damage**.
- **Dependent pressure and abdominal content pressure** decrease expansion of the dependent lung, which also receives a majority of the blood flow. Thus, the lung which is able to expand receives less perfusion, thereby compromising ventilation.
- **Pressure on the abdominal vessels** decreases circulation, and pooling of blood can occur when the extremities are in a dependent position. Vena cava compression occurs in the right lateral position.
- **Injury to the eye and ear** can occur in this position. The ear is to be laid flat on the table and the eye is to be closed.

Jackknife Position

The jackknife position is achieved by placing the patient in the prone position and then flexing the center of the table. The legs, head, and arms are in a dependent position.

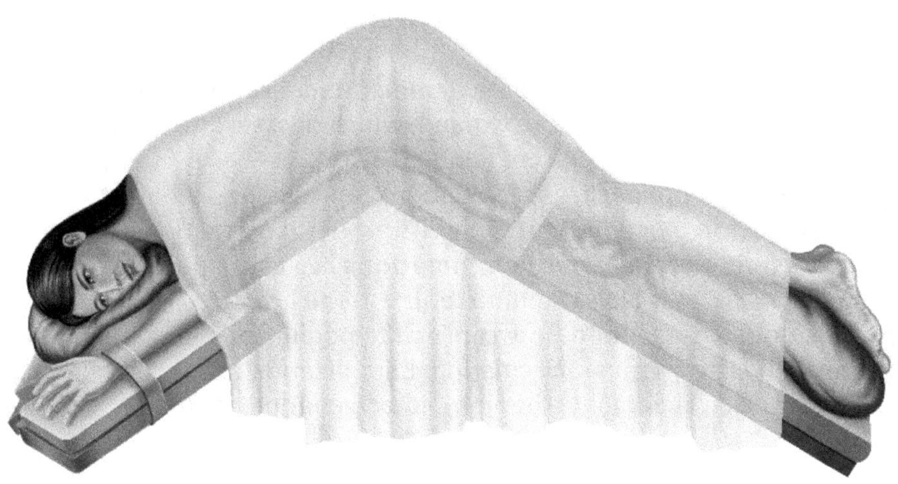

Considerations include the following:

- **Proctology procedures** are performed in this position.
- This position is not often desired due to its potential **positioning side effects**.
- A **decrease in blood pressure** occurs due to extreme pooling of blood in the legs and chest, decreasing cardiac output. The chest cannot expand well in this position, which decreases ventilation.
- The **arms** are positioned on arm boards next to the head with the palms down and are secured.
- The **table strap** is placed over the thighs as in the prone position.
- The **head** is turned to the side.

Interventions for Patient Emergencies Involving Patient Positioning

The following are some nursing interventions that can be undertaken to prevent/respond to patient emergencies involving patient positioning:

- Know what positions are **appropriate** for certain procedures. Improperly positioning a patient for a procedure necessitates repositioning the patient, which provides potential for an emergency to happen.
- Know how to place the patient correctly in the proper position, using proper **body mechanics** to avoid a fall or injury to the patient or staff.
- Perform a proper **assessment** and identify any potential **factors** that may hinder positioning or induce complications. This may necessitate a change in position or additional equipment to prevent injury. Thus, knowing how to assess whether the patient is adequately padded or supported is important to prevent injury.
- When an emergency does occur, the nurse should know how to properly **respond** according to institutional guidelines.

Potential Complications Related to Positioning

Respiratory and Circulatory Compromise Related to Positioning/Anesthesia

The following are some factors that can contribute to respiratory or circulatory compromise in the surgical patient related to positioning/anesthesia:

- Trendelenburg positioning causes the **lungs to engorge with blood**, which prevents alveolar expansion/ventilation.
- Some positions or factors that contribute to **mechanical restriction of the thorax** can inhibit the rib cage from being able to expand, which decreases the lung's ability to expand and prevent adequate ventilation from taking place.
- **Anesthetics** interfere with normal vasodilation/constriction and often decrease blood pressure. A decrease in blood pressure inhibits proper oxygenation and circulation.
- Placing the patient in certain **dependent positions** can cause pooling of blood to occur and a decrease in intravascular blood volume return to the heart.
- Positioning that **obstructs blood flow** can lead to pooling of blood and possible thrombosis, which can further restrict proper circulation. Embolization of a thrombus can lead to a pulmonary embolus, which can further inhibit oxygenation of blood.

Neuromuscular Compromise Related to Positioning/Anesthesia

The following includes factors that can contribute to neuromuscular compromise in the surgical patient related to positioning/anesthesia and how to prevent them:

- Anesthesia prevents normal **neuromuscular protection** by inhibiting a patient's ability to warn against painful positioning. The anesthetized patient cannot move to prevent injury when excessive pressure is being placed against the body. Reduced muscle tone inhibits normal mechanical protection of the neurovascular system. Adequate padding, prevention of hanging of extremities, and slowly positioning the extremities in unison helps to prevent joint dislocation and injury.
- **Pressure injuries** can occur to extremities when equipment in the operating room is adjusted and rests on the extremities or if surgical members rest against the patient's body. It is important to prevent such injury by adjusting equipment and tables carefully and keeping personnel from resting on the patient's body at all times during surgery.
- **Nerve injury** is caused by prolonged stretching or compression of the nerves. Nerve injury is evident by loss of sensation, paralysis, numbness, tingling, or pain.

Injury to Nerves by Positioning/Anesthesia

Damage to Facial, Suborbital, Brachial Plexus, Ulnar, or Nerves

The following are some situations in which facial, suborbital, brachial plexus, ulnar, or medial nerves can be damaged in surgery by positioning/anesthesia and how these injuries can be prevented:

- **Buccal branch (facial) nerve injury** results when nerve compression occurs. Facemasks must appropriately fit to prevent this injury.
- The **suborbital nerve** can be injured by endotracheal tube connectors causing numbness in the forehead.
- Improper positioning of the arms can lead to **brachial plexus injury**. Hyperextension or hyperabduction of the arm can cause this injury. Shoulder braces, when positioned laterally or medially can cause compression of the plexus and should not be used unless necessary.
- **Compression of the ulnar or medial nerves** by the epicondyle can occur when the arm slips off of the operating table and rests against the metal edge or is compressed by a team member resting against it. Securing the arm with a sheet can prevent this injury. A blood pressure cuff that stays inflated too long and/or does not allow for recirculation to occur can also injure the ulnar nerve.

Damage to Lower Extremity Nerves in Lithotomy Position

The following are some situations in which lower extremity nerves can be damaged in the lithotomy position and how they can be prevented:

- The **lithotomy position** can put compression/extension/stretch on the peroneal, posterior tibial, femoral obturator, and sciatic nerves. Injury to these nerves can cause foot drop, numbness of the foot, and paralysis/numbness of the calf muscles. These injuries can be prevented with proper positioning and padding.
- The **peroneal nerve** can be injured when compressed by a stirrup bar placed laterally and compressed against the fibula.
- The **posterior tibial nerve** as well as the femoral obturator nerve can be injured if popliteal knee supports are not adequately padded and compression of the nerves occurs.
- The **sciatic nerve** can be injured when the legs are fully extended in the high lithotomy position and/or the thighs are flexed more than 90 degrees toward the patient's torso.

Friction and Shearing Injuries

Friction and shearing injuries, how they are caused, and how they can be avoided in the surgical patient, are described below:

- **Friction injury** occurs when a patient's skin rubs across surfaces such as linens, or simply by objects frequently rubbing the skin. Abrasions, blisters, or pressure ulcers may result. Proper and careful movement of the patient when repositioning, and removing objects that rub the patient's skin or padding skin prone to rubbing can prevent these injuries.
- **Shearing injury** occurs when the surface of the skin and the structures beneath move at different rates/velocities/directions. Subcutaneous capillaries and tissues can be damaged or separated and affect circulation in these areas. Shearing injuries can occur when the patient is being repositioned quickly or when the patient is in a position to allow the patient's body to slide via gravity down a surface such as on the operating room table. Lifting the patient upward to reposition them and proper positioning in surgery can prevent this type of injury.

Pressure Injuries

Pressure injury occurs when excessive amounts of pressure are placed on a particular body part, or when small amounts of pressure are exerted for long periods of time. Excessive pressure results in ischemia and eventually necrosis of tissue. Removal of items putting pressure on the body and repositioning the body every 2 hours (if possible) help to prevent pressure ulcer formation. At higher risk for pressure ulcer formation are those with previous impairments in their integumentary and circulatory systems, and those who are scheduled for surgery lasting more than 2.5 hours in length. Elderly, obese, malnourished, immunocompromised, diabetic, and hypertensive patients all fall into this high-risk category.

Deep Vein Thrombosis and Sequential Compression Devices and Antiembolic Stockings

Sequential compression devices (SCDs) and antiembolic stockings are used to prevent deep vein thrombosis (DVT) in patients before, during, and after surgical procedures. When a patient is immobilized, anesthetized, and/or positioned in certain dependent positions, blood can pool and has a higher potential for clotting. Vasodilation caused by anesthesia can cause endothelial damage, which is a precursor to development of a thrombus. SCDs and antiembolic stockings help to prevent pooling by shunting (through squeezing the muscles and vasculature) the blood back through the venous system back to the heart. Risk of DVT increases in more lengthy procedures, patients over the age of 40, patients with a previous history of DVT, and patients who have vascular disease.

PREVENTING INJURY RELATED TO POSITIONING

The following are some things the perioperative nurse can do to prevent injury in a patient who has a diagnosis of potential for injury related to positioning:

- Use proper **padding** over potential pressure point areas in surgery.
- Keep edges of equipment from creating **pressure points** against skin, nerves, and tissues either by padding or proper positioning.
- Make sure limbs are not **hyperextended** or **flexed**.
- When stands or items are raised or lowered, make sure all limbs are free from potential **crush injury** related to the position they are in. Additionally, do not rest against the patient's body/limbs during surgery.
- Prevent **shearing injury** by lifting the patient instead of scooting them.
- If the patient is **prone**, close their eyes, turn their head to the side, and use eye pads for protection.
- Maintain **safety straps** on the patient at all times to prevent sliding off the operating room table.
- Make sure enough staff and the right equipment are available for **positioning** the patient to prevent injury during the positioning process.

Surgical Site Preparation

Use of Antiseptics in Skin Preparation Prior to Surgery

The following are some important things for the perioperative nurse to remember regarding the use of antiseptics in skin preparation prior to surgery:

- AORN guidelines recommend patient **preoperative bathing** the night prior to invasive procedures using soap or an antiseptic solution (often in the form of wipes or clothes). The nurse must perform the preoperative bath on patients unable to do so effectively themselves.
- The patient's skin is **cleaned** prior to antiseptic application. The nurse may have to clean the surgical area to remove hair, skin, oil, and bacteria. Hair must only be removed if indicated and must be removed by the nurse (not the patient).
- The most common **antiseptics** include iodophors, chlorhexidine gluconate, and alcohol preparations. While recommendations vary, alcohol (with or without CHG) is largely the most recommended first line antiseptic unless contraindicated. Contraindications include specific surgical sites (mucosa, ears, eyes, or areas with dense hair), preterm infants, and those with allergies to any of the ingredients). Generally speaking, any antiseptic should have the following properties:
    - Ease of use
    - Cleans effectively, reduces microorganisms quickly, and maintains residual protection
    - Broad spectrum
    - Nontoxic, not irritating to the skin
- Prior to the skin prep, the patient should be questioned regarding **potential allergies** to preparation solutions; alternative ones should be used if an allergy is identified.
- **Preparation areas** should include the site of incision, secondary incisions, and drain sites, and should include a wide area surrounding each area.
- When **alcohol** is used in the prep, it must dry completely before the procedure begins to prevent ignition of fumes.
- **Surgical site infection (SSI) bundles** are often utilized by facilities in effort to decrease incidence of SSI and include specific skin antisepsis protocols. The nurse must be familiar with the entire bundle and follow facility protocols.

Performing Basic Skin Prep

Important things for the perioperative nurse to remember when performing the basic skin preparation include the following:

- Only the area that is to be prepped is to be **exposed**.
- Sterile technique must be utilized.
- The prep is performed using **circular motions** working from the site of incision outward and is repeated several times as back-and-forth motions can pick up bacteria from the outer edges of the prep and deposit them in the center, toward the area of incision.
- The **applicator sponge** used to apply antiseptic/cleaning solution is used only once, and then thrown away. It is never reused.
- **Pooling of antiseptic/cleaning solution** is not allowed. Towels or other linens can be used to absorb excess solution used in the prep as excess amounts can potentially cause chemical burn on the skin.
- Cleaning/prepping an area occurs from the **cleanest** area desired to the **dirtiest**/most likely to be contaminated.
- **Warm** prep solutions should be used instead of tepid preps.

Prepping the Patient with Hair at Site of Operation

Some important factors for the perioperative nurse to remember when preoperatively prepping a patient who has hair at the site of operation include the following:

- Hair should only be removed if leaving it would **interfere** with the surgical procedure, wound closure, or ability to appropriately drape the surgical site.
- Hair should be removed **outside of the operating area.** If hair must be removed in the operating room, it should be removed **wet** to prevent contamination of other sites, including the sterile field.
- Hair removal should occur with **clippers** when possible to prevent nicking the skin, and inspection of the skin should be done to prevent nicking of moles, warts, or other raised areas of skin.
- **Depilatory creams** may be used; however, they may cause irritation of the skin and are often not used for this reason.
- Hair should be removed as close to **surgical procedure time** as possible.

Skin Preparation for Unique Circumstances

Some important things for the perioperative nurse to remember when performing the skin prep for the eyes, traumatic wounds, limbs, malignancy, and for areas such as stomas, axillae, and the umbilicus include the following:

- Use a **nonirritating solution** for the eyes. Start from the nose and work outward towards the cheeks. Use warm sterile water to rinse.
- Large quantities of solution are used to remove **debris** in traumatic wounds.
- Normal saline is used to prep **burned** or denuded skin.
- A **second person or a device** is necessary to hold a limb for prep around the entire limb.
- With malignancy, **gentle motions** should be used to prevent spread of cells.
- The umbilicus, stomas, axillae, vagina, and anus are prepped **last** and/or **separately** from other body parts.

Surgical Draping

Drapes

Drapes are used to create a field in which bacteria cannot invade the surgical site. They are used to cover the patient, to cover tables holding surgical instruments, and to cover equipment to prevent contamination. In order for a material to be sufficient as a drape, it must be resistant to penetration by fluids, durable, free of lint or particulate matter, flame resistant, and must not hold memory shape. Drapes may either be reusable or disposable.

- **Reusable drapes** must be inspected for integrity as repeated washings deteriorate fabrics over time.
- **Clear plastic drapes** are applied directly over the incision site and the incision is made through the drape. These drapes are sometimes impregnated with iodophor.
- **Polyvinyl drapes** are used to drape equipment in the operating room that cannot be sterilized to help prevent spread of contaminants to the patient.

Types of Drapes

The following are the various types of standard drapes used in surgery:

- **Flat sheets** are used to drape standard tables and the patient.
- **Mayo stand covers** are used to drape Mayo stands.
- **Sterile towels** are used to drape the patient's incision site.
- **Fenestrated drapes** have openings and come in various shapes and sizes depending on the area intended to be draped.
- **Aperture drapes** are a specific type of fenestrated drape used in eye/ear operations.
- **Equipment drapes** are plastic drapes used to cover equipment used in the operating room that cannot be sterilized. The drape prevents contamination by the instrument in surgery.
- **Stockinette drapes** are used on the hands/feet.
- **Legging drapes** are used when the patient is in the lithotomy position.

Nursing Considerations for Sterile Draping

The following are some important considerations for the perioperative nurse to remember regarding draping in the surgical area:

- Only **intact** drapes are appropriate for use.
- Drapes should be **handled** minimally.
- Drapes should not be **shaken** or forcefully placed. Shaking can potentially contaminate a sterile area by allowing air currents to pick up contaminants and deposit them elsewhere.
- Drapes should always be held **higher** than the area that they are intended to drape to prevent contamination of the drape.
- Draping is performed from the site of operation toward the **periphery**.
- Drapes are not **repositioned**. If they are inappropriately placed, they are removed by a non-scrubbed person and replaced.
- The edges of the drape are not touched by a sterile person to avoid **contamination**. When placing drapes, the area away from the edge is used to position.
- **Towel clamps** that penetrate drapes must be removed after the procedure is completed.
- If the **sterility** of a drape is questioned, it is removed.

Anesthesia, Pain, and Medication Management

Common Preoperative Medications

The following are commonly used preoperative medications:

Medication	Dosage	Timing
Midazolam (Versed)	0.5-2 mg IV (based on patient response) administered over 2 minutes, 0.5 mg at a time	Used immediately preoperatively to sedate patient
Diazepam (Valium)	≤10 mg IV (0.03-0.1 mg/kg)	Used immediately preoperatively to sedate patient and relieve anxiety
Lorazepam (Ativan)	1-4 mg IV (0.02-0.04 mg/kg)	Same as above
Ondansetron (Zofran)	4 mg IV over 2-5 minutes	Administered immediately preoperatively to reduce postoperative nausea and vomiting
Famotidine (or other H2 blockers)	20 mg IV	Administered 40-90 minutes preoperatively to reduce risk of aspiration
Antibiotics (many different medications)	Cephalosporins (1st gen) 250-1500 mg IV Cefuroxime 750-1500 mg IV Cefepime 1-2 g IV	Administered within 60 minutes preoperatively to prevent infection

Perioperative Antibiotic Use

The three main factors to consider when using **perioperative antibiotics** include when the antibiotic should be given, which antibiotic to use at what dose, and when it is appropriate to use antibiotics. Studies have shown that the most appropriate time to administer antibiotics is approximately 60 minutes before surgery begins. The effectiveness of prophylactic antibiotic therapy decreases once the surgical incision is made, and the initial dose of antibiotics should not be given after that time. A broad-spectrum antibiotic that will kill the bacteria commonly responsible for causing SSIs should be used. This is usually a cephalosporin unless this is contraindicated because of direct allergy or penicillin allergy. Vancomycin is usually used in those cases. This should be given in a large dose, not low dose, to provide appropriate coverage. Many surgeons use antibiotics for all invasive procedures, but the type of surgery should also be considered. For surgeries that have a very low risk of infection, the risks and benefits of antibiotic use should be considered based on the patient.

Review Video: Antibiotics: An Overview
Visit mometrix.com/academy and enter code: 165628

Labeling Medications to Be Used in a Sterile Environment

Medication safety requires proper **labeling of drugs** used in the sterile environment, which avoids costly mistakes that result in incorrect medications being given, as well as breaking sterile technique. When labeling medications in the sterile field, the circulating nurse first verifies the five patient rights: right medication, right patient, right time, right dose, and right route to be given. The nurse also verifies with the surgeon that the medication is indeed the medication the surgeon intended to order. The medication is transferred to the sterile field via transfer tubing, syringe, or another sterile device. The scrub person or nurse who is in the sterile field labels the medication using labels and sterile markers that have already been placed in the sterile field. The information on the label includes the medication name, strength, and amount, as well as its expiration time. Each medication should be transferred to the sterile field and labeled one at a time. The medication is then verified again before its use.

Anesthesia

Types

The four types of anesthesia are described below:

- **General anesthesia** occurs when the central nervous system is depressed to the point of obtundation or unconsciousness. The patient will have amnesia, analgesia, and the musculature will be relaxed.
- **Moderate sedation/anesthesia** (conscious sedation, monitored anesthesia care) is used for patients who cannot tolerate general anesthesia, or for procedures that require small lengths of time for anesthesia to occur. Intravenous medications are given to provide sedation and analgesia, and local anesthesia is often used in conjunction. The patient will have amnesia, analgesia, and relaxation of the musculature. However, they will often awaken very quickly after discontinuation of the medication.
- **Regional anesthesia** occurs when a particular nerve is anesthetized, preventing pain conduction to and from the area. The patient remains awake but cannot feel pain during the procedure. Sedation is often induced to reduce anxiety during procedures that use regional blocks.
- **Local anesthesia** is essentially regional anesthesia to a much smaller area.

Inhaled Anesthetics

Inhaled anesthetics provide rapid induction and emergence from anesthesia:

- **Nitrous oxide** acts quickly, but lacks potency. Recovery is fast and has few side effects. Too high of an inhaled concentration may cause hypoxia.
- **Halothane** is a cardiopulmonary and hypothalamic depressant. Thus, hypotension, bradycardia, and hypothermia, are some of the potential complications. It can also sensitize cardiac muscle to catecholamines and prevent their use together. Halothane metabolites may also affect liver function.
- **Enflurane** induces anesthesia without affecting heart rate but may cause hypotension. It provides good muscle relaxation.
- **Isoflurane** is a good muscle relaxant and does not greatly affect the cardiovascular system.
- **Desflurane** provides good muscle relaxation. Heart rate/blood pressure may increase. It has a foul taste and is often not used for induction of anesthesia.
- **Sevoflurane** provides the quickest induction of anesthesia. It does not irritate the respiratory tract or myocardium.

Intravenous Anesthetic Medications

Intravenous anesthetic medications include the following:

- **Narcotics** are used in the preoperative to early operative phase to provide pain relief. They provide good analgesia with few cardiovascular side effects. Respiratory depression is a significant side effect.
- **Benzodiazepine tranquilizers** are used as adjuncts to other amnesic agents, as their use reduces the amounts needed of other amnesic agents. They do not provide analgesia. Respiratory depression is a common side effect, and flumazenil is the reversal agent for benzodiazepines.
- **Neuromuscular blockers** are used to ease intubation and provide muscle relaxation necessary for the handling of tissue intraoperatively. They are paralytics and prevent motor impulses from reaching skeletal muscle. They are either depolarizing or nondepolarizing. Depolarizing agents work faster and emergence is faster, and nondepolarizing agents are used for longer desired effect. Pyridostigmine and neostigmine are reversal agents for nondepolarizing paralytics and are often used with atropine or glycopyrrolate to counteract the muscarinic effects of the reversal agents. Because they do not sedate the patient, the patient must be adequately sedated prior to the administration of a neuromuscular blockade.
- **Barbiturates** are often used to induce anesthesia, but only provide sedation, not analgesia. They are short acting and easily progress from sedation to anesthesia. Hypotension and respiratory depression are side effects of barbiturate use.
- **Propofol** is a nonbarbiturate agent that is a hypnotic sedative. It is a lipid emulsified agent and must be used quickly after preparation to prevent bacterial growth. It has a rapid emergence and minimal aftereffects.
- **Etomidate** is a nonbarbiturate agent that is short acting and has minimal cardiovascular side effects. It is a sedative and does not provide analgesia.
- **Ketamine** is a dissociative agent that provides amnesia and analgesia. The patient can move around and appears awake. It does not depress respirations and can be used in procedures where muscle relaxation is not necessary. Hallucinations are a common side effect in the emergence phase.

Review Video: Muscle Relaxants
Visit mometrix.com/academy and enter code: 862193

Noninvasive Monitoring Devices for Patients Receiving Anesthesia

The following are some noninvasive monitoring devices that can be used for patients receiving anesthesia to monitor oxygenation, ventilation, circulation, and body temperature:

- **Precordial stethoscopes** can be used to monitor heart rate and rhythm, as well as breath sounds for air movement and the presence of adventitious breath sounds.
- An **electrocardiogram** (EKG) can be used to monitor heart rate and rhythm and check for proper cardiac perfusion. Decreased myocardial perfusion or myocardial infarction is picked up on EKG.
- **Pulse oximetry** is used to measure oxygen saturation of hemoglobin in the arterial system. Percentages below 95% indicate inappropriate oxygenation.
- **Blood pressure cuffs** can be used to measure the patient's blood pressure and pulse, which can be altered during anesthesia secondary to vasodilation.
- **Capnography** measures the amount of carbon dioxide exhaled with mechanical ventilation and checks proper endotracheal tube placement.
- The patient's temperature can simply be measured via a noninvasive **thermometer**. Hypothermia can occur with overexposure of skin and can be due to the cold operating room environment.

Role of Perioperative Nurse in Monitoring and Evaluating Effects of Anesthesia

One of the major roles of the perioperative nurse is to monitor and evaluate the **effects of anesthesia** on the patient to ensure that comfort and safety are maintained. During the procedure, the nurse assists the anesthesiologist as necessary to ensure that the patient remains stable, such as by monitoring vital signs, urine output, or the patient's position. Afterward, the nurse continues to monitor vital signs, as anesthesia can impact breathing and circulation. The nurse should remain with the patient during recovery from anesthesia, as this can be startling for the patient and assistance may be needed. The nurse ensures the patient remains comfortable by giving medications to control pain or nausea. The nurse must assist the patient with mobility, whether this is helping the patient to turn in bed, or to sit up. The nurse must provide assistance the first time the patient tries to get up after surgery, as anesthesia can impact perception of space and time.

Postoperative Pain Management

Methods of postoperative pain management include:

- **Comfort measures**: Careful positioning of the patient to relieve tension on incision lines and application of warm blankets may provide some relief of discomfort.
- **Analgesia**: Multimodal analgesia (such as opioids, paravertebral block, and TENS) may be most effective with severe postoperative pain. The WHO pain ladder may be used to provide the most appropriate analgesia for the patient's level of pain. In many cases, the combination of acetaminophen and an NSAID may be as effective as opioids, especially if pain is not severe. PCA may be appropriate for opioid administration.
- **Alternative physical therapies**: These may include acupuncture, massage, heat, cold, and TENS. They may be used alone or as an adjuvant to analgesia.
- **Cognitive-behavioral approaches**: Guided imagery, self-hypnosis, music therapy, and relaxation methods may all help to reduce the patient's anxiety and perception of pain.

Environmental Factors

Impact of Environmental Factors in Operating Room

Environmental factors that must be considered in the operating room include the following:

- **Temperature**: Operating room temperatures should usually be maintained at 68-75 °F (20-24 °C) to help prevent hypothermia while maintaining comfort level for staff. The decontamination area is kept cooler at 60-65 °F (16-18 °C) to discourage growth of microorganisms. Temperatures in the PACU and cardiac catheterization lab are higher at 70-76 °F (21-24 °C).
- **Humidity**: The ideal relative humidity varies based on the type of surgery being performed but it should generally be kept below 60%. Maintaining humidity at a low level helps inhibit the growth of mold and bacteria. A relative humidity of 50-60% reduces the production of static electricity associated with electrosurgery.
- **Air exchanges**: Because the OR environment and air are contaminated by dust, respiratory droplets, and surgical smoke, air exchange should be done at a minimum of 20 air exchanges per hour with up to 25 recommended. The PACU should have 6 air exchanges per hour, and the sterile storage area should have 4 air exchanges per hour.
- **Noise**: Noise may be distracting to team members and may interfere with communication and the ability to hear alarms. The OR door should be kept closed, conversation carried out in low tones, and music (if used) kept at low volume.
- **Medical gases**: Compressed medical gases should be stored based on regulatory requirements and secured when transported. Valves should be tightly closed when not in use to prevent leakage. AORN guidelines recommend maintaining an emergency supply of oxygen that would last one day in the case of an emergency.

Traffic Patterns of Instruments into and out of Operating Room Area

Contaminated items are not moved through the same areas that clean and sterile items move through. Contaminated items move from the operating room to a separate holding area and are transported safely out of the room to prevent contamination of clean/sterile areas. Items being delivered to the operating room are removed of their outside coverings before entering the operating room. This way, any contaminants on the outside packaging are removed, thus decreasing the likelihood of contamination of the internal operating environment. Likewise, instruments being delivered to the operating room from other departments in the hospital must be delivered in an enclosed container to prevent contamination en route to the operating room.

Restricted, Semi-Restricted, and Unrestricted Areas

The operating suite is divided into various zones/areas based on their level of sterility and personnel allowed:

- **Restricted areas** are where surgery takes place and the sterile supply is located. Operating rooms, procedure areas, scrub sinks, and sterile storage are included in restricted areas. Personnel must be in scrub attire with hair covering, long sleeves, and masks.
- **Semi-restricted areas** store clean and sterile supplies, areas for instrument cleaning/processing, and hallways to restricted areas. Scrub attire, hair covering, and long sleeves are also required in semi-restricted areas.
- **Unrestricted areas** are where interaction occurs between personnel in the operating suite and other departments, families, etc. Supplies are received from other departments in unrestricted areas. Street clothes may be worn in unrestricted areas.

Movement by personnel from **unrestricted to restricted areas** takes place through specific areas to prevent large amounts of traffic into and out of restricted areas.

Preventing Contamination using Environmental Factors

The following are some environmental factors implemented in the operating room that prevent **contamination**:

- **Separate ventilation systems** are in place for the operating room as are air filtration systems.
- **Airflow** in the operating room occurs from ceiling to floor. Positive pressure is used to prevent potential contaminated outside air from other rooms and departments from entering the operating room.
- **Laminar airflow systems** that utilize high-efficiency particulate air (HEPA) filters are used to circulate air over the patient in the operating room. The air in this system is unidirectional, and items that are not sterile are not permitted to be stored in the airflow of this system.

Operating Room Lighting

There are usually two lights in the operating room. Once the patient is in the operating room, but before they have been given any anesthesia, the operating table should be positioned so that one light is shining down on the patient's head and one on their feet. This allows the lights to be in a position so that they can be moved during surgery to illuminate just about any surface of the patient's body. The operating room lights have handles that are covered with sterile covers so that they can be manipulated during surgery. Generally, the lights are always positioned above the patient to shine down on the surgical site. In surgeries involving the head and mouth, the light may be positioned behind the surgeon and assistants and angled to shine up into the surgical site. With some deep surgeries or surgeries that take place within a small area, a small light may be attached to the surgeon's head to shine down on the area where he is focused.

Aseptic Technique

Pathogenic Organisms

Pathogenic organisms that cause infection are becoming increasingly resistant to antibiotics. Methicillin-resistant *Staphylococcus aureus* (MRSA) and Vancomycin-resistant *Enterococcus* (VRE) are two of the most common resistant strains of bacteria causing nosocomial infections in the hospital. The more resistance these organisms acquire to antibiotics, the more difficult they are to treat. Organisms with endotoxins in their outer cell membranes are more virulent than other organisms and thus cause an infection with fewer amounts of bacteria present than other organisms. Treatment for inoculation of these organisms becomes difficult, lengthy, and costly. Strict maintenance of aseptic technique prevents nosocomial spread of these bacteria and demonstrates the importance of maintaining this technique at all times.

Surgical Hand Antisepsis

The scrubbing procedure for surgical hand antisepsis is as follows:

1. All jewelry is removed from the hands and wrists, and a surgical mask is donned. A scrub sponge/brush is selected, the water is turned on, and the hands are first washed with **soap and running water**.

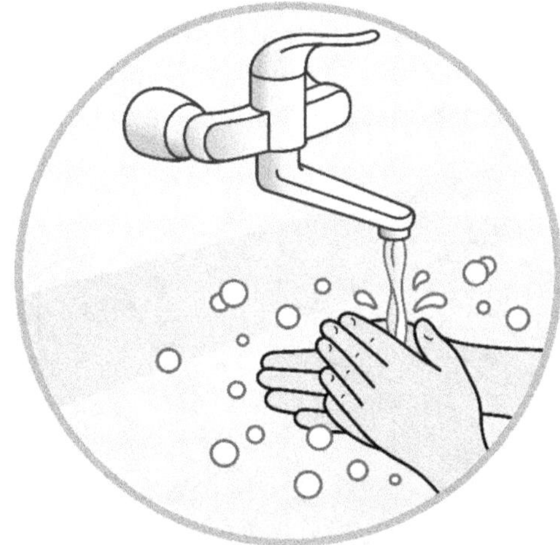

2. The scrub brush is opened, and the nail cleaner is used to clean in and around **nails** under running water and repeated on the other side. The hands are then rinsed.

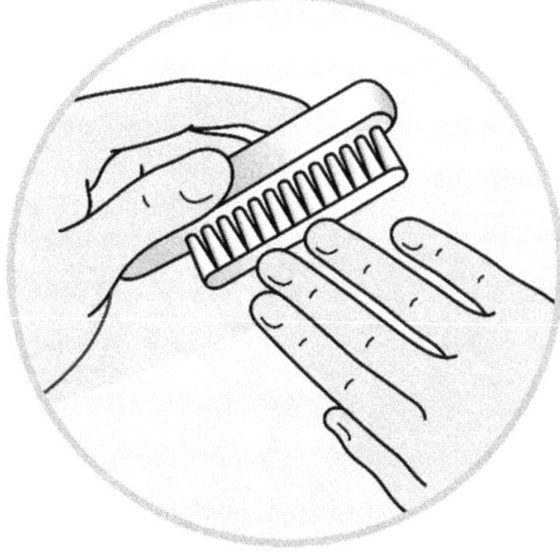

3. The scrub brush is moistened and the arms are held in the flexed position with hands held up above the elbows and water running toward the elbows. With the arms in this position, the nails, fingers, hands, wrists, and arms are scrubbed according to facility requirements (either timed or surface scrubbed a certain number of times) from the **fingertips** down to the **elbow**. The hands are then rinsed.

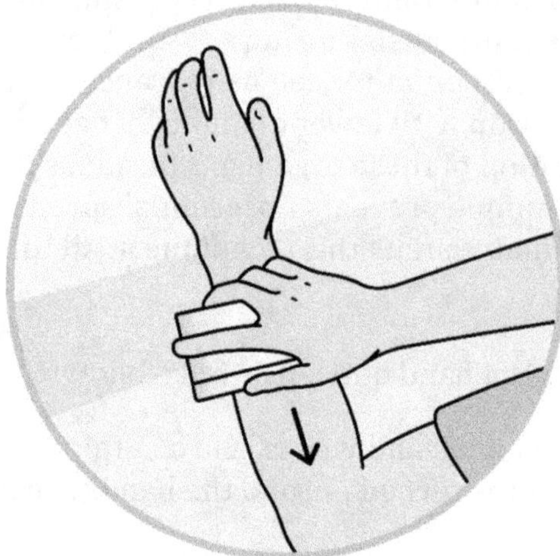

4. The sink is then turned off using the elbow. If an **alcohol-based rub** is to be used instead of scrubbing, hands are dried after washing on a clean towel, and then the rub is applied to hands and forearms, which are rubbed until the product and hands are dry.

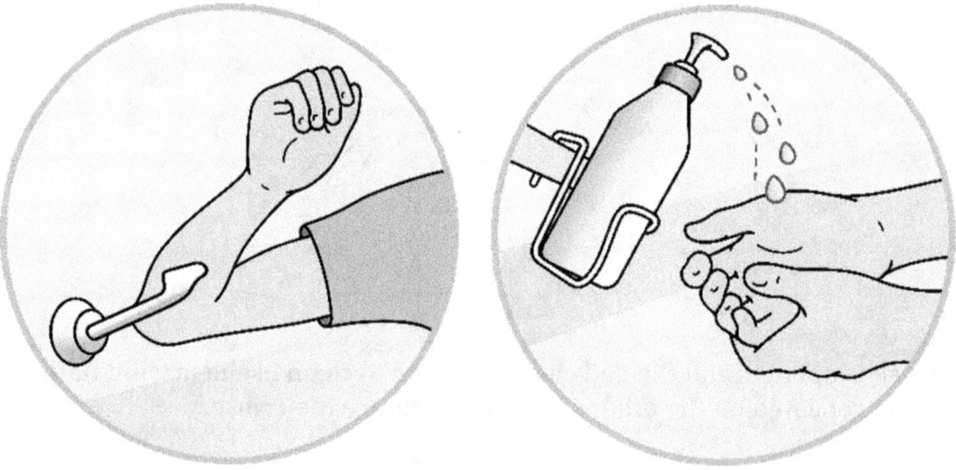

Gowning and Gloving Using Surgical Antiseptic Technique

When gowning and gloving using surgical antiseptic technique, the nurse must take into account the following considerations:

- Care is taken by the scrubbed person to maintain a **sterile field** while gowning and gloving.
- Reusable gowns must be **inspected** for wear as they lose protective qualities with repeated washings.
- If the gown does not have a removable pull-tab, a sterile instrument can be used by the scrubbed person and handed to the nonsterile person to wrap the **tie** around.
- One must use **latex-free gloves** when a patient has a latex allergy.
- Gloves should be free of **powders** as powders can cause inflammatory reactions if introduced under the skin.
- When using the open-gloving technique, the bare hands should only touch the **inside** of the glove. Unwrapping of the cuff should be done by the sterile, gloved hand.

Gowning and Gloving Procedure

The gowning and gloving procedure, maintaining surgical asepsis, is as follows:

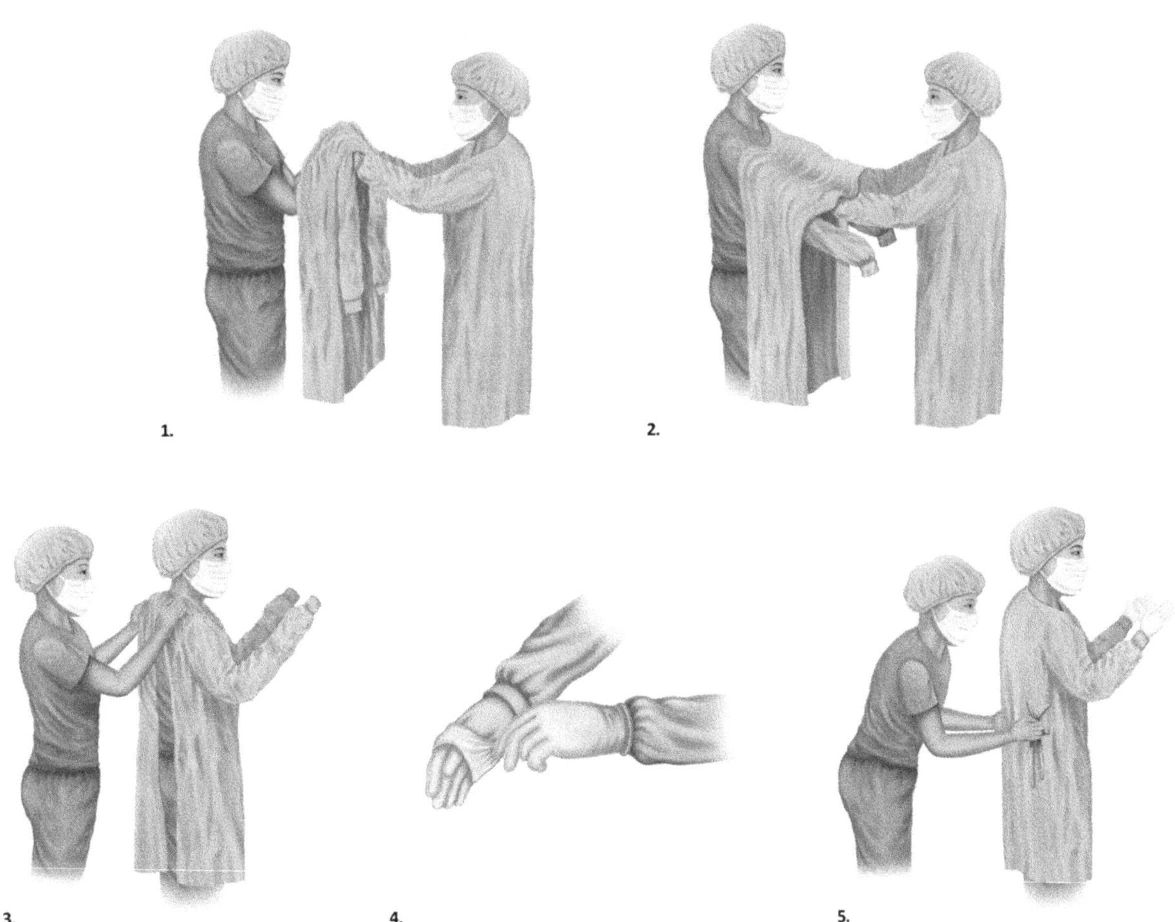

1. The gown is handled by the **neckline** by the **sterile scrub person**, lifted off and away from the sterile field, and allowed to unfold down.
2. The **armholes** are identified and both arms are inserted into the corresponding holes simultaneously to prevent dragging of the gown on the floor. The hands are inserted up to the cuff if a closed-gloving technique is required, through the cuff for open gloving.
3. A **nonsterile scrub person** fastens the gown at the neck and at the waist.
4. **Gloves** are donned in a sterile manner, pulling the gloves over the cuffs of the gown. Gloves can also be donned through **assistive gloving**, in which the scrub person holds the glove open and the sterile person inserts their hand into the glove, only touching the inside of the glove. The glove should completely cover the cuff of the sterile gown.
5. Using the pull-tab that is easily removed without contaminating the gown, a nonsterile member pulls the **tie** around the gown so the sterile person can grab the end and tie it around the waist.

Glove Contamination and Perforation

Specific protocol must be established and enforced with regard to glove contamination (with blood, bodily fluids, or hazardous material) and glove perforation. During invasive surgical procedures AORN guidelines recommend that gloves are changed under the following circumstances:

- After sterile draping
- After manipulating instruments/objects with sharp or rough edges (including body parts such as bones)
- After the procedure and every 90-150 minutes when relevant
- In the case of perforation, actual or suspected (If perforation occurs in the outer glove, it should be removed and the inner glove examined.)
- After touching contaminated objects (surgical helmet/hood/visor, fluoroscopes, or eye pieces of surgical microscopes)
- After touching hazardous materials (methyl methacrylate, specific medications)

Gloves should be changed away from the sterile field and with the helped of an unscrubbed team member (to remove the glove) and a scrubbed team member (to don the new glove)

Prepping and Maintaining Sterile Field

A new sterile field is prepped for each procedure, immediately prior to the patient's arrival at the procedure room. Hand antisepsis and sterile gown/glove donning should be performed prior to setup. In order to maintain a sterile field and prevent its contamination the following must be taken into consideration:

- **Basins** for holding solutions are held at the edge of the field to prevent splashing of the sterile field.
- Constant monitoring of a **sterile field** should take place to prevent potential contamination of the field without notice. Therefore, it is best and easiest to monitor when the field is created as close to surgery time as possible.
- **Furniture and equipment** that are part of the sterile field are often covered to prevent contamination.
- **Talking** is kept to a minimum to prevent droplet contamination of the field.
- **Movement** within the sterile field is done in a manner that preserves sterility of the field. Personnel pass each other back-to-back to prevent potential contamination of one's back to one's sterile front side. Standing persons should remain standing, and sitting persons should remain sitting.
- Only personnel who are **scrubbed** and who don hats, gowns, and gloves are to operate within a sterile field. Only the chest down to the sterile field of the person is considered sterile and the gloved hands to two inches above the elbow. Areas of potential perspiration and edges are not considered sterile.
- Sterile **drapes** establish and maintain the sterile field.
- Any **items introduced** to a sterile field must be sterile. Any items thought to be contaminated are not introduced and/or are removed to prevent contamination. Proper techniques are used to make sure that items are transferred to the sterile site appropriately. Packaging is thoroughly inspected for punctures or other threats to the sterility of the item. Wrapped items are unwrapped with the furthest item unwrapped first and the closest last. Items not able to be dropped or flipped onto the field are to be picked up by a sterile scrubbed person. Heavy items are to be carefully placed to prevent rolling, dropping, etc.

Maintaining Sanitation of Operating Room

Before and During the Procedure

The following are some standards the operating room personnel utilize to maintain sanitation of the operating room area **before and during the procedure:**

- All persons who may potentially come into contact with blood or body fluids must wear **personal protective equipment**.
- All furniture and equipment are **damp dusted** in the operating room before the first procedure to reduce dust and particulate matter in the room.
- Patients with **latex allergies** are often scheduled as the first case of the day as latex products used later in the day may deposit latex particles in the operating room.
- All contamination is **confined, cleaned, and disinfected** during the procedure as much as possible.
- **Large spills** are soaked up with a cloth, and the remaining residue cleaned with a germicidal agent.
- Soiled **disposable items** are thrown away. Soiled **reusable items** are wiped with an antiseptic agent and placed in a leak-proof container.
- All **tissue specimens** are placed in leak-proof containers and sealed. If indicated, the outside may be wiped with a germicidal agent.

After the Procedure

The following are some standards the operating room personnel utilize to maintain sanitation of the operating room **after the procedure**:

- All items on the sterile field after the procedure are considered **contaminated.**
- **Disposable items** are put into hazardous waste bags/receptacles.
- **Infectious waste fluids** can either be poured into a sewer drain or placed in appropriate leak-proof containers and placed in a hazardous waste bag/receptacle.
- All **sharps** are considered infectious waste and are put in appropriate sharps containers.
- All other **instruments that are reusable** are cleaned and processed for reuse. They are put in appropriate transportation containers to cleaning areas.
- All **furniture/equipment**, including the floor, in the operating room is wiped down with an appropriate germicidal agent after the procedure. At the end of the day, all furniture, equipment, and surfaces are terminally cleaned.
- Periodic cleaning of areas just **outside the operating room** takes place to prevent contamination into the operating room. Locker rooms, cabinets, walls, restrooms, etc. are included in these areas.

Instruments, Supplies, and Equipment

Inspection of Instrumentation Before Use

The following are various ways to properly inspect instrumentation before **use** to ensure adequacy:

- Check that **two-halved devices** have aligned tips and do not overlap. Jaws with serrations must align perfectly and not allow light to pass through when closed.
- **Teeth** at the tip of instruments should align so that they do not rub/stick on one another.
- **Joints, box locks, hinges, and ratchets** must open and close easily and hold firmly. Loosening of joints or ratchets may prevent them from holding and compromise the surgery. Stiff joints may need lubrication.
- **Cutting edges** should be sharp and free of dents and nicks.
- **Holders** should be free of wear.
- **Plated instruments** should have intact plating to prevent microbial contamination.
- Instruments with **lenses** should be clear.
- Instruments with **moving parts** should be smooth, and sheaths and cords should be intact from wear and bending.
- **Cameras** should function properly.
- Instruments with **multiple parts** should have all parts present.

Tourniquet Use

Tourniquet use during surgery is generally indicated in procedures where local anesthesia is to be confined to a certain area of an extremity or when bleeding to the surgical site needs to be controlled/minimized for visualization and efficiency purposes. Pneumatic tourniquets are an alternative to manual tourniquets and maintain the appropriate compression required without excess, but they have been associated with complications such as skin breakdown, VTE, nerve damage, burns, and compartment syndrome. The following are some important things to remember when applying a tourniquet on a patient for surgery:

- **Inspection** of the tourniquet (and its subsequent cuffs, tubings, etc.) should take place to make sure the integrity of the tourniquet is intact.
- The **patient should be thoroughly assessed** (skin, perfusion, circulation) prior to application to ensure safety and/or risk factors.
- If **gas** is used to inflate the tourniquet, there should be enough available for the entire procedure.
- The **widest cuff possible** should be used, as they occlude using smaller amounts of pressure. If the extremity has extreme tapering, then contoured cuffs should be utilized when available.
- The length should permit adequate **overlap** to provide appropriate circumferential pressure.
- A **Webril or stockinette** only should be placed on the skin of the extremity to protect it from the tourniquet unless specified otherwise. It should not fold or bunch when pressure is applied. Traction of excess skin in obese patients before inflation should take place to prevent folding and bunching of skin.
- The tourniquet should be placed at the point of **maximum circumference** to protect against nerve/blood vessel injury with tubing on the side of the extremity that is away from the sterile field.
- **Fluids** should not be allowed to pool underneath the tourniquet.

Procedure

The procedure for applying a tourniquet for surgery is described below:

1. The extremity being prepped for surgery is **elevated** to allow as much blood to displace (exsanguination) from the extremity as possible.
2. An **Esmarch bandage** may then be wrapped around the extremity distally to proximally to further displace blood.
3. While the Esmarch bandage is in place, the tourniquet is applied on the extremity well **above** the site of surgery.
4. The tourniquet is either **tied** or, if it is a pneumatic tourniquet, **inflated** to the appropriate pressure to inhibit blood flow to the extremity. AORN guidelines do not recommend a standard pressure, and instead reinforce that pressure be patient-specific. Limb occlusion pressure can be determined using Doppler or the arterial occlusion pressure formula if time allows. This is an evidence-based approach to determining appropriate tourniquet pressure for the individual patient to minimize damage to the extremity.
5. When the procedure is completed, the tie or air from the bladder of the tourniquet is released and blood is allowed to **redistribute** into the extremity.
6. The patient should be closely monitored after removal of the tourniquet, ensuring vital signs are stable, reperfusion to the limb is appropriate (checking pulses and temperature), and pain level is assessed and managed.

Considerations for Tourniquet Use During Surgery

The following are some important things to remember when a tourniquet is used on a patient during surgery:

- **Inflation** of the tourniquet and amount of time for tourniquet inflation should be to the surgeon's desired specifications. Usual inflation time is 60 minutes for an upper extremity and 90-120 minutes for a lower extremity. The nurse should report inflation time to the doctor periodically during the procedure.
- The nurse should periodically check the **pressure indicator** on the tourniquet to assure adequate pressure is maintained throughout the procedure.
- If 2 cuffs are used for bilateral extremity surgery, **1 cuff should be deflated at a time** with significant time in between to prevent excessive metabolite buildup.
- If a tourniquet **loses pressure** during the procedure, the cuff should not simply be inflated as thrombosis can occur in vessels engorged in blood with additional pressure application. The tourniquet should be deflated, the extremity allowed to re-perfuse, and the process for re-applying the tourniquet should be employed.

Clamping Devices

Clamps are used to hold tissues, structures, or tools. They include hemostatic clamps, noncrushing vascular clamps, occluding clamps, and grasping clamps. They all have finger holes, shafts, joints, and tips, but all vary within their specific categories as to whether they are straight, curved, or angled.

- **Hemostatic clamps** have serrated jaws and are used to stop bleeding. They can also be used to separate tissue.
- **Noncrushing vascular clamps** have fine serrations and are used in occluding vessels, but do not crush the vessel like a hemostatic clamp might.
- **Occluding clamps** are used to occlude tissue or vessels and have very fine vertical serrations that prevent crushing and tissue trauma.
- **Grasping clamps** are used for retraction of tissue and may be used for suturing. Some grasping clamps have serrations, and some do not.

Cutting, Holding, and Suction Devices

There are various cutting, holding, and suction devices used in the operating room, including the following:

- **Scalpels** are used for cutting and have a handle and a blade. They are handed off with the cutting-edge away from the palm of the receiving person. The blades are to be inserted with a needle holder and should never be handheld.
- **Scissors** are used for cutting and come in a variety of different shapes and sizes used for different procedures.
- **Osteotomes, chisels, rongeurs, and curettes** are used for cutting bone. Periosteal elevators are used for separating tissue from other tissue or bone.
- **Blunt dissectors** are used for separating tissue without cutting.
- **Forceps** look like tweezers and are used for holding and lifting tissue. Some have teeth for holding thicker tissues and some do not.
- **Retractors** are used to move tissue and organs away from the field that the surgeon would like to visualize.
- **Suction devices** remove fluids from the operative site.

Forceps

Forceps are used for grasping and picking up objects. They are held in the hand like a pencil and are very helpful and easy to use once one becomes comfortable with the feel of them. There are several different styles of forceps. The length can vary, as well as the width. The tips can be smooth or have a series of teeth that provide a better grip for grasping. Forceps without teeth are generally used on more delicate tissues, while forceps with teeth are used on more sturdy tissues that are not as susceptible to damage. Care should always be taken to avoid grasping tissue too firmly because of the risk of tissue damage. Grasping too firmly can also cause the forceps to slip off the tissue which can lead to tissue injury. Tissues should be held with the forceps for as short a period as possible to avoid damage from excessive compression.

THUMB FORCEPS

There are several different types of thumb forceps available, and they have many different uses to help with manipulating tissue during surgery. They are available with a smooth tip or a tip with teeth for stronger grasping capabilities. There are also different types of thumb forceps which are specially designed for a specific procedure. The tips of the thumb forceps extend from the thumb and from the ends of the other fingers. This tends to give an effect as if the thumb and fingers were extended, which can help with fine grasping skills. They are easiest to use when held like a pencil. Thumb forceps are used for grasping tissue that needs to be lifted or removed. They are valuable when used in conjunction with a needle holder while suturing. Thumb forceps are also used to grasp the needle while suturing and a longer version can be used to pack and remove sponges in the operative site.

SUCTION TOOLS

Suctioning is used to remove blood and other body fluids from the operative site. Suction tools come in various shapes and sizes and will vary depending on the type of surgery being performed and the amount of blood loss expected during the surgery. Suctioning should be performed very carefully to avoid any trauma to the tissues within the area. Most suction devices have an opening on the shaft portion of the tool that is covered with the finger to increase the amount of suction provided. To avoid tissue damage while suctioning, suction should not be applied at full force directly against organ tissue. If organ tissue is absorbed into the suction tip, the suction should be discontinued and then the device removed from the area. Never force the suction tip off tissue while the suction is being applied because this can result in significant tissue trauma. Some suction devices may have small, removable parts that should be monitored during surgery to prevent them from being lost in the operative site.

FLEXIBLE ENDOSCOPES

AORN guidelines detail explicit procedures and protocols for the processing, use, transportation, cleaning, sterilization, and storage of flexible endoscopes to prevent complications related to patient-to-patient disease transmission. Guidelines are as follows:

- **Processing**: Flexible endoscopes should be processed in a designated area for endoscope processing that minimizes risk for contamination and has appropriate ventilation and temperature per regulatory guidelines. There should be 2 air filters for the processing areas, the first graded 7 minimum efficiency reporting valve (MERV) and the second, 14 MERV. There should be at least 2 decontamination sinks and handwashing sinks in the decontamination area/room. Clean surgical attire and head coverings should be worn in the processing room and procedure rooms, in addition to appropriate PPE. Individuals conducting instrument processing should be appropriately trained, educated, and vaccinated.
- **Point-of-use treatment**: Equipment and accessories should be immediately precleaned at point-of-use to prevent drying of organic material. Precleaning should include rinsing, suctioning, flushing, and visually inspecting. The instrument should then be transferred to the processing room in a closed container and processed as soon as possible.
- **Leak tests**: Flexible endoscopes should have leak tests performed before first use of new equipment, after each use (and before manual cleaning), and after repairs or returns from loaned uses. It should then be manually cleaned per manufacturer's guidelines as soon as possible after the leak test. If the leak test is failed it should be removed from use and repaired.
- **Sterilization**: After the leak test and manual cleaning, the flexible endoscope should be disinfected and sterilized per the manufacturer's guidelines. Accessories should be appropriately taken apart. Critical water should be used in mechanical processing, then the manufacturer-recommended solutions for disinfecting and sterilizing. AORN guidelines discourage the use of skin antiseptics, hypochlorites, phenolics, and quaternary ammonium compounds in processing. The parts are then rinsed and dried with a cloth or sponge.
- **Storage**: Flexible endoscopes should be stored in designated drying cabinets located in the processing room or a separate room (not the procedure room) that minimizes exposure to contaminants, per manufacturer's guidelines. Valves should be open, and removable parts should be detached and stored in the same drying cabinet. Visual labels regarding the date/time of sterilization availability for use should be applied. Gloves should be utilized when handling processed endoscopes. Records for processing should be maintained with the details for the period of time designated by the facility.

IMPLANTS

The US Food and Drug Administration defines a surgical implant as a device or item that is placed inside a patient, through a naturally or surgically formed opening, to remain for 30 days or more. Implants are placed inside patients in order to restore, replace, or assist with a bodily function that does not take place without it. Because an implant is placed inside and remains in a patient's body, it must be sterile to avoid introducing infection. Implants should be sterile in their packages when prepared. Often, they are pre-packaged so they can be opened when needed. However, there are times when implants need to undergo sterile processing. The manufacturer's instructions should be followed, but in most cases, the implant can be steam sterilized and then packaged and labeled. Once ready, the package is opened onto the sterile field during surgery, where it remains until it is implanted into the patient.

Explants

Explants are devices that have been removed from patients when they were previously used as implants. Explants are sometimes returned to patients; however, this sometimes cannot be done because of contamination and safety issues. Whether an explant is returned, the process of cleaning it must be determined by authorities of the facility. If the explant is returned to the patient, it must be thoroughly cleaned and decontaminated first. Explants typically are not sterilized before being returned, and the decontamination process alone may not remove all biohazardous material. Therefore, when returning it to the patient, it should be cleaned and decontaminated as well as possible and then placed in a biohazard bag and labeled for the patient. In some cases, the explant cannot be returned to the patient because it is required to be returned to the manufacturer. In these cases, it should be explained to the patient that it is not possible to have the explant returned.

Sponges

The following are some various types of sponges used in surgery and their uses:

- **Lap pads** (tapes, lap packs) are square/rectangular gauze pads used to soak up moderate amounts of blood. They are x-ray detectable.
- **Gauze sponges** (Ray-Tec, swabs, 4×4s, 1×1s) are used to soak up small amounts of blood. These are also used for swabbing/cleaning.
- **Peanuts** are small sponges used to soak up small amounts of blood or are used on forceps when dissection is being performed.
- **Kittner dissectors** are rolls of cotton tape used for absorption/dissection.
- **Tonsil sponges** are balls of cotton-filled gauze used in tonsil surgery. They have a long tape attached to them, which is used for identification/removal.
- **Cottonoid patties** (neuro sponges) are small cotton sponges used on delicate structures. They are x-ray detectable.
- **Pledgets** are small felt pieces used for support underneath sutures in patients with friable tissue.

Sponge Counts

The following are some important things to remember when performing sponge counts:

- All sponges are **counted** by the scrub person and circulating nurse before surgery begins, and numbers are **documented**. If sponges are added later, that is also documented.
- **Packaging** that encloses sponges is to be removed, and sponges are counted regardless of numbers documented on the packaging (as packaging errors can occur).
- Sponges should **never be cut** or manipulated in shape as this may increase the risk for retainment of some or all of the sponge.
- As sponges are used, they are **audibly counted** by the scrub person and circulating nurse, placed in leak-free packages/bags or a pocketed sponge holder, and **discarded** in appropriate containers.
- All sponges are **left in the room** until the procedure is done, counts are accurate, and the patient leaves the room.
- All sponges are counted upon **closure of the surgery** to make sure counts are accurate. If inaccurate, a search is performed on the patient, sponges are recounted, and if still inaccurate, an x-ray of the patient is taken to recover lost counts.
- Packing of wounds should not be done with **x-ray detectable sponges**.

Sharps/Instrument Counts

The following are some important things to remember when performing sharps and instrument counts:

- All sharps and instruments are **counted and documented** by the scrub person and circulating nurse before the procedure.
- Sutures with needles are **left in packaging** until used in the procedure to prevent excessive needles on the field. When opened, the scrub person/circulating nurse verifies the count.
- When a sharp is **broken**, care must be taken to ensure the entirety of the sharp is located and removed.
- All sharps and instruments are **kept in the room** until the entire procedure is finished, counts are accurate, and the patient leaves the room.
- Sharps are contained on **magnetic strips** to prevent movement and subsequent injury to the patient/staff.
- Sharps are **disposed** in leak-proof, puncture-resistant, and appropriately labeled containers.
- Although rare, instruments can be left **inside a patient**, especially when the procedure involves a large/deep area. The final instrument count should occur after the wound has been closed and all instruments have been returned to the scrub person. When counting instruments should be assessed for any signs of breakage/fragmentation or lost parts.

Suturing Equipment

SUTURE SELECTION, SIZE, AND RETENTION

Factors that influence suture selection, suture size, and when retention sutures are used include the following:

- Predicted wound **healing time**
- Presence of wound **contaminants**
- **Location** of wound and desired presentation outcomes or aesthetics
- **Tissue type** involved
- **Nutritional status** of patient
- **Surgeon** preference or familiarity
- **Suture size and type** used
    - **Suture sizes** range from 7 to 11-0. Size 7 is the largest diameter and size 11-0 is the smallest. Sizes 5-0 to 11-0 are smaller than a human hair and are very fragile. Heavier tissues may require larger diameter sutures. Delicate surgeries require small diameter sutures.
    - Tissue that heals rapidly is usually closed with **absorbable sutures**. Tissue that heals slowly may require **nonabsorbable sutures**.
    - **Retention sutures** are used in areas of suturing that require extra support, usually for closures of the abdomen. They relieve tension placed on the smaller sutures holding the wound closed.

NATURAL ABSORBABLE SUTURES

Absorbable sutures are broken down by the body in the healing process and gradually lose tensile strength until completely absorbed by the body. These sutures are either natural or synthetic. Characteristics of natural absorbable sutures include the following:

- **Plain surgical gut** is a natural absorbable suture that loses tensile strength in 7 days and absorbs in 70 days.
- **Chromic gut** is also natural and is treated with chromium salt to allow it to retain tensile strength from 10-14 days. It fully absorbs in 90 days.
- **Phagocytosis** produces enzymes that digest plain gut, chromic gut, and collagen sutures.
- **Absorption** is altered based on altered nutritional statuses, inflammatory responses, and types of tissue involved.
- **Gut sutures** require an alcohol/water solution to keep them pliable. If sutures dry, they must be moistened with sterile water to restore flexibility, but over-moistening can lead to a decrease in tensile strength.

Synthetic Absorbable Sutures

Characteristics of synthetic absorbable sutures include the following:

- **Synthetic absorbable sutures** are made from lactic and glycolic acid and polyester.
- **Hydrolysis** causes these sutures to break down, which involves less tissue reaction than natural suture absorption via phagocytosis.
- **Absorption** is not affected much by patient nutrition, tissue involved, or inflammatory response.
- **Synthetic sutures** have greater tensile strength than natural sutures.
- They are to remain **dry** as moisture reduces tensile strength.
- These are often used on those who have **delayed healing**.
- They are sometimes coated with **triclosan** to prevent bacterial growth/contamination of the wound.

Monofilament and Multifilament Suture Materials

The characteristics/differences of monofilament and multifilament suture materials include the following:

- **Monofilament sutures** contain a single strand of suture material. They have little drag on tissue due to their smooth structure and bacteria do not easily cling to them, which reduces infection rates. The only drawback to the smoothness is that they are more difficult to maintain a knot, and have less tensile strength.
- **Multifilament sutures** contain multiple strands that are either twisted or braided together. They have greater tensile strength and hold knots well. However, they have greater drag on tissue and are more prone to harboring bacteria due to capillarity (allowing of wound fluid to be carried along the suture). Coating of these sutures reduces their drag and capillarity characteristics.

Nonabsorbable Sutures

Characteristics of nonabsorbable sutures include the following:

- **Nonabsorbable sutures** are permanent and are natural or synthetic.
- **Cotton** is natural, twisted multifilament and is somewhat reactive in tissue. Moisture increases tensile strength.
- **Silks** are natural, twisted/braided multifilament strands and are usually black. Even though considered permanent, tensile strength is lost after 1 year. These may exhibit spitting and are somewhat reactive with tissue.
- **Synthetic sutures** include nylon, polyester, polyethylene, polybutester, polypropylene, or stainless steel. These are less irritating to tissue and hold tensile strength longer than natural sutures.
    - **Nylon** is smooth, has high tensile strength, and does not react with tissue.
    - **Polyester** is braided and is coated to reduce drag.
    - **Polybutester** is monofilament and exhibits much flexibility/elasticity.
    - **Polypropylene** does not react with tissue, is monofilament, and has a good tensile strength. It also has memory and must be gently stretched to straighten.
- **Stainless steel** does not react with tissue, has the highest tensile strength, and is used in the closure of bony structures such as the sternum.

Alternatives to Suturing Devices and Drain Use for Wounds

Alternatives to suturing devices include stapling, skin tapes, and adhesives. Drain use for wounds including passive, active, and sump devices are described below:

- **Stapling devices** utilize stainless steel or titanium staples, which are used to approximate wound edge tissue.
- **Skin tapes** also approximate wound edge tissue. They come in varying sizes and have adhesive backing that adheres to the skin. They can be used alone or in conjunction with other skin closing devices.
- **Skin adhesives** actually glue the skin/wound edges together. They prevent bacterial contamination of the wound by sealing it off. In addition, there are no suture/staple tracks/scars left after healing is complete.
- When a wound is closed and has areas of known or potential dead space that may delay healing, **drains** are inserted to eliminate this area. They are used to drain off dead tissues, fluid buildup, or to determine whether hemostasis is adequate beneath the epidermis.
    - **Passive drains** work via gravity or capillary action.
    - **Active drains** utilize negative pressure.
    - **Sump drains** are hooked up to a suction source.

Eyes of Suture Needles

The eye of the suture needle is the location where the suture material is attached to the needle. There are three different types.

- The **closed-eye needle** has a hole that is threaded with the suture material, similar to a regular sewing needle. The edges of the eye are very smooth to prevent fraying of the suture material. This type of needle can be sterilized and reused.
- The **French-eye (split-eye) needle** has a spring mechanism that allows for easier threading of the suture material. They are not commonly used because needles with this type of eye are generally very small and only used in very specialized surgeries.
- **Swaged (atraumatic) needles** do not have an eye, and the suture material is attached to the end of the needle without any break in the contour of the needle. This is the most common type of suture needle used and is disposable. There is a type that allows the needle to be broken off to prevent accidental needle sticks when suturing is completed.

Needle Shapes

Suturing needles with a slight curve, such as one-quarter circle needles and compound curved needles, are primarily used in eye surgeries. The one-quarter circle needle may also be used in microscopic surgeries. The one-half circle and five-eighths circle needles are more curved and require more manipulation of the wrist to properly "bite" the tissue when creating sutures. These are useful when in a deep, crowded space because it is possible to completely visualize the tip of the needle after initially inserting it into the tissue that is to be sutured. The most commonly used suture needle is the three-eighths circle needle. It provides a slight curvature but is comfortable for creating sutures and is commonly used for basic skin lacerations and surgical closure of the skin. The straight needle is rarely used because of its decreased flexibility and limited use, along with the increased risk of needle stick injury associated with it.

Shaft of the Suture Needle

The shaft, or body, of the needle is the main section of the suturing needle between the eye and the point. It can vary in width and even in shape. It may also be straight or curved depending on its use. Some needles can vary in shape. For example, there may be an indented area of the body of the needle in the area where it would be gripped for suturing. Curved needles can vary from forming a quarter of a circle up to curving into over one-half of a circle. The degree of curvature will affect the degree of difficulty the user will have in creating the sutures. The more curved the needle is, the more dexterity is necessary to manipulate the needle when placing the sutures.

Points on Suture Needles

Suturing needles can have points that are sharp, cutting, tapered, or blunt. The cutting needles have a triangular-shaped body and are very sharp. They are frequently used for penetrating thicker tissues, including connective tissue and some bone. Sutures can be placed in tendons using this type of suturing needle. The tapered-point suturing needles have a round body. They are used throughout the GI tract as well as for suturing muscle and fat tissue. Surgeries performed in the oropharyngeal cavity may include sutures using this type of suturing needle. The blunt-point needles have a round body, also. They have been used more frequently to prevent the risk of needle stick that can occur with the sharp suturing needles. It is used primarily for organs of the gastrointestinal tract as well as in connective tissue. There has been some concern that blunt needles may cause some minor tissue trauma when used.

Needle Holders

Needle holders are used for exactly what their name says, to hold the needle while suturing an incision. They are available in different sizes and weights. The important part of selecting an appropriate needle holder for suturing is to ensure it is the correct size and will not damage the needle. Needle holders are usually blunt tipped and have ringed hands and the ability to ratchet closed. The needle is grasped just distal to the eye of the needle. The needle should be positioned within the needle holder so that the curvature of the needle is perpendicular to the straight edge of the instrument. Once positioned correctly in the needle holder, the handles are ratcheted to secure the needle in place. Holding the needle holder, the needle is directed through the patient's skin at about a 90° angle, and the needle holder is rotated to drive the needle back out through the skin. The exact technique for placing sutures using needle holders will vary depending on the type of suture to be used.

Electrosurgery Equipment

Electrosurgery

Electrosurgery involves applying an electric current to tissue that is bleeding to provide hemostasis. Excessive tissue damage can occur, though, if the electrocautery device is set with an energy level that is too high or if nonbleeding tissues are treated with the device. When bleeding is present within the surgical site, pressure should be applied, and the exact source of the bleeding should be identified. The electrocautery device should than be applied to the area, using the lowest voltage of electricity necessary to effectively provide hemostasis. A mistake that is frequently made is that electrosurgery techniques are applied over an entire area when there is bleeding instead of just the specific identified vessel that requires cautery. For tissues that tend to bleed quite heavily, such as organ tissue, the electrocautery device may be used for creating the surgical incision. This prevents massive bleeding and the potential resultant effects upon the patient.

Evolution of Electrosurgery

In the 1920s the first electrosurgery generator was developed by a biophysicist named William Bovie. This machine used high frequency electrical current that passed through the patient's tissues. Neurosurgeon, Dr. Harvey Cushing, was the first to use the "Bovie" as it became called to assist in removing a brain tumor. The instrument consisted of two small metal pieces that conducted electricity and were separated by air. This is similar to the function of a spark plug. Dr. Cushing performed over 500 cranial procedures using this device. As more surgeons became familiar with the use of an electrosurgery device, the popularity of the device increased. This new technique allowed the surgeon to perform surgery in less time, with less blood loss, lower infection rates, and decreased tissue damage. Electrocautery is now standard in every operating room around the world.

Electrocautery Machines

Electrocautery ("Bovie") machines are described below:

- Ground-referenced generators used for electrocautery require an **adequate ground** to be placed from the generator to the earth.
- Newer, isolated systems allow a **transformer** within the unit to accept the ground.
- A **continuous-frequency waveform** causes cutting to occur.
- An **interrupted-frequency waveform** causes coagulation to occur.
- The **active electrode** is the part that delivers the current to the operative site and is controlled by a foot pedal or handpiece controller. These can be monopolar or bipolar.
    - **Monopolar electrodes** are used in combination with a dispersive electrode attached to the patient.
    - **Bipolar electrodes** have the dispersive electrode next to the active electrode.
- **Dispersive electrodes** may be disposable or reusable and may attach directly to the patient or may be a pad underneath the body of the patient. Some reusable dispersive electrodes have weight requirements in order to be used.

Bipolar Electrosurgery

Bipolar electrosurgery is accomplished by using a device that contains both positive and negative poles that are located close together. This allows the electric current to pass from one pole to another, rather than through the patient's body. This also prevents a grounding device from being necessary. The instrument is designed like forceps so that the electric current passes through the tissue that is grasped. Bipolar electrosurgery is not very effective against larger bleeding vessels. It is commonly used in surgeries that do not have a large amount of bleeding, such as some neurosurgical procedures. Because the electrical current is contained and not traveling through the patient, it has been recommended with electrical implants, such as a pacemaker or automatic internal cardiac defibrillator. When using a bipolar electrosurgery device, ensure that it is connected correctly to the generator to prevent delivery of a monopolar electric current with resultant tissue damage to the patient.

Electrocautery Pencil

The electrocautery pencil is a relatively small, handheld device that contains a battery which supplies a direct, or simple, current of electricity. This prevents the electric current from leaving the device to travel through the patient. The electrocautery pencil consists of a looped wire at the end of the instrument that is heated by electricity delivered from the battery. This is then used to cauterize bleeding tissue. Because this is based on a simple current of electricity without transmission of the electric current to the patient, a grounding device is not necessary. The drawback to an electrocautery pencil is that it is effective on only small amount of bleeding and cannot be used on larger bleeding tissue. It is frequently used in surgeries that involve small amounts of bleeding, such as eye surgeries. The ease with which the wire loop on the end of the pencil can become adhered to tissue is another drawback to using this device.

Pros and Cons of Using Electrocautery for Hemostasis

Some pros of using electrocautery include the fact that cutting and coagulation occur rapidly, which may reduce the amount of time needed to perform the surgery. Power settings can also be adjusted for appropriateness for the surgery to be performed. Some cons in using electrocautery include the fact that electrocauterized tissue produces free radicals that must be reabsorbed by the body, and sloughing of tissue may occur in the wound when excessive amounts of tissue are cauterized, inhibiting the healing process.

Fulguration utilizes sparks from the electrocautery unit to char tissue, wherein the electrode does not come in direct contact with the tissue, causing initial coagulation and further necrosis. It can be used to remove masses of tissue or to stop heavy bleeders. **Desiccation** is used more frequently and consists of the active electrode coming into contact with the skin and coagulating tissue without causing the same degree of necrosis as fulguration.

Supply and Material Management

Preventative Maintenance of Surgical Equipment

Preventive maintenance for surgical equipment includes the following:

- **Organizing**: Checklists should be prepared for different types of equipment to ensure that preventive maintenance is done consistently, following the same procedures, so that no steps are missed.
- **Cleaning/storing**: The appropriate manner of cleaning (including the correct cleaning solution), drying, sterilizing, and storing surgical equipment should be utilized to prevent damage. Blood and body fluids should be removed within 20 minutes of surgery if possible, to prevent corrosion of metal.
- **Inspecting/testing**: All equipment should be examined with each use to ensure it is intact and operating correctly. Cords of all electrical equipment must be inspected and the equipment removed from service with any sign of fraying or breakage. Routine testing should be carried out.
- **Maintaining**: According to manufacturer's guidelines, all routine maintenance procedures should be scheduled, carried out, and documented.
- **Repairing**: Damaged equipment should be immediately repaired or discarded if unusable. Replacement parts should be readily available to prevent extended down time.

Managing Materials

The perioperative nurse is first of all responsible that the materials in the operating suite are kept in appropriate containers and locations to prevent contamination. Material counts are very important to ensure that there are adequate numbers to be able to perform surgery; the nurse must do this frequently. The nurse must also check the integrity of the materials in the operating suite. They must be free from visible evidence of potential contamination and have evidence of sterility via outside labeling. When the nurse is preparing for an operation, he or she must assemble the appropriate materials for the procedure and have them in the room ready to go. During and after the procedure as materials are used, proper disposal, cleaning, and packaging is important not only to maintain safety of the environment, but also to keep materials in good working order to maintain their integrity and preserve cost containment.

Services or Material Shortages

As with staffing shortages, service or material shortages also sacrifice patient care. Once the shortage is identified, the nurse should immediately place calls to the institution's supply acquisition department. If supplies are not in-house, it is sometimes necessary to send a staff member to a local medical supply store to pick up supplies. If the shortage is not able to be fixed, or when certain services are not able to be rendered to the unit, it may pose some potential complications. All staff members should be notified of the shortage and when it is expected to be corrected. Sometimes, depending on what is not available, the staff can make some minor adjustments in what materials they use or can perform some of the services not available for that day. However, sometimes staff cannot make up for the shortage, and it may be that certain procedures must be canceled and rescheduled.

Specimen Management

Obtaining and Labeling Specimens in the Surgical Environment

When obtaining a specimen during a surgical procedure, care is taken to avoid contamination or damage throughout the process of handling the specimen. The correct size container must first be made available, depending on the size and type of specimen. The container must be leak- and puncture-proof. The surgeon obtains the specimen and it is transferred to a sterile container. The scrub nurse may assist with the container and add a fixative or preservative, if required. The nurse then labels the container. The specimen should be labeled appropriately, including two patient identifiers (name, DOB, MRN) and hospital number, type of specimen and its site of removal, the date and time, the type of preservative, and the name of the physician. The nurse should verify the type of specimen by reading aloud the type and having another member of the team verify that it is correct. If required, a specimen requisition form should be completed and the specimen label verified against the form.

Preparing a Specimen for Transportation

Cerebrospinal fluid	Collect in 3 tubes and keep at room temperature with immediate delivery to lab. Cerebrospinal fluid must be processed within 60 minutes to avoid degradation.
Gastric fluids	Place in sterile container at room temperature.
Nasopharyngeal secretions	Place swab in tube with transport medium.
Serous fluids	Place in sterile container for C&S, EDTA tube for cell counts/smears, and oxalate or fluoride tubes for chemistry tests.
Synovial fluid	Place in ETDA or heparin tube for cell counts, smear, and crystal identification, sterile tube for C&S, and plain tube for chemistry and immunology tests.
Tissue samples	Place in correctly labeled sterile container that identifies the type of specimen and the location where it was obtained (e.g., left breast). Large specimens (such as a kidney) may be placed in a basin and handed off to the circulating nurse, who will place it in an appropriate container. Directions vary according to the type of sample, but some require preservatives (such as formalin) while others must remain dry. Multiple samples should be numbered consecutively.

Special Considerations

Certain specimens require special considerations for collection and transportation:

- **Breast cancer specimens**: Specimens must be kept moist prior to fixation and transported to the lab as quickly as possible in a puncture- and leak-proof container. The date and time of specimen collection and time of fixation must be recorded.
- **Placental specimens**: Procedures for collection and transportation must follow facility guidelines and adhere to local and federal regulations, which generally require a release form and conditions for collection (specimen is non-infectious and in a fresh state). Prior to wasting the specimen, the patient's preference for this process must be confirmed, as some cultures may not view placental tissue as medical waste. Placentas that are not disposed of immediately should be refrigerated.
- **Radioactive specimens**: Handling is dictated by local and federal guidelines. Sentinel lymph node localization procedures are considered radioactive and require standard precautions, placing as much distance between the perioperative staff and the radioactive tissue as possible by using special instrumentation, and following proper containment, transportation, and cleaning procedures. Radioactive seed localization procedures also require standard precautions. AORN guidelines recommend the use of a collection sock in the suction cannister to ensure all seeds are collected (by forceps) before closure, instrument breakdown through the use of a radiation detection device or radiograph, and immediate notification in the case of a lost seed. Proper emergency equipment must be nearby for emergent radioactive seed retrieval and annual training on radiation monitoring and emergency procedures provided to all staff.
- **Forensic evidence specimens**: The appropriate chain of custody for specimens for forensic evidence must be established in facility protocol, which includes input from both perioperative staff and other medical staff (emergency department, pathology, and risk management) in addition to local law enforcement and local security. Standardized forensic evidence kits must be utilized for collection. Evidence must be collected as soon as possible using appropriate PPE. Clothing should be collected with minimal disruption (do not shake or ball up) and put into a paper bag. Linens from the stretcher should be collected in a paper bag. Invasive collection, such as bullet fragments/shrapnel should be grasped with rubber forceps and contained individually (unless they are fragments of the same bullet in which case they can be collected together).
- **Highly infectious specimens**: Patients should be screened for highly infectious diseases such as Ebola or COVID-19 prior to specimen collection so that staff can be prepared with the appropriate PPE. Standard precautions are used during transport after the specimen is placed in a rigid and leak-proof container, which is then labeled and put into a second container with the required documents attached to the outside of the second container. Specimen handover to pathology staff should include alerting the staff of the infectious status of the specimen.

Universal Protocol

Elements of Universal Protocol for Surgery

Pre-Procedure Verification and Site Marking

The Joint Commission's Universal Protocol for surgical error prevention (wrong site, wrong procedure, or wrong person) consists of the pre-procedure verification, site marking, and surgical time out. The **pre-procedure verification** is performed first, and involves confirmation of the patient, the procedure, and the site. When possible, the patient should be involved in this process. Additionally, documentation is reviewed, ensuring consent was gathered, instruments/equipment required for the procedure are summarized and confirmed as available, and labs and baseline vitals reviewed.

Site marking with an appropriate surgical pen, which is required by CMS, occurs prior to the procedure, often prior to the patient entering the procedure room. The surgical pen should be such that the ink does not interfere with or disappear with surgical skin antiseptic agents. The site marking should be visible after the patient has been draped.

Surgical Time Out

The pre-surgical/procedural time out is the final part of the Joint Commission's Universal Protocol for preventing surgical/procedural errors. The **time-out procedure**, which should follow a standard format, includes the following elements:

- A designated team member initiates the time-out before beginning an invasive procedure/incision.
- All team members who will participate in the procedure must be present and all must communicate during the time-out.
- The entire team must agree that they have the correct patient and the correct site and must agree on the procedure that is scheduled.
- If a patient is scheduled for more than one procedure, a time-out must be called prior to the beginning of all subsequent procedures.
- If those performing the procedure change during the procedure, for example if another physician takes over, another time-out must be called.
- Each time-out must be documented.

Hospital National Patient Safety Goals (2021)

The Joint Commission has issued the 2021 Hospital National Patient Safety Goals, intended to improve patient safety. Goals include:

- Identify patients correctly: Two identifiers are necessary.
- Improve staff communication: Test results should be reported immediately to the correct person.
- Use medicines safely: Ensure proper labeling, verify anticoagulant dosages, review and report medications.
- Use alarms safely: Respond quickly and appropriately.
- Prevent infection: Use appropriate handwashing and guidelines to prevent difficult-to-treat, post-surgical, central line-associated blood, and catheter-associated urinary tract infections.
- Identify patient safety risks: Assess for suicidal ideation.
- Prevent surgical mistakes: Ensure correct surgery on the correct patient, mark surgical area on the patient, and carry out a surgical time-out prior to beginning the surgical procedure.

WHO SURGICAL SAFETY CHECKLIST

The World Health Organization (WHO) published the Surgical Safety Checklist to improve safety. It has 3 components.

Prior to induction: Sign in	Confirm identify, site, procedure, consent, and site marked. Complete anesthesia safety check, monitor pulse oximetry, check allergies, assess aspiration risk or difficult airway and determine if equipment is available, and assess risk of bleeding (>500 mL or 7 mL/kg in pediatric patients), IV access, and availability of fluids.
Prior to incision: Time out	Team members are introduced and roles are explained; patient, site, and procedure are confirmed by the team; the surgeon reviews steps, duration, and anticipated blood loss; anesthesia team reviews patient-specific concerns; determine if antibiotic prophylaxis given within 60 minutes and if essential imaging is displayed.
Prior to transfer: Sign out	Nurse and team confirm name of procedure recorded; instrument, needle, and sponge count correct; specimens properly labeled; and key concerns reviewed.

OBTAINING SURGICAL CONSENT

Surgical consent must be informed, which means the patient is aware of the procedure, as well as its risks and benefits. It is the physician's responsibility to explain the information so the patient will understand. The nurse is not responsible for this part of the consent, although he or she may sign the form as a witness. The nurse should ensure that the patient actually understands what is being signed and is that the patient is competent. The patient who is having the procedure should be the person to sign the consent. However, if the patient is unable to sign due to being a minor or due to not having the capacity to make the decision, then another person must sign for the patient. In the case of a minor, this person is a parent or guardian. If the patient is an adult who cannot sign, then a designated proxy, such as a power of attorney must sign.

ADVANCE DIRECTIVE STATUS

It is essential for the health care staff to know the status of a patient's advance directive before surgery. The advance directive is a legal document that explains the patient's wishes for care as well as appointing a person to make decisions if that patient should become unable to do so. If something were to happen during the surgical process, the advance directive would indicate the patient's wishes, but in most cases the physician must translate that directive into an actual hospital order, such as a Do Not Resuscitate (DNR) order if indicated and if the physician felt that was appropriate. Prior to surgery, the patient should notify the physician that he has an advance directive, as well as give a copy of the advance directive to the admitting nurse. The patient should have a copy of the advance directive, and if there is a designated power of attorney for medical decisions, that person should have a copy as well. During surgery or admission to any inpatient facility, a copy of a patient's advance directive should be kept on the chart, and all involved in the care of the patient should be aware of directives.

Management of Hemodynamics

Hemostasis

The body performs a natural method for hemostasis in the event of injury to a blood vessel, when platelets become attracted to the site, adhere to the surface, and create a plug which occludes the injured area, preventing bleeding. The **coagulation cascade** then takes over. Platelets break down releasing thromboplastin, which combines with prothrombin and calcium in the blood to form thrombin. Thrombin combines with fibrinogen, which forms fibrin, which forms a framework for the clot to form. As blood loss decreases, a negative feedback system prevents the clot from forming further. This process is sufficient for small wounds. In surgery, large bleeding must be controlled through artificial methods, whether chemical, mechanical, or thermal.

Artificial Chemical Hemostasis

The forms of artificial chemical hemostasis include the following:

- **Thrombin** is an enzyme that is used on superficial bleeding sites for controlling capillary bleeding. It is only used topically, never injected. It is a dry white powder that can be premixed and applied with a gelatin sponge, or sprinkled on the site directly. It lasts for 3 hours.
- **Absorbable gelatin** is either supplied as a powder or a pad (Gelfoam). It is used for capillary bleeding and when placed at the site, fibrin deposits into the pad, the pad will swell, and clot formation ensues. It can soak up to 45 times its weight in blood. If left in the body, it will be absorbed in 20-40 days. The powder form is mixed into a paste and applied to the site. Once hemostasis occurs, the paste or pad is often simply removed to prevent excess undue pressure on the site.
- **Oxidized cellulose** (Oxycel, Surgicel) is a gauze/cotton pad that is specially treated and can absorb 7-8 times its weight in fluid. In the presence of blood, it swells, forms a gel, and causes clot formation. It is absorbable in the body in 7-14 days. Care should be taken as swelling may cause undue pressure on surrounding structures.
- **Microfibrillar collagen** (Avitene, Instat) is a fluffy, white material, also available as pads, sponges, or felt. It is applied dry over the source of bleeding. Platelets and fibrin adhere to the collagen to form a clot. It is often used around friable tissue. It is absorbable, but should be left at minimal amounts to absorb.
- **Styptic sticks** constrict blood vessels. Epinephrine, silver nitrate, tannic acid, or a combination of phenol and alcohol are common styptic agents. They are usually used topically on very small injuries/vessels.

Artificial Hemostasis Using an Argon Beam Enhanced Device

Argon beam electrosurgery coagulates tissue rapidly. Characteristics of artificial hemostasis using an argon beam enhanced device include the following:

- This technique uses **argon gas and electrical energy** to achieve hemostasis. When delivered to the desired site of coagulation, the ionized argon gas removes liquid blood, which allows for greater visualization of the surgical site, and the electric energy creates an eschar on the tissue and coagulates the tissue.
- The system is composed of a **generator**, a **handpiece**, and a **dispersive electrode**.
- The **dispersive electrode** must be used to dissipate energy as in monopolar electrocautery.
- Argon beam devices cause **less tissue damage**, so less plume and odor are created as well.
- It can be used in **open procedures** or **endoscopically**.

Artificial Hemostasis Using an Ultrasonic Energy Device

An ultrasonic energy device cuts and coagulates tissue through ultrasonic motion instead of electric current:

- The ultrasonic motion causes **protein denaturation** and **coagulation** of tissue.
- The system is composed of a **generator**, a **handpiece**, and a **foot pedal**.
- This device is useful in **open procedures** and **endoscopically**. It is also safer than electric current for use around delicate organs.
- **Cutting and coagulation** are dependent on 4 factors:
    - If more tension is placed on the tissue, cutting is faster and coagulation is slower. The opposite occurs with less tension.
    - A blunt blade coagulates more; a sharper blade will cut more.
    - If more power is used, cutting speed increases and coagulation is decreased. The opposite is true with less power.
    - Time is also a factor. If the device is allowed to stay on the tissue longer, more coagulation occurs. If not, more cutting occurs.

Mechanical Forms of Hemostasis

Various mechanical forms of hemostasis can be utilized to control bleeding:

- **Clamps** can be used to occlude a vessel, which is usually followed by a means of maintaining hemostasis such as a tie (material tied around the vessel/structure), suture ligature (tie with a needle to tie through the structure), or a ligating clip (metal clip used to permanently close off the structure and left in the patient).
- **Bone wax** is used for hemostasis to bony structures. It is made from beeswax and is rubbed over the area until hemostasis occurs.
- **Pressure** is applied with sponges/gauze to control bleeding from small sources. Pressure is sometimes used to blot large areas of blood in order to be able to identify the source of bleeding, and then additional methods of hemostasis can be employed.

Permanent Hemostasis Techniques

Vascular clips	Used in place of suture ligatures, especially when many small vessels need to be ligated. Most are made of titanium although absorbable vascular clips are also available. The clips are applied with a special clip applicator.
Vascular staples	Vascular staples are applied to occlude vessels with a stapler and are especially useful for difficult to reach areas with laparoscopic or minimally-invasive procedures.
Aneurysm clips	Titanium clips are placed about the neck of an aneurysm to prevent rupture or further bleeding for aneurysms located in the brain. This procedure requires a craniotomy to locate and visualize the aneurysm.
Aneurysm glue	Aneurysm glue is introduced to the aneurysm through a femoral catheter in an outpatient procedure. When the glue is released at the aneurysm, it solidifies and strengthens the wall of the vessel.

Ligation Methods

Suture Ligature

Suture ligature (AKA stick tie) involves the use of an instrument-held suture to tie off a vessel or other hollow tube or structure. Suture ligatures are utilized during surgery primarily to permanently occlude a large blood vessel, such as may be needed with vein stripping or other surgical procedures where large blood vessels are cut. For a common procedure, the vessel or other structure is first clamped and then an atraumatic needle with a piece of suture material is threaded through the vessel beneath the clamp, back through again, and then the needle removed and the suture pulled tight. The suture is then tied in the front and then brought back around and tied again in the back. This results in a double ligation. The clamp is removed and the vessel/structure assessed for any further bleeding. Commonly used suture ligature material includes silk and catgut but absorbable sutures, such as Vicryl may also be used.

Free Tie, Reel, and Instrument Ligation

Ligating methods include the following:

- **Free tie:** The surgeon or RNAS-C wraps a length of suture material about the vessel to be ligated and then ties the suture into a surgical knot, pulling it tightly to occlude the vessel. The vessel may be clamped, but the suture material is handled manually. A common procedure is to simply wrap the ligature material about the vessel below a clamp and knot the front and back.
- **Reel**: This dispenser contains a long continuous length of absorbable or nonabsorbable suture material, such as Vicryl, and can be used to quickly tie off multiple vessels or to suture tissue without needing to request more suture material or look away from the operative site. Typically, the surgeon pulls the length needed, uses the suture to tie off a vessel, and the assistant cuts the suture, and then the process repeats. Reel sutures are commonly used on superficial bleeders.
- **Instrument**: A length of suture material is loaded on to an instrument, such as a Crile hemostat or Adson clamp, to ligate vessels that are not easily accessible by hand, such as deep veins that are clamped with a hemostat.

RNAS-C's Role in the Hemostasis Response

The role of the RNAS-C in **hemostasis response** for noncritical tissue bleeding and routine bleeding includes:

- Monitoring blood loss through observation of sponges, suctioning, and wound appearance.
- Monitoring urinary output for a decrease that may indicate hypovolemia.
- Monitoring changes in vital signs, especially blood pressure and heart rate.
- Alerting the physician to indications of excessive bleeding.

Interventions by the RNAS-C may include:

- Applying compression to the site of bleeding.
- Using instrumentation, such as hemostats, to clamp bleeding vessels.
- Utilizing temporary and permanent hemostatic devices, such as vascular clamps, vascular staples, vessel loops, tourniquets. and umbilical tape.
- Using suture ligatures to control bleeding.
- Utilizing an electrosurgical device for coagulation to control bleeding vessels.
- Assessing the need for chemical hemostasis and selecting and utilizing the appropriate method, which may include silver nitrate, topical gelatin matrices (Gelfoam), thrombin sealants (Thrombin-JMI), fibrin sealants (Evicel), oxidized regenerated cellulose (Fibrillar), microfibrillar collagens (Instat), and various other surgical glues.

Surgeon's Role in the Hemostasis Response

When a bleeding and coagulation emergency occurs during surgery, such as critical tissue bleeding, massive bleeding (blood loss of more than a normal circulating volume in 24 hours), and DIC, the **surgeon's role in hemostasis** response includes:

- Initiating a call for extra surgical staff to assist.
- Directing the notification of the blood bank and activating the protocol for massive blood transfusion or articulating the need for multiple transfusions if there is no established protocol.
- Exploring and assessing to determine the cause and source of the bleeding.
- Identifying the need for anticoagulation reversal.
- Directing large IV access with rapid infusion sets to facilitate transfusions and fluid resuscitation.
- Monitoring vital signs, hemoglobin (to maintain >6 g/dL), and coagulation status.
- Utilizing appropriate hemostatic measures and considering the need for recombinant coagulation factors for coagulopathy.
- Assigning a surgical staff member to monitor ordering and administering transfusions.
- Monitoring for adverse reactions to transfusions, such as hypervolemia, TRALI, hypocalcemia, hyperkalemia, and hypothermia, and directing corrective measures.

Fluid Replacement

Colloids

Colloids are solutions (usually isotonic saline but available with glucose and in hypertonic solutions) with dissolved, high-molecular-weight (large), non-crystalline molecules and electrolytes. Colloids stay in the intravascular space more readily than crystalloids, so they are effective volume expanders. They are used primarily for fluid replacement with severe intravascular deficits, such as from hemorrhage and in conditions with severe hypoalbuminemia or where protein loss is probable, such as severe burns. Colloids are derived from plasma proteins or synthetic glucose polymers. Colloids obtained from plasma contain albumin (5% or 25% solutions) and plasma protein fractions (5%). Jehovah's Witnesses may object to receiving these solutions. Colloids obtained from synthetic glucose contain hydroxyethyl starches and gelatin. Colloids have more safety concerns than crystalloids. Allergic reactions (including anaphylaxis) may be caused by dextran, hydroxyethyl, and (to a lesser degree) albumin. Bleeding may also result from a reduction in platelet aggregation, factor VII, von Willebrand factor, and prolonged partial thromboplastin time, so colloids should be avoided in patients with coagulopathies.

Crystalloid Solutions

Both colloids and crystalloid solutions (or a combination) are used as intravenous fluid therapy during surgery. Crystalloids are solutions of inorganic small molecules, glucose, or saline, dissolved in water. There are many **types of crystalloid solutions**:

- **Hypotonic solutions** are maintenance solutions used to replace water loss. Dextrose in water (D5W) is commonly used when patients have a water deficit and for those with sodium restriction.
- **Hypertonic solutions** are used for hyponatremia (3% saline) and severe hypovolemic shock (3–7.5% saline).
- **Isotonic solutions** are replacement solutions for loss of water and electrolytes. Isotonic crystalloids, such as normal saline (0.9%), Ringer's lactate (contains potassium), and Plasmalyte (contains potassium) are most commonly used. Different solutions contain different electrolytes (e.g., sodium, chloride, potassium, calcium, lactate, magnesium), so monitoring electrolytes is essential.

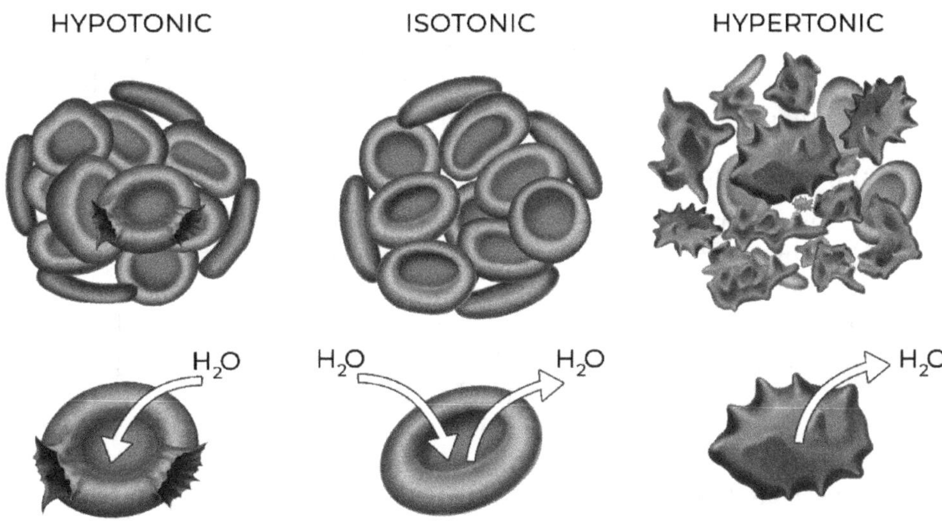

Crystalloids are effective in restoring fluid volume, but blood replacement requires 3:1 administration of crystalloids, while colloids are 1:1 replacement, and rapid crystalloid administration may result in tissue edema. Crystalloids are usually given as initial resuscitation fluid in emergencies. Glucose in some solutions may prevent ketosis and hypoglycemia.

Hypertonic Saline Solution

Hypertonic saline solution (HSS) has a sodium concentration higher than 0.9% (normal saline) and is used to reduce intracranial pressure/cerebral edema. Concentrations usually range from 2–23%, but 3% solutions may be used with cardiac surgery patients to treat total body fluid overload. HSS draws fluid from the tissue through osmosis. As edema decreases, circulation improves. HSS also expands plasma, increasing cerebral perfusion pressure, and counteracts hyponatremia that can occur in the brain after injury, causing increased intracranial pressure. Peripheral administration can only tolerate a concentration up to 3% of HSS in a large bore (18-gauge) catheter. Higher concentrations of HSS must be administered via central line.

HSS can be administered continuously at rates varying from 30–100 mL/hr. Rates must be carefully controlled. Fluid status must be monitored to prevent hypovolemia, which increases the risk of renal failure. **Laboratory monitoring** includes the following:

- Sodium (every 6 hours) is maintained at 135–155 mmol/L. Higher levels can cause heart, respiratory, and renal failure.
- Serum osmolality (every 12 hours) is maintained at 320 mOsm/L. Higher levels can cause renal failure.

Mannitol

Mannitol is an osmotic diuretic that increases excretion of both sodium and water and reduces intracranial pressure and brain mass. Mannitol may also be used to shrink the cells of the blood–brain barrier to help other medications breach this barrier. Mannitol is administered by intravenous infusion. It may be used during cardiopulmonary bypass to control blood pressure. Additionally, 20% mannitol at 5 mL/kg is given with furosemide, 1 g, and dopamine, 2–3 µg/kg/min, to produce diuresis within 6 hours of onset of oliguria. Fluid and electrolyte balances must be carefully monitored as well as intake, output, and body weight. Concentrations of 20–25% require a filter. Crystals may form if the mannitol solution is too cold, and the mannitol container may require heating (in 80 °C water) and shaking to dissolve crystals; the solution should be cooled to body temperature or less before administration. Mannitol cannot be administered in polyvinylchloride bags as precipitates form. Side effects include fluid and electrolyte imbalance, nausea, vomiting, hypotension, tachycardia, fever, and urticaria.

Intravenous Fluid Warmers

Intravenous fluid warmers warm fluids to body temperature to avoid inducing or worsening hypothermia, especially in geriatric patients. In cases of severe hypothermia, warmed fluids (104–108 °F) may be administered to raise core temperature. Also, medications are absorbed more effectively in warmed fluids. There are numerous types of fluid warmers. Simple warmers warm fluid in the tubing as the tubing passes through the warming device. Some units are disposable and battery powered, some are approved for both blood and fluids, and some units require special tubing or equipment. All must be monitored carefully. Special heating chambers may heat a number of IV fluid bags at one time in a cabinet-type structure. Intraoperative warming of IV fluids may prevent anesthesia-associated hypothermia.

Wound Healing

Phases of Wound Healing

Closed Wounds

There are three main phases to closed wound healing:

- The **inflammatory phase** begins within seconds of wound formation. This is the process by which platelets and clotting proteins form a clot at the wound site. Immune cells travel to the area and begin releasing substances that will destroy bacteria and dead tissue cells.
- The **proliferative phase** begins a few days after the wound is created and lasts for about 3 weeks. This is the stage at which healing is evident with scab tissue being replaced by soft skin and connective tissue. The wound edges close during this phase and protein is used to form collagen and create a strong base for the wound to enter its final phase of healing.
- The **maturation phase** occurs for months and is the stage in which the wound forms a scar and gains added strength. Once complete, the wound has reached its maximum strength.

Open Wounds

The healing process that occurs with an open wound is similar to that of a closed wound, except it may take longer for the proliferative phase to occur. Once the inflammatory process has completed, the inflammatory cells leave the area. They are replaced by cells that promote tissue growth and the development of granulation tissue within the wound bed. After just a few days, the wound edges begin to contract and continue doing so for approximately 2 weeks. At this point, the wound can be left to heal by secondary intention or, if possible, the wound edges may be drawn together and secured with sutures or staples which would be considered tertiary intention. Once the granulation tissue has filled the wound, the body will lay down collagen over the area of new tissue to help increase strength and begin scar formation. This final phase can continue for several months.

Primary Intention Wound Healing

Wounds can heal by primary intention if they are caused by a clean cut. This would include a surgical incision or a traumatic cut made by a knife or piece of glass. They are generally not dirty wounds nor caused by rough trauma, and can be cleaned adequately using irrigation with sterile saline. This type of wound has edges that can be well-approximated with slightly everted edges and closed using skin glue, sutures, or surgical staples. There are generally no gaps in the incision line while healing occurs because the incision is a clean cut and the edges will draw together evenly. This type of wound usually heals without any complications, though infection can occur. This is more likely with traumatic wounds caused by a clean cut that may have a very small foreign body or bacteria trapped inside. Copious irrigation with sterile saline is essential to ensure the wound is as clean as possible before the edges are pulled together and sealed.

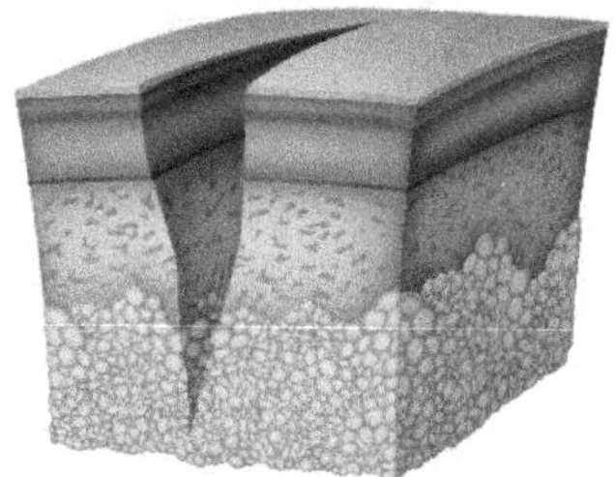
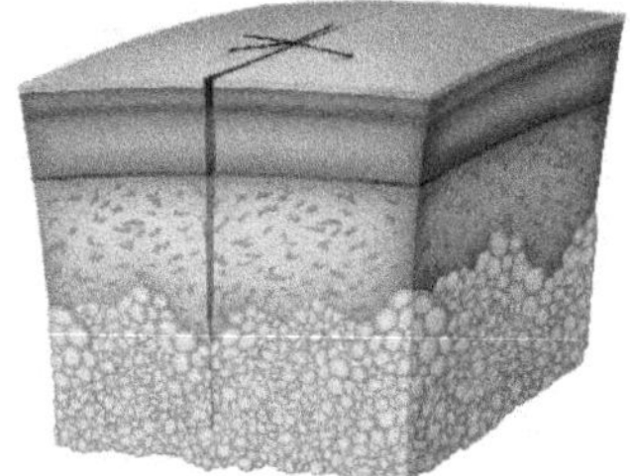
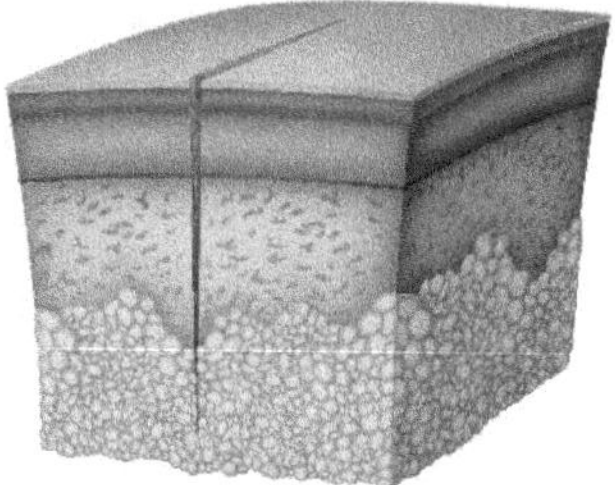

Secondary Intention Wound Healing

Wounds that heal by secondary intention are characterized by excessive tissue loss that prevents the use of sutures or staples for wound closure. These wounds are wide and left open to heal. If kept clean and moist, granulation tissue will form along the bottom of the wound and gradually fill in. This will be followed for the formation of scar tissue over the superficial surface of the wound, though the scar will be wide and not as cosmetically pleasing as the scar that is left behind after a wound that has healed by primary intention.

Tissue that has undergone excessive debridement may be left open to heal by secondary intention. This is necessary in a situation where an infection is present to avoid trapping bacteria within the wound. Traumatic wounds may also be left open to heal by secondary intention because there may be loss of tissue that prevents the wound edges from being well-approximated for suturing or stapling.

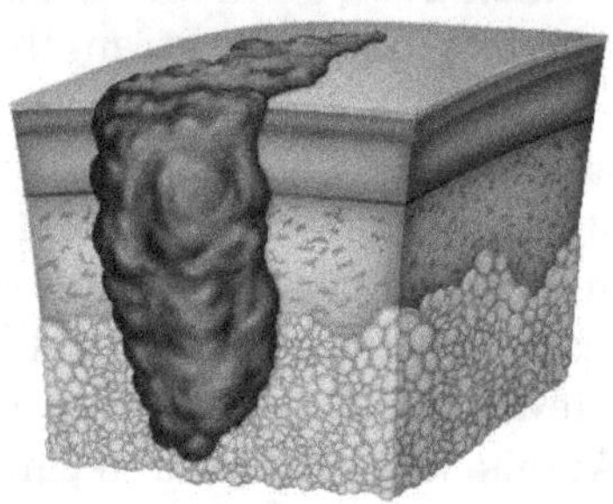
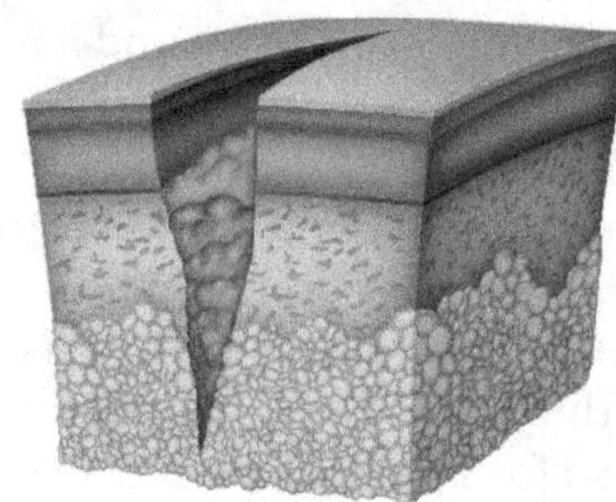
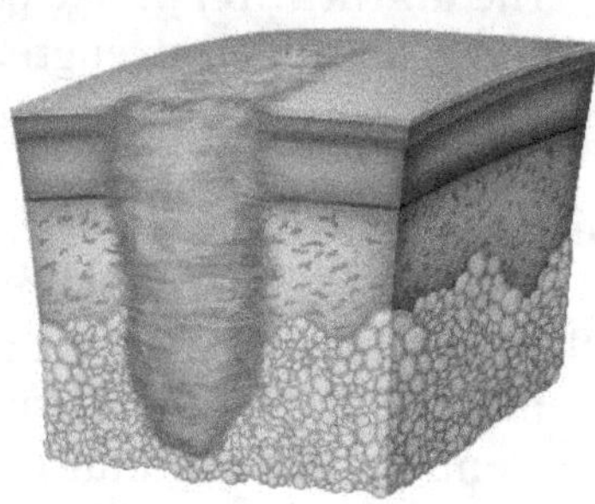

Tertiary Intention Wound Healing

Tertiary wound healing is similar to healing by secondary intention, except that the wound edges will be pulled together and sealed using sutures or staples after several days of healing. As the wound begins to heal and granulation tissue forms in the wound bed, the wound edges tend to draw slightly together. If enough of this contraction of the wound edges occurs, they can be pulled together to close the wound. The advantage of tertiary wound healing is the prevention of infection. The wound will not be left open for an excessive period of time, which decreases the chance of bacteria growing within it, leading to a wound infection. There can be more scarring with wound healing using the tertiary method, but it cannot be avoided if the wound is very wide with excessive tissue loss. This most frequently occurs with traumatic wounds or wounds that are widened due to removal of tissue from debridement.

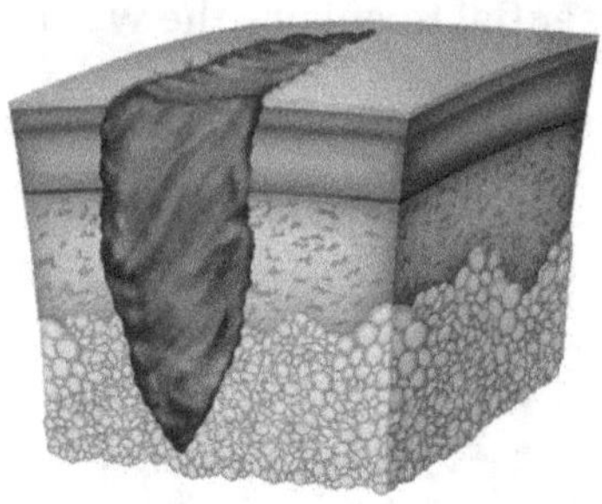
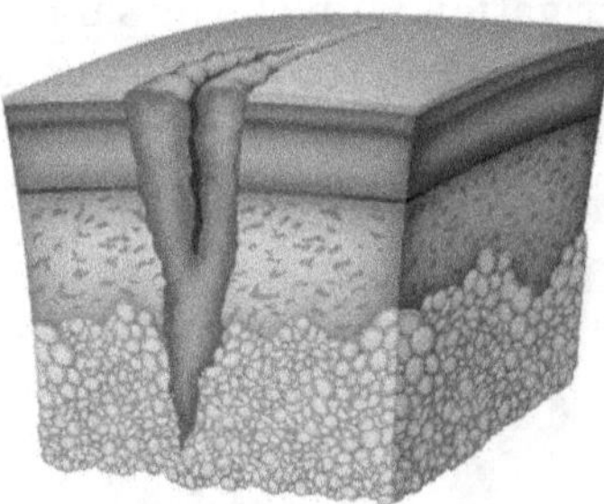
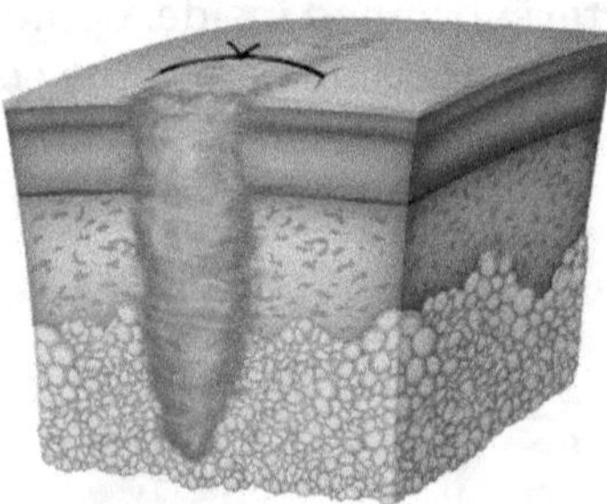

Preoperative Factors Contributing to Wound Healing

A patient's risk factors should be identified and addressed before surgery to prevent any complications of wound healing. Consideration should be given for appropriate administration of prophylactic antibiotics prior to surgery. It is recommended that antibiotics be given parenterally (IV) no more than 2 hours before surgery begins. Most patients only need one dose of antibiotics, but patients undergoing more complicated surgeries may require more than one dose. Another factor to consider preoperatively is the length of time that the patient has had an open wound. If this is a traumatic injury and several hours have passed since the time of injury, it may be necessary for the patient to undergo extensive debridement and irrigation for proper removal of contaminated tissue. It may even be advisable to let the wound heal by secondary intention to prevent closure of a wound that could possibly be contaminated with bacteria. This would depend on the nature of the injury.

Skin Grafts to Promote Healing

Skin grafts are used to form the superficial layer of the wound when there is extensive tissue damage that prevents wound healing. The skin is either from a donor or can be harvested from the patient. The graft is a very thin layer of skin that does not contain its own blood supply. The graft can be split thickness which involves the outer layer of skin and part of the dermis, or second layer, or it can be a full thickness graft which includes all of the first two layers of skin. The graft is placed over the open wound and the blood supply from the recipient will function to heal the wound by incorporating the graft into the layers of tissue. The first few days of healing following placement of the skin graft are crucial to ensure the graft is not moved and that the blood supply is not compromised. Collections of blood can form under the graft so a small drain may be placed to prevent this complication.

Drugs That May Interfere with Proper Wound Healing

Various medications can interfere with wound healing; therefore, their benefits must be assessed against their risks, with the patient being closely monitored for wound healing complications:

- **Anti-inflammatories** will suppress the body's immune response, which can help to decrease pain but also hinders wound healing. The immune response is necessary to activate specific immune cells to phagocytize bacteria in the area and induce proper wound healing and scar formation. Anti-inflammatories will interfere with this process. This class of medications can also interfere with the formation of protein which is necessary for cell and tissue formation.
- **Anticoagulants** will decrease the body's ability to stop bleeding, and may lead to excessive bleeding within the wound. This can develop into a hematoma. Immunosuppressant medications, including steroids can suppress the immune system and impair wound healing.
- **Steroids** can also increase the risk of bleeding and elevate glucose levels which will impair proper wound healing.
- **Chemotherapy medications** can interfere with the formation of protein and disrupt the replication of cells necessary for tissue growth and wound healing.
- **Radiation treatments** can cause changes to skin cells which may prevent cell replication and wound healing.

EFFECTS OF MULTIPLE TRAUMATIC INJURIES ON WOUND HEALING

There are several reactions that occur within the body when multiple trauma injuries occur. The body is triggered to produce more glucose from the glucagon stores within the liver. This is due to the body's increased demands for energy necessary for healing. Electrolyte imbalances are common following tissue destruction and can affect the patient's ability to provide adequate nutrition necessary for wound healing. Oftentimes, there is an increased risk of infection following multiple traumatic injuries because of contaminated wounds. Excessive tissue damage can affect blood flow to an area of trauma which prevents immune factors from entering the region. Excessive blood loss can result in hypovolemic shock and impaired intravascular pressure, which will impair wound healing and could lead to death. Patients who are unconscious following traumatic injury and those who are placed on ventilators are at risk for impaired oxygenation of tissues. Oxygen is necessary for tissue cells to function appropriately, and decreased levels of oxygen may decrease the ability of a wound to heal.

Surgical Wound Complications

Classes of Surgical Wounds

The following are classes of surgical wounds from class I to class IV:

- **Class I** surgical wounds are clean wounds. Aseptic technique is maintained, no inflammation is present; the gastrointestinal (GI), genitourinary (GU), and respiratory systems are not entered, and there is no drainage from the wound. These are closed by primary union.
- **Class II** surgical wounds are called clean contaminated wounds. Aseptic technique is maintained, but the GI, GU, respiratory, biliary, appendix, or vagina is opened/surgically manipulated. No infection is present.
- **Class III** wounds are contaminated wounds. In these wounds, aseptic technique may be compromised, GI spillage occurs in the wound, inflammation is present without purulent drainage, or a wound occurs from a nonsterile object.
- **Class IV** wounds are dirty or infected wounds. In these wounds, necrotic tissue and/or infection are present.

Interventions to Prevent Wound Complications

In order to prevent wound complications, the wound should be carefully inspected regularly with its appearance documented in the patient's chart to record any change. Assess for any erythema, edema, warmth, or discharge. Note whether the wound edges are well-approximated or if there is gapping present. Also describe the patient's pain level using a 0-10 pain scale. If infection is suspected, document the characteristics of the wound discharge and measure the area of erythema or induration surrounding the wound. Record the patient's vital signs to evaluate for an elevation in temperature. Patient education regarding wound dressing changes is important to ensure continuity of proper wound care at home. Verify that the patient or the friend/family member that will be caring for the patient understands how to properly change the dressing and cleanse the wound. Also educate them on the signs and symptoms of infection along with name and phone number of the person to call if an infection is suspected.

Abscess

An abscess is a localized, encapsulated infection. An infection develops at a wound, and borders are formed around the central portion of infection. Bacteria and blood cells wall off the infection into a capsule. The patient will develop a palpable, inflamed mass that is tender. A fever may or may not be present, as well as an elevated white blood cell count. Treatment of an abscess involves incising and draining the abscess and leaving the wound open to drain. This will prevent the re-formation of an abscess in the same location. If it is not treated, the abscess can leak bacterial material into the system and cause sepsis in the patient. Antibiotics may be given if a systemic infection is confirmed on blood cultures or if the abscess has extensive tissue damage and there is risk of re-infection or superimposed infection following incision and drainage of the abscess.

WOUND DEHISCENCE

Wound dehiscence is an opening of the surgical incision. This usually occurs about 1 week after surgery and a serosanguinous discharge is usually present before the wound opens. If a wound becomes dehisced within the first few hours following surgery, it is usually resutured. Nonabsorbable sutures should be used because they provide extra strength to hold the wound closed. If dehiscence occurs after that time, it is usually packed and allowed to heal by secondary or tertiary intention. Tissue debridement may need to be performed as the wound heals. As the wound heals, a ridge will develop along the incision line as collagen and connective tissue cells are deposited. Wounds that do not develop this ridge are more likely to dehisce because of a lack of tensile strength. This is considered a serious complication of surgery and can have a mortality rate up to 30% following some procedures. Fortunately, wound dehiscence occurs in only approximately 2% of surgeries performed.

CAUSES OF NONHEALING WOUNDS

There are multiple forms of cancer that result in nonhealing wounds. These include the lesions commonly seen with basal cell, squamous cell, and malignant melanoma. Leukemia can also cause ulcerative wounds that will have delayed healing. There are situations in which a patient sustains repeated trauma to an area, such as with poor personal care habits that lead to continued skin infections from bacterial invasion. Patients may also have chronic skin infections that can cause pruritus which may lead to wounds that remain chronic and will not heal. Chronic vascular disease, arterial or venous, can lead to skin ulcers that will be nonhealing. When blood circulation is compromised, adequate nutrition and immune factors cannot be present in the area to promote wound healing and tissue growth. The risk for vascular disease is increased in patients with diabetes. Patients who undergo radiation treatments for treatment of cancer can develop dermatitis and damage to the skin. Skin breakdown can occur which may result in wounds that have prolonged healing.

SEROMAS AND HEMATOMAS

A seroma is a collection of blood and immune cells located underneath the surgical incision. It can result from bleeding disorders, increased movement following surgery, or, most likely, from a bleeding vessel within the wound. A seroma contains a clear-yellowish thin fluid while a hematoma contains blood. Depending upon their location, they can compress vital organs or structures around them which can lead to complications. Though these fluid collections are not considered infections of the wound, they can lead to an infection. To prevent this complication, the fluid should be aspirated using aseptic technique. In severe cases, the surgical incision may need to be reopened and drained. If a bleeding vessel is the cause of the hematoma, ligation may need to be performed to control the bleeding. Seromas frequently develop near the surgical incision following mastectomy surgery. This is particularly true if lymph nodes and vessels in the area are removed, which help to facilitate drainage of fluid.

EPITHELIAL CYST

An epithelial cyst usually occurs when sutures are left in place for too long. As part of the healing process, epithelial cells travel to the area where the sutures are placed in the skin. They will line the area around the suture material, but if the suture is in place too long, an excessive number of epithelial cells can congregate in one location which will form a cyst. Epithelial cysts can also occur in non-surgical patients because of an excessive accumulation of epidermal cells in one area. These are usually flesh colored, though some may have a darker colored center. Whether due to a surgical incision or if they occur in a patient who has not had surgery, epithelial cysts are usually left untreated. If they occur in an area that compromises vision or function, they can be surgically removed and covered by insurance. Insurance will not provide payment for removal of an epithelial cyst for cosmetic reasons.

INCISIONAL HERNIA

A hernia is a weakening in the wall of fascia that results in a protrusion of bowel through the opening. An incisional hernia occurs when there is a weakening in the tissue that makes up the incision, allowing protrusion of the underlying tissue. Incisional hernias occur after the wound has healed. An infection can cause a permanent weakening of the tissue around the incision, which can lead to weakening of that area after the healing process has completed. Improper technique with wound closure can also contribute to the development of an incisional hernia. If sutures are not placed properly, the tissue edges may not be well-approximated and the wound may not have adequate tensile strength. Obese patients with an obtunded abdomen have increased stress applied to the abdominal wall which can cause an increased load against the incision. This can contribute to the weakening that results in an incisional hernia.

HYPERTROPHIC SCARS AND KELOIDS

Hypertrophic, or keloid, scars have a predilection for forming in certain populations, especially African-American patients. As a surgical incision or traumatic wound is healing, the body responds by depositing excessive collagen tissue. This results in a large, growth-like mass at the incision site. Keloids can appear as overgrown flesh-colored lesions along the scar. There may be some normal scar formation at an incision along with keloid tissue. Patients who are known keloid-formers may be given steroids during the wound healing phase to suppress the body's natural tendency to form keloids. There has been some success with direct injection of steroids at the incision site, also. Some patients have opted to have the keloids surgically removed, but there is a risk of forming another keloid at the surgery site. There has been success with removing the keloids using cryotherapy, or freezing. Laser therapy can also be effective at decreasing the size of keloid scars.

SUTURE SINUSES AND SINUS TRACTS

A sinus tract can occur due to the sutures themselves or because of an infection. A sinus is defined as an opening, or tunneling, through the skin. A sinus is present when sutures are removed, but these will heal spontaneously when the suture tracts are filled with skin cells. When an abscess occurs due to infection, a sinus tract can form that is a tunneling of infectious material. A cotton-tipped applicator can often be carefully pushed through the sinus to fully assess the depth of the sinus. Most sinus tracts due to infection will heal after antibiotic treatment and/or incision and drainage of the abscess occurs. In some cases, the sinus tracts may be extensive enough that they will need to be opened and irrigated. These will often be left open to heal by secondary intention. Tertiary healing can also be used in sinus tract healing by allowing some granulation tissue to form in the sinus after the infectious tissue is removed and then suturing or stapling the incision closed.

Types of Wound Pain

There are two types of wound pain:

- **Acute wound pain** is present in the immediate postoperative period and is responsive to analgesic medications. It is usually temporary and begins to diminish a few days following surgery, depending on the type of procedure that was performed. Late postoperative wound pain can be chronic and occurs after the surgical incision has healed. This can be due to late development of an infection within the wound, a rare complication of a device or sponge retained in the surgical site, chronic pain following bone fusion or prosthesis placement, or neurologic pain.
- **Neurologic pain** following surgery can resolve with time or may be chronic. It is not unusual for superficial nerve fibers to be damaged during surgery and the patient may describe a sensation of neuropathic pain as these heal. Permanent nerve damage that may be a complication of surgery can lead to chronic pain.

Contracture Following Wound Healing

As a wound heals, the tissue that is reformed may be shortened and less elastic than the tissue that was present before the trauma. This can decrease the range of motion of a joint and there may be obvious deformity at the site. This is frequently seen in areas where there has been tissue damage from a burn. Contractures of muscles and joints can also occur due to immobility. Patients who are immobile for extended periods of time following surgery or trauma are at risk for developing muscle atrophy followed by contracture because of decreased stretching of muscles and use of joints. Contractures can be prevented by having the patient participate in a physical therapy plan that focuses on gentle stretching and mobility exercises while recovery is taking place. If immobility of a specific area of the body will occur during healing, PT can work the patient to gently stretch muscles and joints, if not contraindicated, to prevent contracture formation.

Cellulitis

Cellulitis is an infection that occurs in a wound and involves the surrounding soft tissues. It is characterized by edema, erythema, warmth, and discomfort surrounding the wound. The patient may or not develop a fever with cellulitis. A white blood cell count may be elevated, as well as an elevation in the erythrocyte sedimentation rate, though this test is specific for cellulitis. Cellulitis is usually caused by a form of strep bacteria, though other organisms can also be responsible for the infection. Treatment will include oral antibiotics, though IV antibiotics may be administered if the infection is extensive. Incision and drainage of the infection is rarely used. If significantly extensive, incision and debridement may be necessary if there is concern that devitalized tissue is present. Cellulitis infections can become systemic and lead to sepsis if they are not treated and if the patient's immune system is not able to ward off the spreading bacteria. This can be determined by testing blood cultures for any growth of bacteria.

Tetanus

Though uncommon, tetanus can develop following the infection of a traumatic wound with *C. tetani* bacteria. This can be life-threatening if left untreated. Most patients will develop anxiety and irritability along with spastic and rigid muscles. This first becomes evident in the musculature surrounding the wound. It can progress to include more muscle groups and may even affect the diaphragm which can lead to respiratory arrest. This muscle spasm is what has given the disease the nickname lockjaw. Tetanus vaccination is available and is given by IM injection. Patients can receive a booster of this every 10 years. If a patient suffers some type of trauma and has a wound, ask about their vaccination status. If they are unsure when their last tetanus shot was given, it is advisable to administer a booster at that time. Patients who developed tetanus are treated with tetanus immunoglobulin. They may be intubated with ventilatory support if necessary.

Lymphangitis

Lymphangitis is a bacterial infection that affects the lymph system. Red streaking will be seen under the skin extending off of lymph vessels and enlarged lymph nodes, or lymphadenopathy, will be present. Blistering may also develop in the skin overlying the infection. The patient will usually have a fever with lymphangitis and may develop an elevated white blood cell count as the infection progresses. An abscess may develop in the area of infection or signs and symptoms of cellulitis may be present. Lymphangitis can develop into a serious systemic infection if not treated promptly and appropriately with antibiotics. The source of the infection should be identified and treated, also. Streptococcus is the most common bacteria to cause lymphangitis. It is possible to biopsy a small portion of affected, inflamed tissue to definitively diagnose the bacteria responsible for the infection so that appropriate treatment can be started. However, treatment should not be delayed because of the risk of rapid development of systemic infection.

Gas Gangrene

Gas gangrene is a potentially life-threatening infection that can occur in a wound. It is caused by the Clostridium bacteria. The patient will have dead tissue and muscle present in the wound with a foul-smelling discharge. There may be gas bubbles present in the discharge and they may be palpated around the wound. Patients with gas gangrene can develop septic shock quite rapidly with a decrease in blood pressure, increased heart rate, difficulty breathing, and mental status changes. They may have only a low-grade fever. Treatment of gas gangrene involves emergency surgical debridement. All of the devitalized tissue and muscle must be removed in the area. This can result in an extensive operative wound, but it is imperative that there are clean wound edges to allow for proper tissue healing. This type of wound will often be left open to heal by secondary intention. This is necessary to prevent closure of the wound with possible residual bacteria in the wound bed that can result in reformation of an infection.

Meleney's Ulcer

Meleney's ulcer is a type of progressive gangrene that can involve large areas of tissue with necrotizing ulcers. These ulcers are caused by both Staph and Strep bacteria. The ulcers appear brown at their core with purple and red tissue surrounding the ulcers. They have a foul-smelling discharge. Like gas gangrene, this type of ulcerating infection can become systemic with possible life-threatening consequences. Patients with Meleney's ulcer must undergo extensive debridement and removal of infected tissue. This can leave a wide, gaping wound depending on the involvement of infection. This will be left open to heal by secondary intention with the formation of granulation tissue within the wound bed. Scarring may be extensive after wound healing has completed. Hyperbaric oxygen treatments have been shown to be very effective in promoting healthy, rapid wound healing. Antibiotics may be necessary for treatment if it has been determined that there is systemic involvement.

Actinomycosis

The bacteria *Actinomyces* are usually found in the nose and throat and do not normally cause infections in healthy individuals. When a person undergoes some type of trauma or surgery, such as oral surgery, the bacteria can form an abscess that appears as a hard red-purple mass. This frequently occurs along the jaw line but can occur at other sites as well. The abscess will eventually rupture at the skin surface and residual sinus tracts will be present draining a purulent exudate that contains granules of sulfur. If severe, the wound may need to be surgically debrided and left open to heal. Antibiotics are necessary to eradicate the bacteria, and therapy may last up to one year depending on the extensive nature of the infection. If left untreated, the bacterial infection can spread to the meninges and lead to meningitis or spread systemically and lead to sepsis, which can lead to death.

Creutzfeldt-Jakob Disease

Creutzfeldt-Jakob disease affects the nervous system and is progressive, leading to death. Its presenting symptoms are similar to those seen with mad cow disease, but the exact cause of the disease is unknown. It is viral in nature, and the only known cause is by direct contact with infected tissue. It is thought that after exposure, the virus will sit dormant for a long time, up to 40 years, before symptoms develop. There is a higher prevalence of the disease in certain ethnic groups, such as certain groups of those of Jewish descent, but no known controlled risk factors. There have been documented cases in which transmission occurs through contaminated medical equipment. The virus that causes Creutzfeldt-Jakob disease is very resilient to standard cleansing procedures and can remain on medical equipment used in invasive procedures. It is higher in concentration within the tissues that make up the nervous system, so equipment used during invasive procedures involving this tissue should be sterilized utilizing specific guidelines known to eradicate the virus.

Measures Taken with Instruments and Equipment to Prevent Transmission

Specific measures must be taken during and after procedures on patients suspected to have Creutzfeldt-Jakob disease in order to ensure sterility of the operating suite and equipment:

- **Disposable items** should be used during the procedure when possible, but even these should be sterilized before disposal.
- Any **skin exposure** to the infected tissues should be followed by immediate cleansing of the area with bleach.
- If there is **exposure to blood or body fluids** not found in the tissues in which infection has occurred, the area should be thoroughly washed with soap and water.
- Instruments that are reusable should be **soaked in sodium hydroxide** for at least one hour. These should then be autoclaved before they are handled.
- The **operating room should be cleansed using a bleach solution** to kill any viral cells that may linger on surfaces.
- All **linens** and any other objects that came in contact with the patient should be placed in proper disposable bags so that they are recognized as biohazard materials.

Resource and Personnel Management

Pre-Purchase Evaluation, Product Evaluation, and Cost Containment

Pre-purchase evaluation, product evaluation, and cost containment are important in the operating suite.

- Prior to product purchase, a **pre-purchase evaluation** should be conducted to determine the direct and indirect costs involved with the item, the usability of the item as it relates to the specific facility's procedures, quality reviews, maintenance requirements, storage requirements, and environmental impacts. A plan for implementing the new product should be in place prior to purchase, and all employees appropriately trained.
- **Product evaluation** is conducted to review products for value and assess products for integrity, safety, and ease of use. Products that might injure a patient are dangerous and can lead to expensive recoveries for the patient and hospital. Products that are not easy to use may be left on the shelf instead of used. In addition, the process evaluates whether or not the product is actually necessary and is not a duplication or more expensive than a product already in use.
- Objects that will become obsolete or unavailable soon require further product searching, which increases institutional costs and takes time. Therefore, finding products that are readily available promote **cost containment**. Keeping costs as low as possible helps the hospital to maintain its budget. Maintaining the budget gives flexibility with purchasing when other more expensive or more important items are needed.

Resource Conservation Issues Applicable to Perioperative Nurses

Hospitals and surgical centers generate tons of medical waste every year. Waste is generated from surgical procedures and the use of instruments for practice. Energy is needed for using surgical devices and simply maintaining the hospital or surgical center. Water is used and often wasted during cleaning, sterilizing, and surgical procedures. Perioperative nurses have a responsibility to practice conservation in order to avoid wasting excess materials, energy, and water. When working in the OR, the nurse can practice **resource conservation** by only opening packages that are necessary, reusing, cleaning, and sterilizing those items that can be used again, recycling materials to save on waste production as well as purchasing new items, practicing water conservation to avoid excess waste, following codes that have been devised to keep the organization green, and using environmentally friendly devices. The perioperative nurse should remain aware of the effects of resource use on the environment and continuously seek ways to save time, energy, and products.

Facilitating or Managing Care During Personnel Shortages

With a staffing shortage, patient care is ultimately sacrificed. When the nurse becomes aware of a staffing shortage, he or she should take action. If the institution has a staffing department, calls can be made immediately to try to replace the worker, calls can be made on the unit to see if other staff would be willing to come in, or on-call persons can be called in for replacement. The nurse can be proactive by making calls early, if it is evident that there is going to be a shortage the next day. When there is a shortage, the nurse can notify other personnel in the area to expect that changes may be needed. Good preparation ahead of time for procedures and picking up duties that may not be standard practice (i.e., taking out the trash) can help to pick up some of the slack present with a shortage of personnel.

Supervising Healthcare Representatives, Students, and Others in the OR

The perioperative nurse may have several different roles, depending on the size of the institution and the assigned position for that shift. In the OR, the perioperative nurse may work as the circulator, the scrub assistant, or may otherwise provide coordination during the surgical procedure. When healthcare representatives, students, or others are present in the OR, the perioperative nurse must ensure that patient safety and privacy are upheld. Those present in the OR may need to scrub in or wear protective clothing, such as gowns or shoe covers, even if they are observing. The nurse must assist them with getting ready, show them where to stand so they stay out of the way of the procedure, and guide them in the rules of the OR so that visitors do not break the sterile field or do anything that would otherwise compromise the health and safety of the patient.

Transfer of Care

Monitoring of Postoperative Patients

Surgical patients who are in the postoperative period need careful monitoring of different body systems to avoid complications. The nurse may need to work with a multidisciplinary team to ensure that proper education and follow-up is occurring for the postoperative patient. A wound care nurse may be needed to inspect the patient's surgical incision and to provide teaching for proper care of the incision site to reduce the risk of infection. Assessment of nutritional status is also important to ensure that the patient is receiving adequate nutrients during the healing process after surgery. A dietitian may be needed to consult about the patient's food intake. A case management nurse may also be available to coordinate the efforts of several disciplines. This nurse can review and document that different professionals have assessed or educated the patient. These team efforts are essential for coordinating knowledge of the care areas to focus on for the patient after having surgery.

Assessment Data to Obtain Regarding Discharge Planning

Assessment data a nurse may obtain about a patient with regard to discharge planning include the following:

- Assess **vital signs and stability** of the patient for discharge, including nutritional status.
- Assess wound for presence of **healing/infection** and evaluate wound care needs post discharge. Assess ability of the patient to care for wounds themselves, or assess the need for patients to have home nursing care. (Do patients have insurance coverage for home care, or will payment be out-of-pocket?)
- Assess if patients are able to **care for themselves**, what their rehabilitation needs are, and whether they have family members available for assistance or need other help. Patients may require nursing care in the home or may need to be discharged to a rehabilitation facility, instead of immediately to home.
- Assess **medications** taken, potential side effects that may alter ability of the patient to care for self, and patient knowledge of medication administration.
- Assess the **knowledge of the patient** towards his or her condition and expected process for recovery.
- Assess the patient's ability to **understand** information about discharge needs and follow-up plan.

Making an Adequate Discharge Plan

The following are some important things the perioperative nurse must do to make an adequate discharge plan:

- Make an adequate **assessment** of the patient and family for any potential needs for discharge and educate the family with regard to any areas of information they are not knowledgeable of.
- Coordinate and implement a **discharge plan** including any follow-up needs necessary, while participating in multidisciplinary care planning and implementation of those discharge plans.
- Utilize appropriate and effective **communication techniques** with the family and with other caregivers about the discharge plan.
- **Document** all assessments and the subsequent discharge plan in a manner that relates the needs of the patient and family and plans for meeting those needs.
- Provide any **educational resources** necessary including written discharge and follow-up plans to the patient and family to meet the goals of the discharge plan.

Expected Outcomes Regarding Discharge Planning

The following are the expected outcomes for a patient with regard to discharge planning:

- The patient will have **stable vital signs** and **laboratory values** upon discharge.
- The patient will exhibit **stability of wound and surgical sites** upon discharge.
- The patient will have **adequate resources** for wound management post discharge.
- The patient will have achieved **adequate pain control** upon discharge.
- The patient's **nutritional status** will be adequate prior to discharge.
- **Pain management medications or devices** will be available to the patient upon discharge.
- The patient will be discharged to an appropriate **rehabilitation facility**, if appropriate.
- If the patient is to be discharged **home**, the patient has adequate resources available to them for rehabilitation.
- The patient obtains **adequate social resources** prior to discharge appropriate to his or her needs.
- The patient verbalizes knowledge of **discharge time and plan**.
- The patient verbalizes understanding of **medication administration** after discharge.
- The patient verbalizes understanding of **prescribed follow-up** after discharge.

Patient Knowledge Before Discharge

Important concepts that the patient must demonstrate knowledge of before discharge include the following:

- The patient should demonstrate knowledge of the **procedure** and the expected **response** to the surgical procedure postoperatively.
- The patient should have knowledge of when he or she can be expected to eat after surgery, including what kind of **nutritional needs** they will have postoperatively.
- The patient should know what **medications** they will be on after the surgery and why, including pain management medications and techniques.
- The patient should be aware of the **rehabilitation process** after surgery including length of time in rehab and types of activities to be performed. In addition, the patient should understand expectations about participation in the rehab process.
- The patient should know how to take care of **wounds** after discharge, if necessary, and any planned suture removal, follow-up care for wounds, cleaning, packing, sterile technique, etc.

Patients' Rights and Patient Advocacy

Key Patient's Rights and Responsibilities

People are empowered to act as their own advocates when they have a clear understanding of their rights and responsibilities. These should be given (in print form) and/or presented (audio/video) to parents/guardians on admission to healthcare or as soon as possible:

- **Rights** should include competent, non-discriminatory medical care that respects privacy and allows participation in decisions about care and the right to refuse care. They should have clear understandable explanations of treatments, operative procedures, options, and conditions, including outcomes. They should be apprised of transfers, changes in care plan, and advance directives. They should have access to medical records and information about charges.
- **Responsibilities** should include providing honest and thorough information about health issues and medical history. Patients and guardians should ask for clarification if they don't understand information that is provided to them, and they should follow the plan of care that is outlined or explain why that is not possible.

Review Video: Patient Advocacy
Visit mometrix.com/academy and enter code: 202160

Maintaining Expected Outcomes of Dignity and Comfort for Patients

The following are some things the perioperative nurse can perform in the plan of care for the patient to maintain expected outcomes of dignity and comfort for the patient:

- **Environmental noise** will be reduced to a minimum in the preoperative area, and **excessive lighting** may be turned off.
- **Drapes** may be closed around the patient to maintain privacy.
- The nurse will assess the patient's **level of anxiety** and, using good communication techniques, will appropriately listen to and calm the patient.
- If the patient is in pain preoperatively, **premedications** may be administered to reduce pain. If there are no medications ordered, the nurse will advocate on behalf of the patient to alert the doctor to the need for medication.
- All **positioning activities** taking place while the patient is awake will be explained to the patient.
- The patient will be offered a **warm blanket** and/or sheets for covering during positioning and throughout the preanesthesia phase of the procedure.

Communication and Documentation

Documentation

High Quality Documentation

Because the perioperative nurse cares for the patient in various stages throughout the surgical process, there are many factors to document. The perioperative nurse completes focused assessments through each phase of patient care, and these assessments require documentation to show that the nurse is providing appropriate patient care. AORN guidelines recommend that nursing documentation reflect the nursing workflow from admission through discharge, utilizing the Perioperative Nursing Data Set (PNDS) to standardize language. Electronic documentation is the preferred framework. High quality documentation should include the patient's mental status and ability to understand the needs for and risks of surgery; the patient's surgical history and medical history, including substance abuse; allergies; nutritional status; risk for injury during or after the surgical procedure; fluid and electrolyte status; and any other significant history for the patient. Additionally, the nurse develops nursing diagnoses for each patient and then documents any interventions completed for each diagnosis. The nurse will also document the outcome of any interventions performed before transferring the patient to the next point of care, whether it is an inpatient hospital unit or back home.

Documentation of Patient Information

The perioperative nurse may use various forms to document patient information, including but not limited to the following:

- **Admission forms**: Patient name, admission date and time
- **Medication forms**: All patient medications and allergies to medications
- **Presurgical forms**: Assessment of patient skin condition, positioning, and NPO status
- **Assessment forms**: Head to toe assessment
- **Past history forms**: Past medical/surgical history, any past reactions to anesthesia
- **Operative records**: Information obtained during surgery
- **Nurses' notes**: Pertinent information/observations occurring during perioperative period
- **Vital sign flow sheets**: Vital signs
- **Care plan**: Nurse's documentation of interventions that support the plan of care
- **Implant records**: Location of implants, time, number, and type of materials used
- **Specimen forms**: Type of specimen and location of specimen
- **Chain of custody forms**: In cases dealing with forensic evidence
- **Incident reporting forms**: In the case of an incident occurring during the patient's stay

Elements of Preoperative Documentation

Elements of preoperative documentation include the following:

- **Relevant facts and data regarding patient care considerations**: All information that may affect patient outcomes or are necessary for decisions regarding the procedure must be documented, including such things as allergies to latex, prolonged bleeding time, abnormal laboratory findings, respiratory disease, diabetes, and a history of blood clots.
- **Positioning**: Positioning must allow for access to the surgical site and adequate visualization while preventing trauma and maintaining homeostasis. Any mobility limitations must be documented and reported as positioning is usually carried out after the patient is anesthetized. Documentation should describe the position, padding and support materials used, safety belts applied, position of arm boards, and eye protection applied.
- **Fluids/Medications**: All fluids and medications must be documented, including time, dosage/volume, and any response observed in the patient. Sedation/anesthesia administration should also be documented preoperatively.
- **Sponge count**: The sponge count should be carried out initially before the incision is made and again with the first layer is sutured, when fascia is closed, and immediately before skin closure as well as when sponges are added during the procedure and when there is a change in the scrub or circulator staff. The circulator nurse records the initial and subsequent counts. The count should be done audibly and each sponge separated, using the same sequence for each count. Packs that contain an incorrect number should be removed from the operating room. All sponges that have been counted must remain in the operating room until the end of the procedure.
- **Needles/Sharps**: Includes blades, needles, saw blades, drill bits, and Bovie tips. Procedures are similar to sponge counts. Sharps should be passed to the surgeon one at a time (one-for-one) to prevent miscounting.
- **Instruments**: Counts should be carried out prior to initial incision, before closure of body cavities, with addition of instruments intraoperatively and with change in scrub or circulator staff. Counts for all instruments in surgical packs must be carried out.
- **Aseptic technique and sterilization practices**: The types of aseptic technique required and maintained should be documented. Sterilization/disinfection requirements based on the surgical location and extent and status of patient's exposure to infectious disease must also be documented.
- **Informed consent**: Nursing documentation must confirm that informed consent was collected for both the procedure and anesthesia (if relevant), and time stamped as occurring before the patient leaves the preoperative area.
- **Education**: Discharge education must be provided prior to procedure in ambulatory settings and documented accordingly. This includes possible side effects, complications, restrictions, and follow-up required. If complementary care interventions were recommended, education on the risks and benefits of these interventions should be included.

Documentation Concerning Skin and Surgical Site Preparation

Some important elements in the documentation of skin and surgical site preparation include the following:

- The nurse's **assessment of the surgical site** including skin integrity, location, any considerations for the type of prep to be performed.
- If **preoperative bathing** was required, this should be documented including the product utilized, the time/date, and the duration.
- If **hair removal** was required, document the amount, type, method for removal, and person performing hair removal.
- Document any **allergies or sensitivities** to preparation solutions and the subsequent solutions used for the preparation.
- Document the name of the person doing the preparation and the method/antiseptic used, site prepped, jewelry removed, and any additional information regarding drain sites, etc. prepped.
- Any **additional information** should be recorded, such as if there was an allergic response to the preparation, if the patient tolerated the preparation well, if there were any complications, etc.

Additional Elements of Perioperative Documentation

Additional elements of perioperative documentation must be adhered to with regard to sterilization/infection control, VTE prevention, and autologous tissue management:

- **Sterilization procedures**: Sterilization records should be maintained for all surgical instruments for the amount of time dictated by the facility and/or regulatory body. Each record of use should include the operator's identity, load content and identification, parameters of exposure, and outcome of physical, chemical, and/or biologic indicators. Maintenance records should also be included for each piece of equipment.
- **Infection prevention/control**: Each facility must adopt an approved program for infection prevention and control. The program selection, implementation, and evaluation must be documented.
- **Venous thromboembolism (VTE) prevention**: Precautions to prevent VTE should be documented before, during, and after surgical procedures that present a risk for VTE. Documentation should include patient risk factors, interventions (pharmacologic and/or mechanical interventions, time of intervention, and patient response/compliance to the intervention), a baseline skin assessment, and subsequent skin assessments (requiring the removal of mechanical precautions, visual inspection, and reapplication).
- **Autologous tissue management**: When autologous tissue is removed from a patient, it should be tracked and recorded. Records should include the type of tissue, the date and method of preservation/storage (including temperature), the methods of sterilization/decontamination, and then the date of removal from storage and the indication for removal. For each of these phases, the individual performing the step should be identified in the record.

Documentation Requirements for Instruments and Supplies in the OR

Protocols should be established and followed for the documentation of instruments and supplies used in the operating room, using the following considerations:

- **Implants/prostheses**: The name of the implant and the size, manufacturer, serial number, code number, date of manufacture or sterilization, expiration date, recipient, and date/time of implant.
- **Imaging equipment**: Documentation should include the type of equipment (C-arm, ultrasound, CT), time and purpose of imaging, and any safety measures taken, including use of lead protective equipment.
- **Instrument counts**: Instrument packs, as well as sponge, needle, and instrument counts, must be documented as well as the use of any specialized instruments.
- **Other equipment, such as lasers or electrosurgical units**: The type of device (including the specific type of laser) and the use must be documented as well as the results or any problems observed.

Documentation as a Form of Communication

Documentation is one of the most important forms of communication in the hospital and operating room environment. Documentation is written evidence or proof of the patient's condition and is a reference point for anyone who needs to find information about the patient. Sometimes information in a verbal report is missed or incomplete, and the documented report can provide this information. Since documentation is so critical, it is also important that documentation be done clearly and concisely, using legible writing techniques on the appropriate forms or in the organization's computer program. All patient assessments, the plan of care, interventions, medications, discharge planning, etc. are included in a patient's documented record, and provide for smooth, complete, and multidisciplinary continuation of care by all members of the healthcare team from admission to discharge.

Communication Techniques

Listening Skills and Assertion Skills

Effective communication requires skills in both listening and asserting oneself:

- **Listening skills** refers to the ability of a person to be able to listen to what is being said to them. They must listen in a way that allows them to understand what is being said, so they can respond accurately and efficiently to what a patient or another person is telling them.
- **Assertion skills** refer to the behaviors that a person exhibits, both verbal and nonverbal, to make their needs, desires, and requests known. For effective communication to take place, it is not to be done in a negative manner, but rather, in a manner that does not detract from the situation at hand, demean those to whom the request is being made, and is respectful to all parties involved.

Questions, Direction, Suggestion, and Support Strategies

Questions, direction, suggestion, and support strategies in regards to communication techniques are as follows:

- **Questions** are asked by the nurse in open- or closed-ended fashion to elicit information from the patient. Questions give a platform to provide information, and open-ended questions elicit more information than closed-ended questions.
- **Direction** is used in conversation when a nurse asks about specific aspects of information, trying to focus the conversation regarding a certain topic. Questions or statements can be used to direct the conversation.
- **Suggestion making** should be avoided in the communication process with patients. When a nurse makes a suggestion that something hurts, the patient feels a certain way, etc., it may prevent the patient from making decisions for him or herself, and create subjective emotions or feelings that were not present beforehand.
- **Support** is given to patients as the nurse shares information to help the patient feel confident that the information they are given is accurate, secure, and establishes trust between the nurse and patient.

Silence, Facilitation, and Confrontation

Silence, facilitation, and confrontation in regard to communication techniques are as follows:

- **Silence** refers to remaining quiet long enough to allow the patient to gather their thoughts and relay information.
- **Facilitation** is when the nurse helps to draw out more information from the patient. It can involve body language indicating understanding or confusion by a nod or a quizzical look, or can be verbally implied by saying, "yes," to encourage the patient to further elaborate.
- **Confrontation** refers to simply identifying potential barriers to communication on behalf of the patient as identified by the nurse. For instance, if the patient appears to be worried about a situation, the nurse can say, "You seem worried," to indicate that the patient's feelings are okay and that he or she can feel free to discuss further beyond their feelings. This should not be done forcibly, and the patient should not be required to share information they are not comfortable with.

Therapeutic Interviewing Techniques

Both verbal and nonverbal responses should be observed during an **interview**. Patients may look away or become tense if they are not telling the truth or don't want to answer a particular question. Information elicited during an interview should include not only facts but also the patient's attitude and concerns. Using therapeutic questioning technique is essential for eliciting information:

- Ask **information questions** (as opposed to yes/no) with "who," "what," "where," "when," and "how," but avoid questions with "why" if possible:
  - Instead of "Why do you continue to eat sugar?" ask, "What sugar substitutes have you tried?"
- Ask brief **clarifying questions**: "How long were you in the hospital?"
- Provide a **list of options**: "Is your headache throbbing, stabbing, or dull?
- **Rephrase/reflect** to encourage clarification:
  - Patient: "My husband had the same surgery and died a month later."
  - Nurse: "You're afraid you might die from this surgery?"

Assessments to Help with Effective Communication

Perioperative nurses should assess for the following factors that influence communication:

- The person's **age, developmental status, understanding of the language, language barriers, and educational level**
- **Mechanical factors,** including the ability to hear due to presence of noise, need for hearing aids, need to communicate via sign language, voice enhancers, etc.
- **Verbal and nonverbal clues** as to the patient's willingness to communicate
- The other person's clarity of **speech**, patterns of speech, grammar usage, tone of voice, etc.
- **Privacy level** of the immediate environment, which should also be free of distractions, if possible
- One's **own body language** to avoid giving signals of inattention to or disinterest in what the other person is saying and to instead give good eye contact, reassurance, support, etc.
- The other person's **understanding** of the information provided after communication has occurred

Communicating Through Conflicts

In order to effectively communicate through conflicts, the nurse must consider the following:

- **Conflict resolution skills** can be used to identify a potential or real conflict and handle or resolve the conflict in a way that maintains respect, dignity, and relationships of all persons involved.
- **Collaborative problem-solving skills** are those skills that a person utilizes to problem solve or resolve conflict by involving others in the decision-making process. In the hospital setting, it is often interdisciplinary.
- **Skill selection** refers to a person's ability to utilize certain skill sets when communicating with others and determine which skills are appropriate and under which circumstances to effectively communicate and resolve conflict. These skills may include actively listening, facilitating response, and properly offering support to a patient in the perioperative area.

Communicating with the Family Before, During, and After Surgery

Communicating with the family establishes trust between the staff and family members, and enables them to have a sense of control over a situation in which they have little control.

- **Before surgery**, the nurse/doctor can speak with family members in the preoperative area/waiting room. Phone numbers can be exchanged at that time.
- **During surgery**, the family frequently has a lot of anxiety, and calls can be made during the procedure to update the family, or a nurse/doctor may be able to leave for a period of time to talk with them in the waiting room.
- **After surgery**, the nurse/doctor should notify the family about the end of surgery, any highlights about the surgery, ("the procedure went well," "there were no surprises," etc.) and the patient's condition. Sometimes, the nurse/doctor can make a quick call indicating this and then ensure the family that a follow-up consultation will occur once the patient is stable.

Maintaining Confidentiality While Giving Family Updates During Surgery

Each patient has a right to confidentiality according to the **Health Insurance Portability and Accountability Act** (HIPAA). Through HIPAA, healthcare staff cannot access or share a patient's confidential health information if they are not directly related to the patient's care. The patient also can request that his health information not be shared with certain people. However, when a patient has surgery, the patient's family will often visit or wait while the surgery is performed. The surgeon typically speaks with the patient's family to give updates. Under HIPAA, a surgeon may share information with a patient's family regarding a surgical procedure if the patient gives permission for family members; if the patient is awake, present, and consents to the information; or in an emergent situation when the surgeon feels it is in the patient's best interest. The surgeon may share patient surgical updates through a face-to-face meeting, over the phone, or in writing.

Importance of Transcultural Nursing in the Process of Communication

People understand issues and facts based on a series of mental and emotional filters. For some, certain aspects of life and certain issues are very easy to understand, and for others, these can be very difficult. Often this is due to many **cultural, spiritual, and other belief systems** that are in place in the person's life. Other contributing factors may include age, race, educational level, spiritual beliefs/practices, desired food choices, etc. When nurses are **transculturally aware**, they are more able to offer a more culturally competent nursing plan for the patient, one in which the patient is more comfortable and more willing to participate. Nurses may also learn to delay communicating at certain times due to the person's beliefs about when it is appropriate to receive information, from whom, and about which subjects.

Interdisciplinary Communication and Collaboration

Obtaining, Documenting, and Communicating Assessment Information

The first part of the communication process in the presurgical area begins between the nurse and the patient. First, the nurse must establish clear lines of communication with the patient in order to obtain an accurate and thorough assessment. Second, the nurse then documents that information on standardized forms, including assessment, medication, and diagnosis forms. The nurse must accurately document that information on those forms or in the appropriate computer software in the appropriate manner, as recording the information inappropriately may cause other personnel to miss pertinent information. Third, the nurse may also be required to verbally communicate pertinent information to certain members of the surgical team in order to facilitate timely and appropriate care to the patient either preoperatively or intraoperatively.

Information Communicated to the Surgical Team

There is a plethora of information that the nurse communicates to the rest of the surgical team before, during, and after surgery. Pertinent allergies, NPO status, skin condition, potential complications with positioning, and medication usage can all be reported before surgery takes place, along with any other pertinent information that may impact the surgical procedure. During surgery, the nurse may need to report to the surgical team assessment of the patient's vital signs, skin integrity, availability of materials, surgery time, and patient response to therapy. After surgery, the surgical team may need to be notified of the patient's condition, response to anesthesia and recovery time, potential needs for discharge, wound condition, etc.

Modalities Used to Communicate

The perioperative nurse can communicate with other personnel, families, and outside facilities using a variety of modalities. These may include:

- Verbal communication **face-to-face** to other nurses, doctors, or ancillary staff.
- Verbal communication via a **telephone** or cellular telephone to other departments, outside facilities, or on-call staff members outside the hospital.
- Verbal communication through an **interpreter** to patients with language barriers in person or over a special interpreting telephone.
- Written communication via **email**.
- Written communication via **documentation** in a patient chart, on a requisition form, memorandum, or in a letter format to other personnel in the hospital, other departments, outside facilities, etc.
- Nonverbal communication via **body language**.
- Nonverbal communication using **sign language** to a deaf patient.

SBAR Verbal Reporting System and Taking Verbal and Telephone Orders

The SBAR verbal reporting system is an effective template for taking and communicating verbal and telephone orders. SBAR stands for situation, background, assessment, and recommendation and provides a framework with which to develop concise, clear reporting between members of the healthcare team.

- **Situation** describes the patient and the problem/concern, **background** provides pertinent findings to support the concern, **assessment** describes the nurse's identification of the problem, and **recommendation** provides any suggestions for correction.
- When verbal or telephone orders are taken, the information should be **written down**, and then **read back** to the provider as written. Ask the provider for confirmation of the order as written.
- Only **authorized personnel** should take orders on behalf of a patient.
- In addition, reading back an order should be by **number verbatim**, meaning multi-digit numbers are read back by digit (e.g., 50 is read as "five zero" rather than "fifty").
- Current guidelines by CMS state that verbal orders are to only be used in **emergency situations**, and that a practitioner must sign those orders promptly, within at least 48 hours.

Importance of Effective Communication During Emergencies

When an emergency situation presents itself, it often requires some very specific interventions to take place in a very efficient manner. Emergencies usually require or involve multiple persons from multiple specialties who have different capabilities and knowledge about situations. In an emergency, it is important that all members are aware of the situation, know their own and respective colleagues' abilities, and perform in a manner conducive to solving the problem. Effective communication is essential to notify all appropriate members, properly delegate appropriate tasks to personnel, and help all persons involved in the emergency know which aspects of care have been accounted for and which ones need to be addressed. When all members accurately communicate together, all aspects of care can be attended to, and the emergency can be resolved effectively.

Assessing the Effectiveness of Communication in the Hospital

Assessment of the effectiveness of communication can be made based on the outcome of the communication process. When communicating needs with other departments about the need for services or materials, whether or not those are obtained is usually a good indicator as to the effectiveness of communication for those needs. Communication with the surgical team is more difficult and involves more specific and intimate information, but seeing how they respond to the information (making changes to solutions used due to allergic responses, changing of surgical gown due to contamination via nonsurgical field, etc.) will indicate whether they received the information. Body language and potential responses to those requests often indicate the effectiveness of the communicator to deliver the information in an appropriate or inoffensive manner. Effective communication with the patient is evident when they can reiterate what was told them or perform a specific task as indicated for discharge.

Barriers to Effective Communication

Some common barriers to effectively communicating with people might include some of the following:

- Making critical evaluations or critical comments about or toward a person
- **Prejudice** towards the person giving information, stereotyping, or name calling
- **Domineering or commanding** behaviors and communication, including telling someone what they should or should not do
- **Threatening** body gestures or statements
- **Excessively praising** someone to the point of seeming fake or sarcastic
- **Closed-ended questioning** that becomes inappropriate or unclear as to what the interviewer is looking for with their questions
- **Not staying on track** with the conversation being discussed
- **Arguing** with someone about what is the right thing to do
- Telling someone that what they are feeling or experiencing is **wrong** or **inappropriate**

Roles of Interdisciplinary Team Departments

The surgical interdisciplinary team includes various departments that contribute to the goals of the procedure being performed:

- **Radiology**: Imaging modalities that may be used to assist with surgical procedures, such as neurosurgical procedures, include standard x-rays, CT, PET, and MRI (including CT, PET, and MRI angiograms). Radiology is essential in helping the surgeon to determine the need for surgery, to isolate the incision site, and to guide excision. Radiology is commonly used with minimally-invasive procedures. Many surgical suites now include medical imaging devices, such as C-arms and CT scanners.
- **Ultrasound imaging**: Images, including intravascular ultrasound, are used to determine the need for surgery, such as breast biopsies, and to guide excision, tracking instruments throughout the surgical procedure in some cases.
- **Pathology**: Pathology is of critical importance in not only identifying the need for surgical procedures (such as with examination of tissue samples to identify cancerous cells) and determining the need for follow-up treatment, but also during surgical procedures (such as MOHS) to determine the extent of excision needed.

Infection Prevention and Control

Operating Room Precautions

Standard Precautions and Universal Precautions in the Operating Room

The **2007 CDC isolation guidelines** include both standard precautions that apply to all patients and health situations and transmission-based precautions for those with known or suspected infections. **Standard precautions** should be utilized for all patients because all body fluids (sweat, urine, feces, blood, sputum) and non-intact skin and mucous membranes may be infected.

Hand hygiene	Wash hands before and after each patient contact.
Protective equipment	Use personal protective equipment (PPE), such as gloves, gowns, and masks, eye protection, and/or face shields, depending on the patient's condition and degree of exposure.
Respiratory hygiene/ Cough etiquette	Educate staff, patients, family, and visitors. Post instructions (language appropriate). Utilize source control measures, such as covering cough, disposing of tissues, using a surgical mask on a person coughing or on staff to prevent inhalation of droplets, and properly disposing of dressings and used equipment. Wash hands after contacting respiratory secretions. Maintain a distance of >3 feet from coughing person when possible.
Safe injection practice	Use sterile single-use needle and syringe one time only and discard safely.
Medical equipment	If reusable, equipment should be cleaned (and sterilized if necessary) per manufacturers guidelines between use.

Universal precautions are more specific than standard precautions and refer specifically to preventing transmission of human immunodeficiency virus, hepatitis B, and other pathogens that can be contained in blood or other body fluids.

TRANSMISSION-BASED PRECAUTIONS IN THE OPERATING ROOM

The 2007 CDC isolation guidelines transmission-based precautions are to be used for those with known or suspected infections as well as those with excessive wound drainage, other discharge, or fecal incontinence. **Transmission-based precautions** include:

Contact	(Appropriate for *Clostridioides difficile,* MRSA, VRE, when exudate is present [abscesses or wounds], and for multidrug resistant organisms) Use personal protective equipment (PPE), including gown and gloves, for all contact with the patient or patient's immediate environment. Maintain the patient in private room or >3 feet away from other patients.
Droplet	(Appropriate for influenza, streptococcus infection, pertussis, rhinovirus, adenovirus, and pathogens that remain viable and infectious for only short distances) Use mask while caring for the patient. Maintain the patient in a private room or >3 feet away from other patients with curtain separating them. Use a patient mask if transporting patient from one area to another.
Airborne	(Appropriate for measles, chickenpox, tuberculosis, SARS, and COVID-19 because pathogens remain viable and infectious for long distances) Place the patient in an airborne infection isolation room. Use ≥N95 respirators (or masks) while caring for the patient.

OSHA PRACTICE STANDARDS

Some practice standards set in place by the **Occupational Safety and Health Administration** (OSHA) include the following:

- **Sharps containers** are to be easily accessible. All sharp objects should be deposited into them after use. Employers are to maintain a sharps injury log. Employers must also identify, evaluate, and implement safer medical devices.
- **Cleaning and disinfecting schedules** should be written and implemented for equipment and hospital environments.
- **Soiled linens** are to be placed in specific, labeled, leak-proof bags.
- Employers must offer **preexposure hepatitis B vaccines** free of charge and postexposure follow-up programs.
- **Training/education programs** are to be put in place for all employees potentially exposed to hepatitis B or human immunodeficiency virus (HIV).
- Job classifications, procedures, and potential exposure to blood or body fluids must be listed by employers for potential employees and current employees within the **job description**.
- **Gloves** are to be worn anytime exposure to blood/body fluids is possible.
- **Masks, face shields, and nonpermeable gowns** are to be worn when splashing of blood or body fluids is possible.
- All **personal protective equipment** is to be provided by the employer to the employee at no cost to the employee.
- **Hand washing** is to commence immediately after exposure to blood or body fluids.
- **Recapping of needles** is allowed only if done by a mechanical device and only when reuse of the needle is necessary for a certain procedure; otherwise, recapping should not occur.

Hand Washing, Surgical Hand Antisepsis, and Properties of Antiseptics

The following are some important things for the perioperative nurse to remember about **hand** washing, surgical hand antisepsis, and properties of antiseptics that make them acceptable for use:

- If hands are visibly dirty, alcohol-based hand rubs cannot **solely** be used. The hands must be washed first, followed by an alcohol-based hand rub.
- **Surgical hand antisepsis** involves hand washing followed by either an alcohol-based antiseptic hand rub or an antimicrobial scrub.
- Hand washing should occur **after** gloves are removed.
- Hand washing removes residue and microbes **mechanically**; the use of antiseptics destroys microbes and prevents their immediate recurrence.
- **Antiseptics** should:
  - Significantly kill/remove microorganisms from the skin quickly
  - Not be irritating
  - Be broad spectrum
  - Have a cumulative effect if used more than once
  - Have a continuing effect of antisepsis after the product has been applied to the skin

Items to Wear or Remove in the Surgical Area to Prevent Spread of Infection

The following are items that healthcare personnel can wear or remove in the surgical area to prevent the spread of infection and their rationale for use:

- **Caps and hoods** are worn to cover the hair and facial hair to prevent contamination of the surgical area with bacteria. Hair contains high numbers of bacteria, which increase with great hair length, curliness, and oiliness.
- **Scrubs** are worn to cover the skin and prevent skin cells from contaminating the surgical field. The shirt should be tucked in to prevent spread as well. Scrub jackets that have long sleeves can also be worn to help prevent spread.
- **Masks** that have a high filtration rate are used to prevent spread of bacteria from the mouth/nose with talking, etc., around the surgical site.
- **Shoe covers** are used when there is a high likelihood of soiling.
- **Jewelry and artificial nails** harbor bacteria and, if removed, can eliminate potential sources of contamination infection.
- **Gloves and gowns** are also worn to protect personnel using standard and universal precautions.

Operation Room Cleaning, Spills, and Turnover

Management of Spills and Room Turnover

Management of environmental procedures includes the following:

- **Spills**: Management should follow recommendations of the SDS for each agent and the spill containment plan of the organization. Staff should have easy access to clean-up and protective equipment, and procedures should be in place for alerting staff to potential dangers. Management of spills may include applying a neutralizing substance (such as sodium hydroxide for glutaraldehyde) and/or absorbent material. If necessary, the area should be evacuated and cleanup staff equipped with respirators or self-contained breathing apparatus. Material from the spill is generally placed in polyethylene bags and then in the appropriate hazardous waste containers for disposal.
- **Room turnover**: When the surgery is over and the patient is transported to the PACU, the procedure room should be cleaned and disinfected. All soiled instruments should be removed and taken to the processing area. The kick buckets should be emptied according to protocol, and the linen hampers, waste containers, and biohazardous waste containers should be emptied and the materials properly disposed of. A room turnover pack should be used to set up the operating room for the next patient. Turnover time is generally 7-10 minutes.

Terminal Cleaning

Terminal cleaning refers to the comprehensive cleaning of the surgical suite at the end of the surgical day in order to prevent the spread of infectious microorganisms. AORN guidelines no longer support terminal cleaning between patients, including after patients with known or suspected infectious diseases. Rather, enhanced environmental cleaning is utilized between patients in this scenario. Terminal cleaning is done on a daily basis for each operating room, whether it was used for surgery that day or not. Every 24 hours, the ventilation system, air ducts, and gas outlets should be dry dusted. All surfaces, tables, cabinets, counters, suction mounts, wall panels, furniture, and the OR table should be first dry dusted and then wiped with a germicidal solution. Other items, such as kick buckets, trash collection frames, and laundry receptacles are wiped clean. The walls, ceiling, and surgical lights are cleaned as needed and when lint or visible debris is noted. The floor is swept and the entire floor is mopped. Any trash or biohazard items that have collected should be removed from the room.

Cleaning Instruments

Spaulding Classification of Devices

The Spaulding classification is a method to categorize and determine what level of sterilization an instrument must be in order to be used. These levels of categorization are critical, semi-critical, and noncritical.

- **Critical**: These items must be sterile because they come into contact with sterile environments or sterile tissues. Any instrument or item that penetrates a mucous membrane must be sterile to avoid introducing new bacteria. Surgical instruments, sutures, needles, catheters, drains, etc., are all included in this classification.
- **Semi-critical**: These items contact mucous membranes that are unbroken; likewise, these items do not break through mucous membranes. They do not have to be sterile, but must be at least disinfected. Thermometers and dental dams are examples of these devices.
- **Non-critical**: These items contact intact skin and do not contact mucous membranes. They require disinfection or simple cleaning. Sphygmomanometers, pulse oximeters, and positioning props are included in this classification.

Medical Device User Fee and Modernization Act (MDUFMA)

Single use devices (SUD), such as surgical drills, catheters, and endotracheal tubes, are manufactured for one-time use, but the reality is that for many years SUDs were reused or recycled with little regulatory oversight regarding methods of disinfecting/sterilization to determine if the SUDs were safe for use. In response to concerns about this practice, the **Medical Device User Fee and Modernization Act (MDUFMA)** was issued in 2002, with requirements for reprocessing. Reprocessed devices are classified according to the Spaulding classification system. The process of validation includes procedures for cleaning and sterilization, the types of materials, and product testing. Studies have shown that properly reprocessed SUDs are equivalent in safety to the original. Reprocessing requires thorough cleaning, sterilization or high-level disinfection, monitoring of automatic reprocessors for contamination, and use of disposable devices for parts that cannot be adequately cleaned.

Cleaning Instruments in the Intraoperative Period

The following are things the perioperative nurse must remember when cleaning instruments in the **intraoperative period**:

- All **contaminated instruments** need to be cleaned as quickly as possible after using them.
- During the procedure, while they are still needed, the instruments should be wiped/rinsed with **lap sponges** or dipped in **sterile water** to keep the instruments clear of large particles.
- If an instrument has a **lumen**, the lumen must be adequately rinsed with sterile water to keep it free of particulate matter. Irrigation is the recommended method of cleaning instruments with lumens. It is important to ensure irrigation of the lumen takes place below the surface of the water to prevent particles from becoming aerosolized.

Cleaning Instruments in the Postoperative Period

The following things the perioperative nurse must remember when cleaning instruments in the **postoperative period**:

- All instruments to be transported should be kept in containers appropriately marked for contaminated items. The containers should be **leak- and puncture-proof.**
- Instruments must be transported as soon as possible to **prevent the drying of soil** and enable a more productive decontamination.
- A **damp towel** (or special soaks or gels) should be applied over the instruments during transport after the procedure to prevent substances from drying to the surfaces of the instruments.
- Make sure to **wash instruments with water**, but to ensure that they do not stay soaking in pools of water (to prevent biofilms from forming).
- Make sure all **joints to instruments are opened** and all instruments that have **multiple parts are disassembled** into single parts to be cleaned.
- Make sure that **heavier items are not placed on top of lighter** ones to prevent shifting of the weight and possible toppling of the container or breakage of smaller items.

Manually Cleaning Instruments

The following are things the perioperative nurse must remember when **manually cleaning instruments**:

- When items need to be cleaned that cannot tolerate mechanical cleaning or when mechanical cleaning is not available, then **manual cleaning** can be considered. It is preferable to use mechanical cleaning when possible to prevent possible injury to the individual.
- Don **personal protective equipment** (gown, gloves, mask, and eye shield) to protect from contamination of blood/body fluids/tissues when cleaning.
- Rinse instruments in **cold water** to remove debris.
- Using a cleaning agent specific for **instrument cleaning**, gently manually clean instruments using a soft-bristled brush (harsh pads and cleaners should not be used).
- When cleaning items able to be immersed in water, make sure that all cleaning is done **below the surface of the water**, especially irrigation to parts that contain lumens, to prevent aerosolizing particulate matter.

Mechanically Cleaning Instruments

The following are things the perioperative nurse must remember when **mechanically cleaning instruments**:

- Instruments must be placed in **trays** for cleaning. The trays must have a wire or mesh bottom to allow for proper drainage and removal of debris from the instrument container.
- When using a **washer-sterilizer**, be aware that debris that is not adequately removed in the washing cycle may be baked onto the instrument during the sterilization phase. Thus, the instrument will have to be decontaminated.
- Even though instruments may go through a washer-sterilizer, they are not considered suitable for patient use after cleaned and dried. At this point they are only considered **safe to handle**.
- Washer-disinfector/decontaminators that do not have a **sterilization phase** are not as likely to leave debris on the instrument or bake it on as a machine with a sterilizer.

ULTRASONIC CLEANER

The following are some important things for the perioperative nurse to remember when using an **ultrasonic cleaner**:

- Instruments should be cleaned of **visible contaminants** before being placed in the cleaning chamber.
- **Ion transferring** may take place when different metallic items are processed in the ultrasonic chamber at the same time, which can damage the instruments. So only similar elements should be placed in the chamber simultaneously.
- **Detergent solution** should be changed daily, when the detergent is dirty, or more frequently if it is required by other guidelines.
- Keep **lid** in place with use as contaminated particles on the instruments can be aerosolized in the ultrasonic cleaner.
- The **ultrasonic cleaning process**, or cavitation, itself does not kill bacteria, but simply removes debris more easily from instruments that are difficult to clean. Proper sterilization/disinfection must still take place.
- Instruments coming out of the cleaner should be rinsed in **deionized water** if not rinsed within the device itself.

CLEANING INSTRUMENTS EXPOSED TO PRIONS

The following are some important things for the perioperative nurse to remember when cleaning instruments that have been **exposed to prions**:

- Prions are **resistant** to disinfection procedures and to most routine sterilization procedures, and instruments contaminated with prions must be cleaned according to specific protocols.
- **Tissues** at high risk for being contaminated with prions are brain, spinal cord, and eye tissue in patients with suspected prion infection. Instruments used on these areas should be kept separate from instruments used on other parts of the body.
- When possible, **single-use instruments** should be used on patients with suspected prion infection or high-risk for prion infection and discarded after use.
- As with other body tissues/fluids, instruments must be kept **moist** until cleaned and cleaning should ensue as soon as possible to prevent drying of tissue on instruments.
- The decontamination process involves using a **steam autoclave** for a prescribed amount of time for instruments easy to clean. Difficult-to-clean instruments can either be soaked in sodium hydroxide for one hour then decontaminated using steam sterilization (prevacuum or gravity displacement) or can be discarded. This is the decontamination process, and proper cleaning, wrapping, and sterilizing should immediately follow.

CLEANING INSTRUMENTS WITH MOVABLE PARTS

Instruments with movable parts or joints create crevices that allow particles and contaminants to hide and potentially be missed in the cleaning process. Care should be taken to inspect each crevice and carefully clean them to ensure all contaminants are removed. Often these instruments require disassembly, if possible, in order to clean them properly. Using a water-soluble lubricant on the joints of the instrument with movable parts is important because it prevents rusting and staining of the instrument. This keeps all moving parts fluid in their movements so that they are easy to use during a procedure. It is important that the lubricant is water-soluble, as water-soluble lubricants are penetrable by sterilizing agents, while oils are not penetrable by sterilizing agents.

Cleaning Specialty Instruments with High Risk of Infection Transmission

Specialty instruments such as ophthalmic equipment and laryngoscope blades/handles should have specific procedures for cleaning due to their risk for transporting infectious agents from one patient to another. Due to the rare but dangerous complication of toxic anterior segment syndrome (TASS) after ocular procedures, special care should be taken to appropriately sterilize ophthalmic instruments after use, as improper sterilization is one known cause of TASS in subsequent procedures. AORN guidelines recommend wiping these instruments with sterile water immediately after use, then bathing them in sterile water in an area away from other surgical instruments. The instrument should then be cleaned with manufacturer-recommended solutions, and thoroughly washed with sterile water. Lumens should be flushed, rinsed, and then dried. Because one source of TASS is improperly decontaminated ultrasonic cleaners, if these are used for decontamination of ophthalmic instruments, the ultrasonic cleaner should be confirmed as disinfected and fully dried per manufacturer guidelines prior to use.

Laryngoscopes are another source of suspected hospital-acquired infections. After utilizing reusable laryngoscope blades and/or handles, these items should be separately and appropriately disinfected per manufacturer's guidelines. Packaging and storing protocols should be established to maintain the sterility of these items after being disinfected.

Inspecting Instruments After Cleaning

After the cleaning process has been completed, instruments are **inspected** for cleanliness and lack of visible contamination, to make sure instruments maintained their integrity through the cleaning process, that all edges remain sharp that are supposed to be, and that the instruments function as they are supposed to. It is important to inspect instruments just after the cleaning process (and not before a surgical procedure) because if the instrument is not suitable for use, it should be removed and not used. Often there is not enough time to inspect instruments before a procedure, especially when it is an emergency procedure. Not inspecting instruments adequately before their use in surgery raises the likelihood that a patient may be injured because the instrument did not function properly.

Handling Hazardous Materials

PPE for Hazardous Materials

Surgical staff who work with hazardous materials should always wear protective equipment to protect themselves from harm. All surgical staff must wear **personal protective equipment** (PPE) at a minimum level of protection for clothing and exposed skin. Examples of standard PPE include gloves and gowns. If working with a substance that could splash, staff should wear protective glasses to avoid getting the substance in the eyes. Masks are already worn during surgery, but if working with a substance that can lead to inhalation of dangerous airborne particles, a specialized filter mask may be necessary. When working with radiation, only employees who must be in the area should remain, otherwise, unnecessary personnel should leave the area while radiation is in use. For those who remain, lead shielding through the use of aprons, eyewear, and thyroid shields offer protection. Pregnant personnel should disclose pregnancy to avoid overexposure of hazardous materials to the fetus.

Handling and Disposal of Hazardous Materials in Operating Room

Handling and disposal of hazardous materials in the OR include:

- **Ethylene oxide** (ETO): ETO is highly flammable and may lead to explosions, so it is diluted with inert gases (such as CO_2) and hydrochlorofluorocarbons (HCFC) to reduce flammability. ETO is easily absorbed through the skin and produces toxic byproducts if mixed with water. ETO sterilized items must be aerated before handling, as EO is a carcinogen. The typical duration of mechanical aeration of EO sterilized items at 50-60 °C is 8-12 hours.
- **Radioactive materials**: Radioactive inserts, such as seeds, should be handled with forceps, tongs, or other devices but never directly handled. Gloves, including those that are radioprotective, do not provide adequate protection. Surgical gloves can only provide barrier protection if radioactive material is liquid or leaks. Seeds are approximately 5 mm in length and 0.5 mm in diameter. A lost seed can be found with a Geiger counter. A safe distance from unshielded seeds is 2 meters (6 feet). Radioactive waste must be placed in special containers and labeled as radioactive waste with the name of the radioisotope, activity, disposal date, and full name and contact information of authorized user.
- **Chemotherapeutic agents**: When administering or handling open containers of chemotherapeutic agents, the nurse should wear double gloves. Per AORN guidelines, when working with chemotherapy, gloves must be changed every 30 minutes. These agents should be transported in warning-labeled, leak-proof, break-resistant containers, and staff should wear PPE as indicated by the type of possible exposure. A gown impervious to chemotherapeutic agents should be worn if the agent may come in contact with the arms or torso, and face shields should be used if a danger of splashing or splattering is present. Manufacturer's guidelines should be followed regarding handling and discarding of hazardous chemotherapeutic agents.

- **Glutaraldehyde (Cidex)**: This high-level disinfectant can cause irritation to the eyes and mucous membranes and should only be used in well-ventilated areas (with a local exhaust ventilation system or air exchanges occurring 7-15 times per hour) and stored in covered containers. Guidelines for safe use must be established by the facility per local and national regulations. Prior to disposal, glutaraldehyde can be neutralized with sodium hydroxide, or concentrated solutions diluted to a non-microbiocidal level (<5 ppm), allowing for disposal in sewage, in accordance with state laws.
- **Formaldehyde**: This high-level disinfectant is a carcinogen and can cause damage upon inhalation or contact. When in use, warning signs must be in place, appropriate PPE worn, exposure times and levels monitored, and the area properly ventilated.

Handling and Disposal of Biohazardous Materials in Operating Room

Medical waste management for biohazardous materials is mandated by federal and state laws, which require that certain types of medical waste be separated from others. This regulated medical waste (RMW) is eventually packaged, transported, and disposed of according to specific regulations for the type of waste material. Separate trash containers, lined with red plastic bags or containers and labeled as "Biohazard," must be provided for RMW, which includes:

- **Blood and body fluids** or **materials contaminated by blood and body fluids**, such as sponges, specimen containers, drainage bags (Hemovac), and contaminated tubing.
- **Creutzfeldt-Jakob disease contaminants**

Additionally, with CJD contaminants, all protective equipment should be single-use disposable and all non-disposable equipment should be masked. One-way instrument flow must be maintained and samples marked with biohazard label and disposed of in biohazard containers. All surfaces must be covered with disposable material. Most chemical disinfectants are ineffective/partially effective and gas disinfectants are ineffective. Boiling, dry heat, and UV or microwave radiation are also ineffective.

Packaging, Transportation, and Storage Techniques

Packaging Process for Instrumentation in the Surgical Area

Important factors to consider when selecting packaging for the sterilization process include the following:

- The package must allow the **sterilizing agent** to penetrate the package.
- The package must allow for **air removal** from the package.
- The package must allow the instruments contained inside the package to be **identified**.
- The package must allow the instrumentation within to be **securely enclosed** inside with a tamper-proof seal.
- The package must be **resistant to soiling** by fluids or particulates, tearing, or puncturing from the outside or by the product contained inside.
- The package must not be **compromised** before use.
- The package must not be **contaminated** with toxic agents.
- The package must allow the user to **deliver** the instrument easily to a sterile environment/field.
- The package must allow for **proper labeling** of the contained product.
- The package must maintain **sterility** of the product until use.

Packaging Agents

Woven Fabric

Some important facts to remember about using woven fabric as a packaging agent for products to be sterilized include the following:

- Woven fabric is suitable for **steam and ethylene oxide use**, not for hydrogen peroxide gas plasma.
- **Muslin** allows for penetration of sterilizing agents, but also allows microorganisms and moisture, and has been replaced by cotton and polyester fabrics.
- **Double layering** is sometimes done in order to prevent microorganisms from being allowed to enter the packaging.
- Some newer woven fabrics do not have to be **double wrapped**.
- **Pressure-sensitive tape** is used that doubles as a chemical indicator.
- Woven fabrics do not exhibit **memory**.
- Woven fabrics must be **inspected** periodically to ensure integrity. Over time, they may require treatment or discarding.

Nonwoven Fabric

Some important facts to remember about using nonwoven fabric as a packaging agent for products to be sterilized include the following:

- Nonwoven fabrics are **single-use items** and are to be discarded after use.
- Nonwoven fabrics are compatible with **steam and ethylene oxide**. In order for hydrogen peroxide gas plasma to be used, polypropylene must be used, as cellulose-based wrappers are not compatible with this process.
- Nonwoven fabrics provide excellent protection against **moisture, dust, and airborne microbes**.
- Nonwoven fabrics may be **single or double-wrapped**, depending on instruments and requirements by the manufacturer.
- Nonwoven fabrics do not need to be **washed**.
- Unlike woven fabrics, nonwoven fabrics demonstrate **memory** that can allow for contamination of a sterile field when the edges fold back in on the field.

Plastic/Paper and Plastic/Tyvek

Some important facts to remember about using plastic/paper and plastic/Tyvek as packaging agents for products to be sterilized include the following:

- Plastic/paper combination wrappers are used with **steam and ethylene oxide**.
- Plastic/Tyvek combination wrappers are used with **ethylene oxide and hydrogen peroxide gas plasma**.
- These types of wrappers are **cheap** to use, are **good barriers** against airborne microbes, allow for **clear visualization** of interior contents, and can be used with certain numbers of **small items**.
- These wrappers display **memory**, which can pose a risk of contamination of a sterile field.
- They are prone to **puncturing**.
- They may be **single or double packaged**. However, when double packaged, the inside pouch must not be folded.
- Instruments packaged this way should be processed **vertically**.

Using Rigid Containers as Packaging Agents for Products to Be Sterilized

Some important facts to remember about using rigid containers as packaging agents for products to be sterilized include the following:

- They are made from a **variety of materials** including aluminum, stainless steel, plastics, etc.
- **Perforations** in the tops allow for entry of the sterilant, but a bacterial filter over the holes prevents invasion from microorganisms.
- The **lids and bases** are held together by some type of mechanical device to keep both together during the sterilization process.
- They can sometimes be heavy and weigh up to **10 pounds**.
- They can sometimes allow for **undesirable condensation** on the outer aspects of the container.
- They must be **cleaned** prior to filling and require routine **inspection** of integrity and maintenance of filters.

TRANSPORTING INSTRUMENTS THAT HAVE BEEN STERILIZED

Transport of sterile instruments must be done carefully to avoid re-contaminating instruments that will be needed for future surgical use. After sterilization, the instruments should be packaged and labeled with the name of the item, the sterilizer used, the load number, and the date. The packages should be handled and placed carefully on the transport system so that the packaging will not be compromised. Before removing the packages from the transporter for either use or storage, they should be inspected again to determine that the packaging is intact. If not, the instruments must be reprocessed before being used. If the package is not compromised, then it can be used or stored until it is needed. In some cases, an expiration date may be added to the package, if applicable. Packages should be routinely checked for expiration dates to ensure they have not expired before being used.

CONSIDERATIONS FOR STORAGE OF ITEMS

Some important things the perioperative nurse should remember when storing items include the following:

- Storage areas for sterilized items should be **well ventilated** and should have good **temperature and humidity control**. They should also be areas without high traffic flow.
- **Sterile and clean** items should not be stored together.
- Areas for storage should be free of **water** and away from sinks. They should also be free of dust and particulate matter.
- Packaging should be stored in such a matter as to prevent **crushing** of the containers.
- If cabinets are used, they must be **well ventilated** and away from floors, fixtures, vents, lights, etc., to prevent contamination.

FACTORS AFFECTING THE SHELF LIFE OF ITEMS IN STORAGE

Some factors that affect the shelf life of an item in storage include the following:

- The shelf life of an item is theoretically considered **indefinite** as long as the item is not contaminated during storage.
- **Expiration dates** may be used on items that have been sterilized, but this is only a guideline as the product may become contaminated at any time between sterilization and the expiration date. Once contamination occurs, the item is no longer considered sterile. Items should not be used beyond their expiration date.
- Frequent handling, poor packaging, longer storage, failure to use dust covers, and storage in a non-enclosed cabinet all increase the chances for an item to be **contaminated**.
- **Inspection** of the instrument and packaging is necessary to identify possible contamination of the item.

Bringing Instruments to Operating Room from Outside the Facility

Most surgical instruments are made from the same type of compounds, regardless of which facility they come from. If a hospital or surgical center brings in surgical instruments from an outside facility, the instruments used are most likely prepackaged from where they were previously sterilized and packaged, or they are new instruments that come from the manufacturer. All instruments that arrive from outside the facility should only be used for their intended purposes. Even if surgical instruments are brand new, they must first be inspected for defects or anything that may make them unusable. If instruments from outside the facility arrive in non-sterile condition, they must be cleaned and then sterilized before being used for the first time. Products should be labeled if they are non-sterile when they arrive. Some manufacturers ship sterile, single-use instruments, which can be used after opening if the packaging is intact and not compromised in any way.

Sterilization Techniques

Sterilization and Disinfection

Sterilization is a process by which all microorganisms on a particular object are killed. This can be performed through various methods. Because sterile objects are introduced into the body and tissues below the mucous membrane, it is very important that new bacteria are not introduced, as it would potentially cause infiltration and infection of the exposed body part. Sterilization effectiveness is measured by the **sterility assurance level**, which perhaps counterintuitively, is the probability that the instrument remains nonsterile after having undergone a sterilization procedure. The maximum permissible value for sterility assurance level may vary for different facilities. Sterilization also kills most, if not all, types of spores on an object as well.

Disinfection is a process that kills microorganisms on an object, but may not be able to kill high numbers of spores on the object. Thus, the potential for transferring spores or microorganisms from an object that has been merely disinfected rather than sterilized is much higher.

Autoclaves

In **gravity displacement** autoclaves, air is displaced by gravity as steam is injected from the top forcing air out through the bottom. Considerations include the following:

- This requires longer sterilization times than other autoclaves.
- A greater length of time is required to displace air from the chamber.
- This is the most appropriate method for sterilizing liquids.
- The object placement within the chamber can affect air removal.

With a **pre-vacuum/high-vacuum** autoclave, a vacuum pump removes air from the chamber before steam is initiated, causing a vacuum in the chamber. Considerations include the following:

- This technique is more efficient than gravity displacement due to the vacuum allowing all areas to be immediately penetrated once the steam is applied.
- Much shorter sterilization times are required.
- Object placement within the chamber has less impact on air removal.
- This requires daily Bowie-Dick/air removal tests to assure seals are adequate in the chamber.

Steam-flush pressure-pulse autoclaves use steam, flushing, and pressure-pulses above atmospheric pressure to remove air from the chamber. In this technique, air leaks do not cause a compromise in sterilization.

Thermal Heat Sterilization

Advantages

- Steam sterilization is cheap and easy to produce.
- Most instruments can be sterilized using this method.
- Steam has no adverse effects to the user or to the environment (as long as care is taken to prevent injury from the heat source).
- The thermal sterilization procedure is faster than other methods of sterilization.

Disadvantages

- Some instruments cannot withstand the heat of thermal sterilization and require other methods to be sterilized.
- Much care must be given to preparation of items to be steam sterilized; otherwise, adequate sterilization will not occur.
- There is quite a bit of variability in terms of how long and how much pressure is to be used in the cycle depending on the number of objects being sterilized, differences in materials being sterilized, etc.

Immediate Use Steam Sterilization (IUSS)

Indications

Immediate use steam sterilization (IUSS) is a sterilization procedure that is used when an instrument is needed immediately for use in surgery. It is not indicated for routine sterilization of instruments, as it is not as effective as other methods. However, in certain circumstances such as during a surgical procedure, an instrument may become contaminated and a suitable replacement is not available. To qualify for IUSS the instrument must be designated as such by the manufacturer. In addition, proper standardized sterilization of the object must not be available (or be too lengthy) in order to consider IUSS. Under these circumstances, although not utilized by certain institutions, IUSS may be undertaken to provide the instruments necessary to complete the procedure being performed. In addition, it is not indicated for use in sterilization of items to be implanted and left in the patient.

Disadvantages

- The cleaning process before sterilization is often **suboptimal** due to immediate need of the object.
- **Inadequate cleaning** due to poor technique, lack of appropriate cleaning supplies in the operating room, etc., may cause sterilization to be inadequate.
- Because there is not a **drying process** in IUSS, the items coming out of the sterilization chamber are wet.
- If the IUSS autoclave is not located in the operating room, methods for transferring the object back to the sterile field become difficult and may possibly **compromise the integrity** of the instrument.
- Flash sterilization is not indicated as a method for sterilization for certain instruments per the **manufacturers**.

Sterilization Process Using Ethylene Oxide Gas

When sterilizing using ethylene oxide gas, items are placed in the sterilization chamber in a loose pattern to allow for proper penetration of the gas. Items are also placed in metal baskets to allow for removal by personnel after the sterilization procedure. Air is evacuated from the chamber and the subsequent items within the chamber are heated, humidity is introduced into the chamber, then ethylene oxide is introduced. This process uses negative pressure in the chamber to prevent release of the gas into the environment.

Advantages

- Ethylene oxide is a potent sterilizing agent that works on all types of microorganisms.
- It can be used on instruments that cannot handle high heat or moisture.
- It is not a corrosive agent and can be used on objects prone to corrosion.
- It permeates materials effectively that may otherwise be too porous or large via other methods.

Disadvantages

- Long sterilization times/high cost are required for use.
- It is a highly flammable gas.
- Hydro chlorofluorocarbons used to dilute the gas for safer administration are being reduced because of their destruction of the environment.
- Items that absorb the gas must be aerated for detoxification after sterilization.
- It is a potential carcinogen and can cause reproductive harm. It is highly regulated by OSHA, and employees are only allowed certain amounts of exposure in an 8-hour period.

Sterilization Process Using Liquid Peracetic Acid

Peracetic acid works by disrupting protein bonds and utilizes oxygen to disrupt cell system processes causing cell death. It is used in a liquid form and is low temperature. Thus, only immersible items can be sterilized in this manner. Sterilization requires a standardized temperature and time for processing. The solution is washed over the instrument and then a rinse cycle ensues. When the cycle is completed, the instrument can be taken in the tray to a sterile scrub person to deliver the item to the sterile field for use. If the instrument is not immediately used and transferred in the tray to the sterile field, it can be dried and stored for future use but is not at that point considered sterile.

Low-Temperature Hydrogen Peroxide Gas Plasma Sterilization

Advantages

- This sterilization process is nontoxic and offers no health risk to its users. Secondary to this, extra time does not have to be taken to aerate the materials, no special equipment is required by personnel to wear, and no monitoring of exposure is required.
- A short length of time is needed to sterilize instruments.
- Because it is a low-temperature unit, the temperature does not need to be adjusted in order to achieve proper sterilization, so it is simple to operate.
- The sterilization unit is mobile due to the fact that all major components necessary are located within the unit.

Disadvantages

- Not all items can be used in the sterilizer. Powder, liquids, linens, papers, and other items containing cellulose are not compatible with the plasma created by hydrogen peroxide.
- Packaging materials for objects to be sterilized are limited to specific containers.

Steam Sterilization

Procedures

Some important factors to consider when using steam sterilizing procedures include the following:

- Instruments are arranged on mesh trays to allow for **penetration of sterilant and drainage**.
- A **towel** may be placed on the bottom of the tray to speed up the drying process.
- Each item should be placed to allow **penetration of the sterilant**.
- All **joints/hinges** should be disassembled.
- **Heavy instruments** are placed on the bottom, lighter items on top.
- **Paper/plastic wrappers** should not be used within wrapped sets, as they cannot be guaranteed to be positioned properly for sterilization.
- Very **heavy/metal items** may need to be processed separately as they may require specific parameters for proper heating of the entire instrument to allow for thorough sterilization.

Using Wood or Reusable Textiles

Some important things to remember when using wood or reusable textiles in the steam sterilization process include:

- **Wood** can be difficult to sterilize as resin from inside the wood can be displaced during the sterilization process. The **resin** can then be deposited on other instruments and can cause a reaction in the patient if it contacts mucous membrane. Therefore, wood items must be sterilized separately or wrapped alone and not included in other instrument sets.
- **Textiles** to be sterilized must be composed of materials that allow air removal, steam penetration, and drying.
- Prior to sterilization, **linens** must be hydrated to prevent superheating during the sterilization process. Superheating will cause the fibers of the textile to be damaged.
- **Reusable textiles** have a limited life span and must be monitored for integrity and tracked to ensure they are not used beyond their intended number of uses.

Using Basins, Bowls, Cups, Rubber Goods, Tubing, and Items with Lumens

Some important factors to remember when using basins/bowls/cups, rubber goods, and items with lumens in steam sterilization include:

- **Absorbent towels or gauze** can be placed between bowls, cups, or basins to allow them to be stacked in the sterilization chamber. The towel/gauze allows for penetration by the sterilant.
- When stacking items in bowls, cups, or basins, they should all be placed in the **same direction**. This allows for proper sterilization, drainage, and prevents air pockets from forming in the chamber.
- **Rubber items** should not be folded. To prevent this, wrapping gauze around rubber surfaces will allow penetration of the sterilant and prevent rubber surfaces from contacting another.
- Items with **lumens** are cleaned and rinsed with distilled water before sterilization. When the item is sterilized in the chamber, the moisture vaporizes and displaces air in the lumen, which allows for sterilization to occur.

Steam Sterilization vs. Ethylene Oxide or Hydrogen Peroxide Gas Plasma Sterilization

The differences that must be considered between steam sterilization versus either ethylene oxide or hydrogen peroxide gas plasma sterilization include the following:

- As opposed to steam sterilization, items being prepared for gas sterilization with ethylene oxide or using hydrogen peroxide gas plasma must be **dry**. Ethylene oxide, a toxic residue, is formed with ethylene oxide use in the presence of water.
- All **oil-based lubricants** must be removed from items before use with ethylene oxide, as it cannot penetrate oil-based compounds. Only water-based compounds can be used.
- Only **polypropylene wrappings** can be used in hydrogen peroxide gas plasma sterilization. Cellulose-containing items (linens, paper, gauze, towels) can prevent proper sterilization of items.

Mechanical Process Indicators

Mechanical process indicators are various forms of devices used to monitor conditions within a sterilization process and maintain quality control of the sterilization process. They help to determine whether a sterilizer is working properly and whether the items within the sterilizer are being appropriately treated for sterilization. There are physical indicators and biological indicators.

- **Physical indicators** measure physical conditions in the sterilization process including temperature, length of temperature achievement, time of use, number of cycles being run in 24 hours, pressures achieved during various cycles, gas concentration, humidity, electricity supply, filters, and troubleshooting for system functionality. Although this information may be printed on a graph, the more common and conventional methods now are printed out in an easy-to-read format.
- **Biological indicators** use microorganisms (most commonly *Geobacillus stearothermophilus* spores) to test the sterilizers effectiveness in killing relatively resistant bacteria. While weekly tests are generally required, daily testing of sterilizers using biological indicators is recommended.

Chemical Indicators

Chemical indicators are to be placed on the outside and inside of all packages. The internal indicator should be placed in the area most difficult to sterilize. Chemical indicators do not guarantee sterility; rather, they only indicate whether the items being processed have been exposed to the measured conditions. When no indicator is present, it should be assumed that the product has not met required sterilization conditions.

Sealing and Labeling of Products for Sterilization

Some important facts to remember when considering sealing and labeling of products for sterilization include:

- All items must be **sealed** before going through the sterilization process.
- **Woven and nonwoven wrappers** are sealed with pressure sensitive tape.
- **Plastic/paper and plastic/Tyvek pouches** are sealed with heat, self-seals, or pressure sensitive tape.
- When packages are sealed with **heat**, resealing must not occur once they are opened.

- All items should be **labeled** as follows before sterilization:
  - Contents
  - Sterilizer identification, type, and cycle used
  - Sterilization parameters
  - Load control number
  - Initials of the assembler
  - Results of process monitoring
- Indelible, nonbleeding, nontoxic labels are to be used for sterilization.
- Felt-tip pens or soft lead pencils may be used for labeling.

IMPORTANT TERMS

Important terms relative to the sterilization process include the following:

- **Autoclave**: A sterilizer that uses steam to sterilize.
- **Bioburden**: The quantity of living microorganisms viable on a certain product.
- **Biofilm**: A film created by clusters of microorganisms that prevents antimicrobial agents from reaching the cells.
- **Biological indicator**: A mechanism used to test a sterilizer's ability to sterilize objects.
- **Bowie-Dick test**: A test that tests the ability of an autoclave to remove air and non-condensable gases from the chamber and measures how well steam is able to penetrate specific objects.
- **Chemical indicator**: An object used to monitor the sterilization process. It works when a chemical change produces a change in the indicator, indicating a chemical change in the environment or exact chemical parameters of the environment.
- **Contamination**: The process of an object being infiltrated with microorganisms.
- **Decontamination**: The process by which an object is freed from microorganisms.
- **Disinfectant**: A solution capable of destroying living microorganisms upon contact; used only on inanimate objects.
- **Disinfection**: The process by which microbes are killed on an object.
- **Flash sterilization**: A process used to sterilize objects quickly for immediate use. It uses steam to sterilize objects.
- **Spore**: The dormant state of a microorganism.
- **Sterile**: Free of all living microorganisms.
- **Sterility assurance level**: The probability that a certain object remains nonsterile despite having undergone sterilization.
- **Sterilization**: The process by which all microorganisms are killed on an object.
- **Washer-disinfector/decontaminator**: A machine used to decontaminate instruments using washing, ultrasonic processing, chemical treating, thermal treating, and rinsing to remove specific microorganisms.
- **Washer-sterilizer**: A machine used to remove microorganisms from instruments using washing, rinsing, and sterilization processes.

Surgical Site Infection Risk Factors

Surgical Site Infections

Three types of surgical site infections according to the tissues involved, frequency, treatment, and severity are described below:

1. **Superficial incisional** surgical site infections involve superficial skin or subcutaneous tissue. They are the most frequent of these types of infections. They are often identified after discharge and are often resolved by removal of sutures and drainage of the area. These are the least severe of all types of these infections.
2. **Deep incisional** surgical site infections involve deep soft tissue and muscle. These are less frequently diagnosed than superficial infections but are more likely to be diagnosed before discharge. Treatment for these may include prolonged hospitalization, antibiotic treatment, and drainage.
3. **Organ/space** surgical site infections involve visceral cavities and organs or anatomic structures not opened during the surgical procedure. Although less frequent, these infections are often quite severe and require prolonged hospitalization and often reoperation.

Factors That Increase Risk of Developing Endogenous Infection

Some individual factors that can increase a patient's risk of developing an endogenous infection include the following:

- **Lengthy surgical time**: This provides more time for bacteria to migrate to surgical site.
- **Extensive preoperative hospital stay**: This leads to increased exposure to hospital bacteria.
- **Very old or very young age at time of surgery**: These populations are more likely to have inadequate circulation or immature immune responses.
- **Poor nutritional status or obesity**: This causes an impaired immune system; in obesity, avascular areas of subcutaneous tissue are more susceptible to infection.
- **Alcohol and drug use**: This causes an impaired immune system, often in correlation with poor nutritional status.
- **Immunocompromised or chronically ill patients**: An already stressed immune system has a lower ability to form defense against microorganisms.
- The presence of an **infection pre-surgery**: This taxes the immune system prematurely; surgery is delayed until infection is gone.
- **Damaged integrity of a patient's skin or internal compartments**: The skin and internal compartments prevent invasion of endogenous bacteria into the rest of the body.
- **Presence of implants and drains**: These devices can allow for migration of bacteria to certain sites.

Factors That Increase Risk of Developing Exogenous Infection

Some environmental factors that present risk to a patient in developing an exogenous infection include the following:

- **A greater number of workers in the operating room** increases risk of infection. People carry microbes on their bodies; the more people, the more microbes are present to threaten infection.
- Increased **talking, coughing, or breathing** around the patient also increases risk.
- Exposure of the patient to **cells** or **hair** shed from the body from hospital personnel increases risk. Shedding of skin cells and hair occurs frequently and is a major source of staphylococcus infection.
- Personnel wearing **artificial nails and jewelry** provide areas for bacteria and other microorganisms to hide. Although good scrubbing techniques can be employed, often bacteria and fungi are not adequately removed from those who wear artificial nails.
- The **operating room and its subsequent instruments** are not able to be sterilized and pose a potential source of infection.
- Instruments that are **exposed to air** are potential sources of infection, especially when they are left out long enough to collect dust.

Role of Perioperative Nurse in Preventing Infection

Even though the perioperative nurse does not do all of the cleaning, disinfecting, packaging, or sterilizing of instruments, he or she plays a big role in maintaining sterilization. The nurse must take care in checking storage of sterile supplies and ensure that they are being used in a manner that prevents newer products from being used first and older products from expiring. The nurse ensures that instruments were packaged in the proper packaging when sterilized and that the sterilization process (through inspection of sterilization indicators) was adequate. Lastly, the nurse may also be responsible for delivering the package to the sterile field, which must be done in a proper manner to assure that the product maintains sterility.

Emergency Situations

Emergency Situations in the Operating Room

Preparation to Prevent Emergencies

When a nurse knows the surgical procedure and the anatomy/physiology involved, he or she can know whether or not the right patient is being prepared for the right procedure. In addition, the nurse can be knowledgeable about potential side effects or complications that may occur with certain procedures, potential medication requirements, or potential emergencies that may arise secondary to that procedure. When the nurse is prepared with this information, she can **respond to an emergency quickly** if one occurs, or **prevent** a potential complication by making accurate assessments of the patient at periodic intervals throughout the procedure, thus avoiding a potential emergency. The nurse can control certain environmental factors in order to be prepared for or prevent potential emergencies by maintaining adequate temperatures, preparing for intervention in case of emergency, and staying aware of traffic patterns, humidity, and the presence of particular materials or emergency equipment to prevent contamination.

Managerial-Type Nursing Interventions to Prevent Emergency Situations

The following are some managerial-type nursing interventions that can be employed to prevent emergency situations:

- Proper **planning** for patient care from entrance into to exit from the operative area can help to prevent emergencies from occurring, as it gives a platform to follow for smooth transition and adequate patient care.
- **Organizing** personnel, equipment, etc., provides the surgical team with the appropriate assistance and materials required to perform surgery and all of the necessary tasks associated with it.
- **Directing** people in an appropriate manner throughout the surgical suite is important to keep the flow of patient care smooth and consistent. Appropriate delegation to the correct people is very important as improper delegation may contribute to patient injury. Having good interpersonal directing skills is important to maintain good communication and prevent potential adverse reactions from staff.
- **Controlling** resources in the surgical environment can help to prevent potential shortfalls in equipment, staff availability, or staff integrity.

Preventing and Responding to Pharmacology/Anesthesia Emergencies

The following are some nursing interventions that can take place to prevent and respond to emergencies involving pharmacology/anesthesia:

- Administer **medications** via the 5 Rights of Medication Administration
- Know the patient's **allergy profile**
- Follow **institutional policy** for preparing and administering mediations
- Know all potential **side effects** of every medication administered and be prepared for possible adverse medication or anesthesia reactions
    - For example, with medications that induce central nervous system depression, make sure that appropriate interventions are being undertaken to monitor the patient's respirations, ventilation, perfusion, etc. If the patient is not being adequately ventilated, emergency intubation may be required. By knowing what equipment is necessary, the nurse can prepare and notify the proper personnel for this action to take place.
- Adequately **assess** the patient throughout the medication administration and anesthesia process to determine how the patient is responding to the medication and be prepared for potential adverse reactions, including malignant hyperthermia, hypotension, hypoxia, etc.

Cardiac Arrest in Operating Room

Roles of Healthcare Providers

If a patient has a cardiac arrest ("Code blue") in the operating room, immediate response is critical. Once an arrest is identified and confirmed by the surgical team, the members generally have defined roles (protocols may vary somewhat):

- **Anesthesiologist/Anesthetist**: Calls for emergency code, provides IV access, orders and administers IV drugs, manages airway/ventilation, and monitors cardiac status and vital signs.
- **Surgeon**: Begins external thoracic compressions, carries out defibrillation if indicated, may order medications and treatment depending on whether the cause is shockable or non-shockable. Opens chest for internal cardiac massage if indicated.
- **Scrub nurse**: Assists surgeon with external thoracic compression, maintains sterile field during resuscitation efforts (especially important with an open incision), provides medications (verifying medication and dosage) as necessary.
- **Circulating nurse**: Gathers supplies as needed, including the emergency "crash cart," and activates timer, opens materials for the scrub nurse, and controls admission of others to the operating room.

Nursing Interventions for Patient in Cardiac Arrest

If a patient is in cardiac arrest, the nurse can begin performing basic **CPR** (cardiopulmonary resuscitation). Additional staff may begin the task or assist, and proper communication between staff members is essential for allowing each member to provide care as necessary. If the patient does not immediately respond to CPR attempts, **ACLS** (advanced cardiac life support) guidelines may need to be employed. In this instance, the nurse must be competent in the appropriate interventions for advanced cardiac care. It is important that the nurse know how to signal for an ACLS protocol to begin and how to obtain or delegate someone to obtain equipment/medications appropriate for ACLS. The nurse may be the manager of the code, keep records of the interventions taking place for the patient, administer medications, take labs, continue CPR, etc., at any time as appropriate during the intervention to restore the patient.

Review Video: Advanced Cardiac Life Support (ACLS)
Visit mometrix.com/academy and enter code: 373365

Malignant Hyperthermia

Screening patients for a personal or family history of malignant hyperthermia can prepare the nurse to take adequate assessments of the patient who might be at risk. If the patient begins exhibiting signs of malignant hyperthermia, the nurse must notify the doctor/anesthesiologist about the patient's vital signs and laboratory values, aid in turning off equipment that is delivering anesthetic agents responsible for the development of malignant hyperthermia, replace the anesthesia machine, prepare cold fluids/baths for cooling the patient, obtain medications for administration to counteract the effects of malignant hyperthermia including proper reconstitution of those medications, and be available for any alternative measures the physician/anesthesiologist may want to employ for proper treatment. The nurse must also assess the patient's responses to such interventions and ascertain their effectiveness.

Care of Trauma Patients

The perioperative nurse plays an integral role in the care of a trauma patient. Many patients who have endured traumatic events have multiple injuries and are complex cases that require surgery. The perioperative nurse may assist with initially stabilizing the trauma patient in order to prepare for surgery. The patient may be unconscious or unable to communicate and the perioperative nurse must understand how to work with the family and the physician to move forward with the required procedures. Because the trauma patient may be physically unstable during surgery, the perioperative nurse must know what to do to assist with resuscitation, if necessary. During the postoperative period, the perioperative nurse provides information through report to the nurse taking over the patient's care. Because there are so many different types of trauma, the perioperative nurse must be flexible and have a thorough knowledge of many different procedures in order to care for the trauma patient.

Barriers to Communication During Emergencies

Physical barriers to communication include those that mechanically or physically alter a person from being able to communicate or receive communication from another individual. These include difficulty hearing voices or seeing gestures, problems speaking, or problems understanding communication.

Emotional barriers are those induced by emotional factors including fear, stress, perception, etc. Planning for a proper delivery of the information, including precise instructions at appropriate intervals using appropriate language, and obtaining feedback from the person to whom the communication is delivered helps to break down barriers to communication through physical and emotional means. Often precise statements given in appropriate situations can help avoid extraneous emotional information that can be read into a statement. Environmental barriers should be reduced because more words are available for misinterpretation in a noisy or busy environment.

Recombinant Activated Factor VII

Recombinant activated factor VII (NovoSeven) activates the extrinsic pathway of coagulation and stimulates production of thrombin, platelet activation, and the formation of fibrin clots, improving prothrombin time. While indicated for those with clotting disorders, factor VII is often given off-label after surgery for those with coagulopathies receiving blood products. Adverse effects include myocardial infarction, cardiac ischemia, supraventricular tachycardia, arterial thromboembolism, cerebral artery occlusion and ischemia, acute renal failure, and pulmonary emboli. Dosage varies. Patients receiving factor VII should be monitored carefully for thromboembolism and coagulation profile. Those with atherosclerotic disease, coagulopathies, or septicemia are at increased risk.

Desmopressin Acetate and Antifibrinolytic Agents

Additional pharmacologic agents used to control bleeding include:

- **Desmopressin acetate**: This synthetic analogue of vasopressin increases blood levels of clotting factors (VWF, FVIII, and t-PA), causes vasodilation, and shortens the clotting time (aPTT). Desmopressin acetate can prevent bleeding in patients with inherited bleeding disorders and platelet dysfunction but can also be used to control or prevent bleeding during surgical procedures. Because of its antidiuretic effect, desmopressin should be used with care in patients with heart failure and fluid overload.
- **Antifibrinolytic agents**: These agents, such as aprotinin, epsilon-aminocaproic acid, and tranexamic acid, inhibit the fibrinolytic pathways and decrease the risk of surgical and postoperative bleeding. Surgery, especially when it requires cardiopulmonary bypass (which impairs hemostasis and increases risk of bleeding), activates the fibrinolytic system, so antifibrinolytic agents are critical to reducing the risk of bleeding and reducing the need for transfusions and are administered with anesthesia.
    - *Aminocaproic acid (Amicar):* An antifibrinolytic agent that prevents plasminogen from binding to fibrin, interfering with the breakdown of clots. It is used in the cardiac patient with postoperative bleeding associated with fibrinolysis. Dosage is 75-150 mg/kg over 60 minutes initially and then a maintenance infusion of 10-15 mg/kg/hr (generally 1 g/hr) for 8 hours or until bleeding is controlled. Adverse effects include thrombocytopenia, dysrhythmias, and thrombosis.

Preventing Injury in the Operating Room

Preventing Safety-Related Injury in Patients in the Operating Room

The following are some things the nurse can do to prevent injury in a patient who has been assessed with a high risk for injury related to safety within the operating room environment:

- Know how to properly **use** a fire extinguisher and the different types of fire extinguishers available according to class (which materials and types of fires each extinguisher is effective against).
- Know the location of **gas shut-off valves** and who is authorized to use them and when.
- Know the location of **SDSs** and how to read them.
- Know **institutional policy** regarding evacuation during particular natural disasters, bomb threats, and terrorist attacks.
- Identify particular **risks** related to electrical and radiation exposure and injury.
- Use proper **policy** regarding maintaining surgical asepsis, prevent contamination of the surgical field, and monitor equipment and traffic within and out of the operating room.
- Monitor patient for signs or symptoms of **potential or real injury** relating to positioning, allergic reaction, response to anesthesia/medication administered, or other common complications with surgery. Know the location of equipment and how to use it in case of an adverse reaction to the procedure.

Natural Disaster or Terrorism

Nursing interventions for a natural disaster/terrorism attack include the following:

- Know hospital policy for responding to a **natural disaster or terrorist attack**, including staffing personnel in the instance of high casualties.
- Know how to **evacuate** in case of a bomb threat or other disaster.

Impaired Colleagues

Nursing interventions for impaired colleagues include the following:

- Know hospital policy for reporting **inappropriate or disruptive behavior**.
- Know hospital policies for **discontinuing an impaired coworker's care** to prevent injury to a patient.

Disruptive Families/Patients

Nursing interventions for disruptive families/patients include the following:

- Know hospital policy for using **restraining devices** for patients.
- Know hospital policy for notifying security of a **potentially dangerous situation**.
- Practice techniques for controlling and maintaining a **calm environment** to help dissipate potential aggravating environmental situations for patients or families.

Professional Accountabilities

Perioperative Nurse Scope and Standards

Core Competencies Within the Domains of the Perioperative Patient Care Model

There are five core competencies within the domains of the Perioperative Patient Care Model:

1. **Safety for the patient**: The nurse must help maintain patient safety in the perioperative area, including making changes necessary to provide for safety for the patient.
2. **Physiologic conditions**: The nurse must have and demonstrate the ability to use the aspects of the nursing process to maintain proper physiologic conditions for the patient.
3. **Knowledge of behavioral responses**: The nurse must be knowledgeable about spiritual, cultural, and psychological responses that a patient or a patient's family may have in the perioperative area.
4. **Patient and family rights and ethics**: Once the nurse is knowledgeable about the psychological, cultural, and spiritual concerns of the patient/family as well as patient rights, then the nurse must support these rights and ethical standards according to the patient's needs.
5. **Results of health system on patient care**: The nurse must be able to demonstrate knowledge of how the health system and administration affects patient care.

Maintaining Competency

The following are some steps the nurse can undertake to maintain competency in their field:

- **Identify strengths, weaknesses, and knowledge deficits** in any area pertinent to patient care including physiological and psychological aspects of care.
- **Practice competencies** necessary for the unit or profession. If new competencies emerge, the nurse can become familiar with them and practice their skills until competency is achieved.
- **Make goals**. The nurse can make goals to develop professionalism on a regular basis, which will help them create a plan to follow.
- The nurse can reach **professional learning goals** by obtaining certifications, taking classes on pertinent subjects, attending conferences on subjects related to the field, taking a college course to learn the newest information, becoming involved in research projects dealing with aspects of the perioperative setting, etc.

Accountability and Responsibilities

The perioperative nurse is accountable to the patient, to himself or herself, to the patient's family, to the organization they work for, and to society for their actions. The nurse has the responsibility to uphold a certain knowledge base and achieve standards of performance to meet the expectations of all groups involved in a patient's care. Thus, nurses have the responsibility to understand what they do and do not know about a particular situation or task. Nurses also have the responsibility to take measures to change their knowledge or skills deficit.

DETERMINING PERIOPERATIVE NURSING ACCOUNTABILITY

The following are various ways to determine perioperative nursing accountability as would be done on a yearly review:

- Have a **peer review** certain aspects of care or performance to ensure adequacy with tasks performed in the perioperative area including tasks that require knowledge of certain standards and ability to perform certain psychomotor skills necessary in the perioperative environment.
- Demonstrate **compliance** with hospital, local, state, and national laws regarding nursing practice including maintaining adequate licensure, competency requirements, classes required to attend, etc.
- Demonstrate the ability to **advocate** for patients regarding safety, physiologic, behavioral, social, cultural, and other needs.
- Demonstrate the ability to accurately and adequately **delegate** tasks using the five "rights" of delegation.
- Develop professional accountability through **continuing education** through a variety of nursing developmental resources (journals, classes, certifications, etc.).

DELEGATION

The five rights of delegation are:

1. The right **task**
2. Under the right **circumstances**
3. To the right **person**
4. With the right instructions, direction, or communication
5. With the right supervision or evaluation

The implementation step of the nursing process is the only one that allows for delegation. The other steps do not allow for delegation because they are part of the nurse's responsibility. The implementation step of the process can be delegated because even in the delegation process, evaluation that the delegated task has been completed successfully takes place. Any of the other steps in the nursing process undertaken by another individual prevents the nurse from being able to accurately assess whether the patient's needs have all been accounted for and whether the tasks necessary to be completed for the patient have been completed.

WHEN NOT TO DELEGATE

Using the five rights of delegation, the following are some situations that can prevent a certain task from being delegated to other personnel:

- The right **task**:
  - The task is too complex for the individual or new to the unit's procedures.
  - The task has high potential risk to the patient.
- The right **circumstances**:
  - The patient is unstable.
  - There is not adequate time to complete the task to allow for proper supervision.
- The right **person**:
  - The person to whom the nurse is delegating is new to the unit/profession.
  - The person to whom the nurse is delegating has not finished their competency requirements.
- The right **instructions**, **direction**, or **communication**:
  - The nurse does not have time to explain various parts of the procedure or certain patient limitations pertinent to the delegated task.
- The right **supervision** or **evaluation**:
  - The nurse does not have time to evaluate the delegated task after it has been performed and/or there are not adequate personnel available to supervise the delegated task

Reporting Disruptive Behavior

Interpersonal Skills in Managing Operating Suite Staff

Because the nurse in the operating suite may be in charge of managing staff actions as well as coaching new staff members, it is often the job of the nurse to give instructions or suggestions that may or may not be desirable or particularly friendly. For instance, if the nurse detects that another personnel's glove or gown has been contaminated in surgery, he or she may have to inform the person of the break in sterility and ask them to change their glove or gown. If done in a non-offensive manner, a quick change and return to the procedure is much more likely to occur without negative repercussions. In addition, new staff members usually have a steep learning curve, and if they are reprimanded in a negative manner, they may not feel as though they can do the job and may quit or become discouraged.

Managing Bullying in the Operative Suite

Bullying usually occurs from doctors to nurses and management to nurses due to the hierarchy of the hospital setting. However, when verbal abuse occurs from staff members to other staff members, it may be more difficult to pin down and deal with. All nurses are responsible for addressing bullying when it occurs. The nurse can say something directly to the person doing the bullying activity, as long as it is done in an appropriate manner. The nurse should identify the disruptive behavior to the person, describe it as violent or abusive, explain that it is not conducive to good staff morale, and insist that it cease. When all members do this, abusive verbal comments will diminish. If it is not taken care of between peers, it may be necessary to talk to management about the issue.

Monitoring Clinical Privileges

An individual who obtains clinical privileges has a particular set of skills or a knowledge base that has properly equipped them for practice in the specific environment that has given them privileges. If the individual loses those clinical privileges, it indicates that they are not able to practice safely or efficiently, due to a breakdown in either practice or knowledge guidelines. The nurses who work in the operating environment know which doctors have clinical privileges that qualify them to perform surgery. If a physician does not have those privileges and attempts to practice in an area without them, the nurse may prevent a potential adverse situation or emergency by following hospital guidelines for informing and disallowing that person from performing a procedure.

Incompetent, Unethical, or Illegal Performance or Provider Impairment

When nurses appropriately report the incompetent, unethical, or illegal performance or the impairment of a provider, they protect the patient by preventing potential or additional injury. Nurses protect the public when they take action on behalf of the facility to prevent the provider from acting inappropriately to others in the future. The impaired provider is also protected from possibly making further inappropriate decisions when nurses give the provider an opportunity to make changes to correct behavior or to withdraw from the situation. The profession is protected in that individuals with impairments like any of those listed above are singled out and detained until corrective actions can be made on behalf of the institution or individual, preventing a charge of incompetent/unethical care.

Identifying and Reporting Individuals Who Mistreat Patients or Who Are Impaired on the Job

Since nurses maintain safety for the patient in the perioperative area, it is their responsibility to make sure that the care they are transferring the patient to is adequate. For this reason, nurses must be able to identify aspects of care provided by others that may affect their patient including mental disability, behavioral problems, inadequate credentials/privileges, or impairment (through a variety of means, including substance abuse). Nurses who identify one of these potential risks to their patient, who is vulnerable in the perioperative setting, must know how to report such impairment and comply with the standards of practice in place as established by the facility or state or local laws. When nurses exercise these standards for the patient, they prevent harm to the patient and become the patient's advocate.

Ethics

Ethical Principles

Autonomy is the ethical principle that the individual has the right to make decisions about his or her own care. In the case of children or patients with dementia who cannot make autonomous decisions, parents or family members may serve as the legal decision maker. The nurse must keep the patient and/or family fully informed so that they can exercise their autonomy in informed decision-making.

Justice is the ethical principle that relates to the distribution of the limited resources of healthcare benefits to the members of society. These resources must be distributed fairly. This issue may arise if there is only one bed left and two sick patients. Justice comes into play in deciding which patient should stay and which should be transported or otherwise cared for. The decision should be made according to what is best or most just for the patients and not colored by personal bias.

Beneficence is an ethical principle that involves performing actions that are for the purpose of benefitting another person. In the care of a patient, any procedure or treatment should be done with the ultimate goal of benefitting the patient, and any actions that are not beneficial should be reconsidered. As conditions change, procedures need to be continually reevaluated to determine if they are still of benefit.

Nonmaleficence is an ethical principle that means healthcare workers should provide care in a manner that does not cause direct intentional harm to the patient:

- The actual act must be good or morally neutral.
- The intent must be only for a good effect.
- A bad effect cannot serve as the means to get to a good effect.
- A good effect must have more benefit than a bad effect has harm.

Nursing Code of Ethics

There is more interest in the **ethics** involved in healthcare due to technological advances that have made the prolongation of life, organ transplants, prenatal manipulation, and saving of premature infants possible, sometimes with poor outcomes. Couple these with healthcare's limited resources, and **ethical dilemmas** abound. Ethics is the study of **morality** as the value that controls actions. The American Nurses Association Code of Ethics contains nine statements defining **principles** the nurse can use when faced with moral and ethical problems. Nurses must be knowledgeable about the many ethical issues in healthcare and about the field of ethics in general. The nurse must help a patient to reveal their values and morals to the health care team so that the patient, family, and team can resolve moral issues pertaining to the patient's care. As part of the healthcare team, the nurse has a right to express personal values and moral concerns about medical issues.

Bioethics

Bioethics is a branch of ethics that involves making sure that the medical treatment given is the most morally correct choice given the different options that might be available and the differences inherent in the varied levels of treatment. In the health care unit, if the patients, family members, and the staff are in agreement when it comes to values and decision-making, then no ethical dilemma exists; however, when there is a difference in value beliefs between the patients/family members and the staff, there is a bioethical dilemma that must be resolved. Sometimes, discussion and explanation can resolve differences, but at times the institution's ethics committee must be brought in to resolve the conflict. The primary goal of bioethics is to determine the most morally correct action using the set of circumstances given.

Ethical Decision-Making Model

There are many ethical decision-making models. Some general guidelines to apply in using ethical decision-making models could be the following:

- Gather information about the identified problem
- State reasonable alternatives and solutions to the problem
- Utilize ethical resources (for example, clergy or ethics committees) to help determine the ethically important elements of each solution or alternative
- Suggest and attempt possible solutions
- Choose a solution to the problem

It is important to always consider the **ethical principles** of autonomy, beneficence, nonmaleficence, justice, and fidelity when attempting to facilitate ethical decision-making with family members, caregivers, and the healthcare team.

Ethical Assessment

While the terms *ethics* and *morals* are sometimes used interchangeably, ethics is a study of morals and encompasses concepts of right and wrong. When making **ethical assessments,** one must consider not only what people should do but also what they actually do, as these two things are sometimes at odds. Ethical issues can be difficult to assess because of personal bias, which is one of the reasons that sharing concerns with other internal sources and reaching consensus is so valuable. Issues of concern might include options for care, refusal of care, rights to privacy, adequate relief of suffering, and the right to self-determination. Internal sources might include the ethics committee, whose role is to make decisions regarding ethical issues. Risk management can provide guidance related to personal and institutional liability. External agencies might include government agencies, such as the public health department.

Ethical Analysis of a Situation

Assessment of the situation is done to reveal the ethical, legal, and professional **conflicts** that are present. Those who are involved are identified, including the patient, family, and healthcare personnel. The decision maker is determined if it is not the patient. Information about the situation is collected to determine medical facts about the disease and condition of the patient, options for treatment, and nursing diagnoses. Any pertinent legal information is included. The patient and family's cultural, religious, and moral values are determined. Possible courses of action are listed and compared in terms of outcomes for the patient using the utilitarian or deontological theory of ethics. Professional codes of ethics are also applied. A decision is made and evaluated as to whether it is the most morally correct action. Ethical arguments for and against the decision are given and responded to by the decision maker.

Professional Boundaries

Gifts

Over time, patients may develop a bond with nurses they trust and may feel grateful to the nurse for the care provided and want to express thanks, but the nurse must make sure to maintain professional boundaries. Patients often offer **gifts** to nurses to show their appreciation, but some adults, especially those who are weak and ill or have cognitive impairment, may be taken advantage of easily. Patients may offer valuables and may sometimes be easily manipulated into giving large sums of money. Small tokens of appreciation that can be shared with other staff, such as a box of chocolates, are usually acceptable (depending upon the policy of the institution), but almost any other gifts (jewelry, money, clothes) should be declined: "I'm sorry, that's so kind of you, but nurses are not allowed to accept gifts from patients." Declining may relieve the patient of the feeling of obligation.

Sexual Relations

When the boundary between the role of the professional nurse and the vulnerability of the patient is breached, a boundary violation occurs. Because the nurse is in the position of authority, the responsibility to maintain the boundary rests with the nurse; however, the line separating them is a continuum and sometimes not easily defined. It is inappropriate for nurses to engage in **sexual relations** with patients, and if the sexual behavior is coerced or the patient is cognitively impaired, it is **illegal**. However, more common violations with adults, particularly elderly patients, include exposing a patient unnecessarily, using sexually demeaning gestures or language (including off-color jokes), harassment, or inappropriate touching. Touching should be used with care, such as touching a hand or shoulder. Hugging may be misconstrued.

Attention

Nursing is a giving profession, but the nurse must temper giving with recognition of professional boundaries. Patients have many needs. As acts of kindness, nurses (especially those involved in home care) often give certain patients extra attention and may offer to do **favors**, such as cooking or shopping. They may become overly invested in the patients' lives. While this may benefit a patient in the short term, it can establish a relationship of increasing **dependency** and **obligation** that does not resolve the long-term needs of the patient. Making referrals to the appropriate agencies or collaborating with family to find ways to provide services is more effective. Becoming overly invested may be evident by the nurse showing favoritism or spending too much time with the patient while neglecting other duties. On the other end of the spectrum are nurses who are disinterested and fail to provide adequate attention to the patient's detriment. Lack of adequate attention may lead to outright neglect.

Coercion

Power issues are inherent in matters associated with professional boundaries. Physical abuse is both unprofessional and illegal, but behavior can easily border on abusive without the patient being physically injured. Nurses can easily **intimidate** older adults and sick patients into having procedures or treatments they do not want. Regardless of age, patients have the right to choose and the right to refuse treatment. Difficulties arise with cognitive impairment, and in that case, another responsible adult (often the patient's child or spouse) is designated to make decisions, but every effort should be made to gain patient cooperation. Forcing the patient to do something against his or her will borders on abuse and can sometimes degenerate into actual abuse if physical coercion is involved.

Personal Information

When pre-existing personal or business relationships exist, other nurses should be assigned care of the patient whenever possible, but this may be difficult in small communities. However, the nurse should strive to maintain a professional role separate from the personal role and respect professional boundaries. The nurse must respect and maintain the confidentiality of the patient and family members, but the nurse must also be very careful about **disclosing personal information** about him or herself because this establishes a social relationship that interferes with the professional role of the nurse and the boundary between the patient and the nurse. The nurse and patient should never share secrets. When the nurse divulges personal information, he or she may become vulnerable to the patient, a reversal of roles.

Legal Issues

Malpractice and Advanced Directives

Recognizing some of the more common legal and ethical issues can help the nurse to be better prepared when preparing for surgery and providing care during surgery.

- **Malpractice** may arise if the health care provider fails to protect the patient from harm or provides care that is below the standard of treatment. Malpractice can occur any time a health care provider is negligent and/or the patient is harmed. Prior to surgery, the patient must give informed consent for the procedure, and ethical or legal issues can arise if the patient is not competent enough to give consent or if it appears that the risk of surgery was not understood but the surgery was performed anyway.
- If the patient has an **advance directive**, it should be followed and the physician should use it to write actual orders that other healthcare providers can follow. Issues can arise if the patient's wishes contradict what has occurred during surgery or if health care staff do not honor the patient's wishes for medical treatment.

Possible Error-Associated Lawsuit Issues

Possible error-associated law suit issues and measures to avoid them include the following:

- **Misidentification**: Two identifiers should be used and the patient's ID band checked with each intervention. The ID band should be checked against the patient's record to make sure they are the same.
- **Incorrect procedure** (such as on wrong site, wrong patient): The surgical site should be properly marked, the procedure verified by the surgical team during time out, and the site/procedure verbally confirmed by the patient if possible.
- **Foreign body (sponge, instrument) left inside patient**: Complete counts before and after use with two people to verify.
- **Burn injuries**: Fire safety and laser safety guidelines must be followed carefully. Heated irrigation solutions and autoclaved instruments must be cooled adequately before use. Electrosurgical units and laser equipment should be tested for proper functioning and electrical equipment properly grounded.
- **Equipment-associated trauma**: All operative equipment should be maintained, serviced, and tested according to manufacturer's guidelines.
- **Loss of patient's personal property**: Any personal property (hearing aid, glasses, or jewelry) remaining with the patient should be removed, documented, and placed in a sealed protective container.
- **Improper delegation**: All delegation should be appropriate and healthcare providers should avoid exceeding authority or operating outside of their scope of practice.

- **Falls/positioning injuries**: Patients should be monitored carefully and siderails kept in raised position on gurneys. Transfers should be done with adequate personnel and safety straps applied as soon as the transfer is complete. Adequate padding should be placed under pressure points, and the patient should be positioned properly for the procedure, taking into consideration any limitations in mobility.
- **Improper handling or loss of specimens**: Each specimen must be immediately identified, labeled properly, and appropriately fixed and processed.
- **Drug errors**: Protocol for placing drugs on the sterile field must be followed: drugs must be clearly labeled with name and dosage information. Medications should be kept separated to avoid confusion and label and dosage verified with each administration.
- **Asepsis**: All precautions (standard, contact, droplet, and airborne) must be used, and careful attention must be paid to maintaining sterile fields and avoiding breaks in sterility.
- **Patient abandonment**: Failing to attend to a patient under care may result in harm to the patient, so the members of the surgical team must always ensure that the patient is properly monitored and care is properly handed over to others.

Quality Improvement and Safety

Reducing Emergency Situations Using Quality Improvement

The following are some things that can be done to reduce potential emergency situations using the principles of quality improvement:

- All workers must know their **job descriptions and capabilities** and how they are to interact with other members of the healthcare team.
- Decisions to **alter the operating room environment** are first taken to management. Management then decides to make changes or not depending on the feasibility of the request. Changes in the operating room system are not undertaken by the staff members without managerial approval.
- Workers are constantly observing methods, procedures, and processes that may not be safe, cost effective, or time efficient and **bringing those issues to managers** in order to allow quality improvement study and implementation strategies to take place.
- All workers **communicate** with each other, whether professional or technical, clearly, and in a reciprocal manner (not one directional).
- When patient care is transferred from one person to another, **clear communication** is undertaken to prevent a breakdown in the provision of proper care to the patient.

Nurse Involvement in Quality Improvement

The following are ways in which perioperative nurses can be involved in quality improvement in their facility:

- **Identify situations** in the perioperative area that require improvement and might benefit patient outcomes (cost containment, incident reporting, etc.) if changed.
- **Identify potential items** that can be measured to be able to test the problem or to be able to monitor patient outcomes.
- **Collect data** on those measurements, and determine current patient outcomes.
- **Analyze the data** and identify procedures, methods, etc., that can be utilized to potentially make positive changes in patient outcomes, doing research if necessary.
- **Make recommendations for changes** to be implemented to determine effect on patient outcomes.
- **Implement recommendations** after approval from administrative personnel.
- **Collect new data** using the same measurements after the implementation of changes, and determine if the changes improved patient outcomes or not.

Role of Nursing Research in Managing Care

Nursing is based on a desire to provide optimum care to patients. Scientific evidence and rationale are critical components of a nurse's knowledge base. Therefore, it is important that the profession maintains nursing research and learns from outside research projects in order to gain information about processes, procedures, and practices that impact the role of nursing. When research is performed on a particular subject, it is done so in a methodical, scientific manner from which valid and accurate information can be derived. Reading research articles is a way to access information that can be applied to any relevant situation on the job.

MANAGING EMPLOYEE SAFETY IN THE OPERATING SUITE

Employee safety in the operative suite is important to maintain because incapacitated or absent employees impact the level and continuity of patient care. Physical dangers (ergonomic injuries, falls), chemical dangers (anesthesia gasses, chemical spills), and biological dangers (contaminated needle sticks) are all potential areas for injury. Perioperative nurses can manage these potential safety hazards by functioning within their scope of practice, maintaining good body mechanics with patient transfers, keeping a watchful eye out for potential dangers in the environment (slippery floors, spilled fluids, etc.), following institutional policy for disposal of sharps and cleaning instruments, and maintaining proper traffic patterns.

PROPER ERGONOMICS AND BODY MECHANICS TO PREVENT EMERGENCIES

Ergonomics refers to fitting appropriate personnel for the appropriate task. When there is a misappropriation of ergonomics in which the person trying to perform a task is not capable of doing so, an environment for injury is created. This is one of the factors contributing to musculoskeletal injuries in the healthcare setting. Ergonomic factors on the part of the worker can be improved through the use of machinery and devices created to help a worker perform a certain task, but they must be used correctly to ensure a positive outcome. When a worker is performing dynamic (moving) or static (stationary) tasks, utilizing proper body mechanics will also help to prevent injury as it prevents overstretching, twisting, and bending activities that can cause harm to the muscles and bones. AORN guidelines present 6 **ergonomic tools** for preventing injury in perioperative staff:

Tool	Details
Lateral transfer of a patient from a stretcher to an OR bed	A flowchart that considers the patient's ability to transfer without assistance, the starting position of the patient, and the weight of the patient. From this information, the number of caregivers and/or use of a transfer device are recommended.
Positioning and repositioning the supine patient on the OR bed	A flowchart that considers the patient's surgical position and the patient's weight and then recommends the number of caregivers and/or use of assistive technology
Lifting and handling the patient's legs, arms, and head while prepping	A chart that determines what type of lift is appropriate (1- or 2-handed lift or holds of <1 to <3 minutes) based on the body part and the patient's weight
Solutions for prolonged standing	A flowchart that considers the perioperative team member's total duration of standing during the work day and whether lead aprons are worn. It recommends limitations and fatigue-reducing techniques accordingly.
Tissue retraction during surgery	A flowchart that considers whether a self-retraining retractor and/or a manual retractor must be utilized, and then makes recommendations on proper ergonomics for manual retraction to reduce injury risk.
Lifting and carrying supplies and equipment in the perioperative setting	A chart that assigns a lifting index (calculated by dividing the weight of the object by the recommended weight limit for two-handed lifting) to commonly lifted perioperative items and then assigns risk (minimal, potential, or considerable) to each item that corresponds with using assistive technology.

Managing Patient Safety in the Operating Suite

Patient safety is maintained in the operating suite through a variety of methods since there are so many potential areas where a breach in safety can occur. The perioperative nurse must first of all be aware of the potential dangers to the patient to be able to prevent them. There are physical dangers (from falling, noisiness of the environment, potential for thermal injury), chemical dangers (from anesthesia, chemical spill, cleaners), and biological dangers (potential contamination sites throughout the environment) that can potentially cause harm to the patient. Practicing within the nurse's scope of practice, maintaining safety checks provided by the institution, keeping an eye out for potential sources of danger, performing accurate and timely patient assessments, etc., all help the nurse manage care for the patient in the operative suite.

Daily Checks

The nurse in the operating suite is responsible for making daily checks of various kinds including:

- **Materials checks** are made for location, ventilation, sterility, number of items in stock, numbers needed for the day, proper storage location, packaging that is free of contamination, proper functioning, etc.
- **Unit environmental checks** are made for temperature, humidity, ventilation, noise, cleanliness, proper traffic patterns being utilized, etc.
- **Biological testing agent checks** are made for potential contamination of surfaces, products, the ventilation system, etc.
- **Activities and personnel checks** are made for procedures to be performed for the day, numbers of personnel available that day, expected procedure times, etc.
- **Patient procedure checks** are made for proper patient identification, proper procedure being performed, proper positioning, etc.

Routine Auditing

In addition to daily checks, quality assurance requires the routine auditing of the following elements to ensure safety of patients and perioperative staff:

- **Environment of care**: Monthly environmental rounds; regular monitoring of adverse outcomes, equipment malfunctions, and hazards related to the environment of care; safety rounds; evaluation of fire safety and fire drill compliance; monitoring chemical and hazardous waste management
- **Environmental cleaning, disinfection, and sterilization**: Process monitoring (compliance with standards and manufacturer's guidelines), reviewing adverse events related to contamination, live audits of cleaning and sterilization procedures, auditing of cleaning and sterilization logs, monitoring high-level disinfection, and auditing instances of breaks in sterile technique and reporting appropriately
- **Instrumentation**: Processing, monitoring, and disinfection of flexible endoscopes; evaluation of instrument cleaning, both manual and chemical; annual evaluations of worker safety with regards to bloodborne pathogens and chemicals; evaluation of instrument preventative maintenance logs
- **Information management**: Reviewing and evaluating privacy practices for maintaining health records, integrating a clinical documentation improvement program, data analysis and management, routine charting audits

- **Moderate sedation/anesthesia**: Audits of adverse events and root-cause analysis as needed, counting of anesthesia medications and reviews of expiration dates, implementation and evaluation of outcome measures (complications, need for reversal, need for deeper sedation, transfers to higher level of care, cases of dissatisfaction)
- **Patient safety**: Auditing of adverse events related to patient positioning, auditing for compliance to patient positioning procedures/protocols, auditing of occurrences of retained surgical instruments (RSIs) and evaluation of RSI-prevention procedures, evaluating near-miss occurrences and implementation of changes to prevent future occurrences, evaluating compliance with surgical smoke evacuation procedures and protocols; auditing implementation and documentation of VTE prevention measures
- **Perioperative staff safety**: Annual or biannual audits of adverse events relating to patient and equipment moving, audits of healthcare worker complications related to hazardous materials and bloodborne pathogens, evaluation of perioperative staff satisfaction

Risk Management in the Operating Room

Risk management is an organized and formal method of decreasing liability, financial loss, and risk or harm to patients, staff, or others by doing an assessment of risk and introducing risk management strategies. Much of risk management has been driven by the insurance industry in order to minimize costs, but quality management utilizes risk management as a method to ensure quality healthcare and process improvement. An organization's risk management program usually comprises a manager and staff, but all surgical team members must participate in risk management procedures:

- **Risk identification** begins with an assessment of processes to identify and prioritize those that require further study to determine risk exposure.
- **Risk analysis** requires a careful documenting of process, utilizing flow charts, with each step in the process assessed for potential risks. This may utilize root cause analysis methods.
- **Risk prevention** involves instituting corrective or preventive processes. Responsible individual or teams are identified and trained.
- **Assessment/evaluation** of corrective/preventive processes is ongoing to determine if they are effective or require modification.

CNOR Practice Test #1

Want to take this practice test in an online interactive format?
Check out the bonus page, which includes interactive practice questions and much more: **mometrix.com/bonus948/cnor**

1. If an operating room is frequently flooded (standing fluids, splashing) during procedures with a patient present, the room should be designated as a:

a. contaminated room
b. wet location
c. flood zone
d. damp space

2. Which type of complementary care can be used for patients without the healthcare professional having formal training, education, or licensure?

a. Visualization
b. Massage
c. Biofield interventions
d. Hypnosis

3. Which of the following is a systemic contraindication to the use of a pneumatic tourniquet?

a. Hyperthyroidism
b. Parkinson's disease
c. Sickle cell disease
d. Diabetes mellitus

4. A patient has been admitted to the postanesthesia care unit (PACU) after surgery and has a persistent Aldrete score of 3 points less than the baseline. What does this indicate about the patient's need for monitoring?

a. Maintain the patient on one-to-one nursing, and check vital signs every 5 minutes.
b. Monitor frequently and check vital signs every 15 minutes.
c. Monitor and check vital signs every 15–30 minutes.
d. The patient is ready for discharge.

5. When transferring a patient directly from the operating room to the intensive care unit (ICU), the nurse should

a. notify the ICU staff when in transit to the ICU.
b. notify the ICU staff before the surgical procedure is completed.
c. notify the ICU staff before leaving the operating room.
d. notify the ICU staff when the incision is closed.

6. If a patient experiences perioperative hypothermia, for what adverse effects should that patient be monitored?

a. Increased blood clotting.
b. Decreased oxygen consumption.
c. Increased vasodilation.
d. Decreased heart rate and BP.

7. A patient with tuberculosis is hospitalized in an airborne infection isolation room (AIIR) but needs surgery. When transporting the patient to the surgical area, the patient should initially be taken to:

a. the operating room
b. a portable plastic-enclosed AIIR
c. a screened-off preoperative area
d. a private room near the operating room

8. On each side of an operating table or procedure chair, the sterile field clear area is:

a. 1 foot
b. 2 feet
c. 3 feet
d. 4 feet

9. When handling hazardous medications, such as chemotherapeutic agents, gloves must be changed every:

a. 15 minutes
b. 30 minutes
c. 45 minutes
d. 60 minutes

10. If a patient has an implantable electronic device (IED), the surgical device that poses the most risk to the patient is:

a. electrocautery
b. bipolar forceps
c. ultrasonic technology
d. monopolar electrosurgery

11. Unless otherwise specified, the beyond-use date of a multidose vial after first use is:

a. 7 days
b. 14 days
c. 21 days
d. 28 days

12. Two days postoperatively, a patient exhibits tachycardia, tachypnea, apprehension, dyspnea, chest pain, slight hemoptysis, and elevated temperature. Although the patient's chest x-ray appears normal, arterial blood gases indicate decreased PaO_2, decreased $PaCO_2$, and increased pH. The most likely cause is

a. atelectasis.
b. pulmonary embolism.
c. pleural effusion.
d. pneumothorax.

13. A key element in product evaluation and selection is:

a. supplier analysis
b. delivery time analysis
c. inventory analysis
d. financial impact analysis

14. The circulating nurse brings a surgical pack upon which the date of sterilization is smudged and unreadable, although the circulating nurse reports that it was with the surgical packs that were sterilized the day before. How should the scrub nurse respond?

a. Consider the pack sterile and use it accordingly.
b. Ask the circulating nurse to verify the correct sterilization date.
c. Use it if the chemical indicators show that the pack was sterilized.
d. Reject the surgical pack.

15. If a patient is to receive a benzodiazepine as part of moderate sedation/analgesia, what reversal agent must be readily available?

a. Naloxone
b. Sugammadex
c. Neostigmine
d. Flumazenil

16. What is generally the maximum duration of time that a pneumatic tourniquet should stay inflated on a lower extremity (adult)?

a. 1 hour
b. 2 hours
c. 2.5 hours
d. 3 hours

17. If using the "3-bucket" venous thromboembolism (VTE) risk assessment model, what prophylaxis is recommended for fully ambulatory patients undergoing minor surgical procedures or observation patients whose hospital stay is expected to be shorter than 48 hours?

a. No pharmacologic prophylaxis
b. Unfractionated heparin
c. Low-molecular-weight heparin
d. Intermittent pneumatic compression device

Refer to the following for questions 18 - 20:

An 84-year-old female patient with an ASA score of 4 and many comorbidities is scheduled for a new pacemaker placement. She is complaining of being cold and is beginning to shiver.

18. It is important for the perioperative nurse caring for this patient to be aware that shivering may lead to which of the following?

a. Cardiac ischemia.
b. Respiratory depression.
c. Hemorrhage.
d. Stroke.

19. Which is the most effective method to deal with this patient's hypothermia in the OR suite?

a. Warmed IV fluids.
b. A forced-air warming blanket.
c. It is not necessary to warm the patient because she will be asleep soon.
d. Regular blankets that have not been warmed.

20. Once the pacemaker procedure is finished, this patient is moved to the PACU area to recover from her anesthesia. The PACU RN should anticipate which of the following routine orders for this patient?

a. Ultrasound of pedal pulses.
b. Blood transfusion.
c. Chest X ray.
d. Additional intravenous line placements.

21. A perioperative team prepares the wrong site for surgery, resulting in a delay while the patient is prepped correctly. In a just culture, the initial response should be to:

a. punish the nurse
b. caution other team members
c. provide education to team members
d. investigate the root cause

22. Perioperative personnel who may experience occupational radiation exposure must receive education regarding radiation safety and verify competency:

a. upon hiring
b. upon hiring and monthly
c. upon hiring and annually
d. upon hiring and biannually

23. When conducting leak testing for a flexible endoscope and the endoscope is pressurized with an automatic or manual pressure tester, the pressure should be maintained for a minimum of:

a. 10 seconds
b. 30 seconds
c. 45 seconds
d. 60 seconds

24. A patient is scheduled for an outpatient procedure, but during the preoperative assessment, the nurse notes what appears to be needle tracks on both arms although the patient denies any recent drug use. What is the appropriate response?

a. Believe the patient
b. Obtain a urine specimen for testing
c. Cancel the procedure
d. Notify the surgeon and anesthesiologist of the observation

25. Unless otherwise mandated by state law, under federal regulations, verbal orders must be authenticated by a responsible physician within:

a. 12 hours
b. 24 hours
c. 36 hours
d. 48 hours

26. The fuel source that is most often associated with surgical fires is:

a. tissue
b. surgical drapes
c. hair
d. GI tract gases

27. A patient is scheduled for the Mohs procedure after the biopsy of the dermatologic lesion has healed. To ensure that the correct site is excised, the safest method is to rely on

a. the surgeon's notes
b. the patient's recollection
c. a photo of the lesion and the surrounding site
d. evidence of scarring from the biopsy site

28. When assessing a patient's airway, if only the soft palate and base of the uvula are visible, this is classified as ________ according to the modified Mallampati classification system.

a. class I
b. class II
c. class III
d. class IV

29. Which of the following statements is NOT true regarding pulse oximetry?

a. Readings under 90% indicate significant hypoxemia.
b. Bright lights can interfere with the pulse oximeter's accuracy.
c. Methylene blue and other intravenous dyes diminish the pulse oximeter's accuracy.
d. Pulse oximetry measures oxygenation and ventilation.

30. Which herbal medication may increase the risk of postoperative bleeding?

a. Fenugreek
b. Echinacea
c. Schisandra
d. Gingko biloba

31. The label for a specimen container must include two patient identifiers, the specimen name, and the:

a. surgeon's name
b. scrub person's name
c. specimen site
d. specimen size

32. Approximately 1.5 hours after initiation of transfusion with packed red blood cells (PRBCs), a patient complains of mild chills, headache, and muscle ache; however, the patient's vital signs are stable except for a 1.2 °C (2.16 °F) increase in temperature. The type of transfusion reaction this likely indicates is

a. a febrile nonhemolytic reaction.
b. anaphylaxis.
c. transfusion-associated graft-versus-host disease.
d. an acute hemolytic reaction.

33. Precleaning processes for flexible endoscopes should be carried out in the:

a. procedure room
b. endoscopy processing room
c. general instrument processing room
d. environmental cleaning supply room

34. Which one of the following disinfectants is appropriate to use for reprocessing flexible endoscopes?

a. Hypochlorites
b. Phenolics
c. Chlorhexidine gluconate
d. 2%–2.4% Glutaraldehyde

35. If using enzymes to target soil, which type of enzyme is effective for organic material?

a. Proteases
b. Amylases
c. Lipases
d. Cellulases

36. During a cardiac arrest, the cardiac monitor shows pulseless electrical activity. What is the emergent treatment?

a. Defibrillation.
b. Cardiopulmonary resuscitation (CPR) only.
c. Amiodarone.
d. CPR and epinephrine.

37. When assessing a patient for ineffective peripheral tissue perfusion, an ankle-brachial index value of ________ is consistent with moderate peripheral arterial disease.

a. >1.4
b. 0.9–0.99
c. 0.5–0.79
d. <0.5

38. Ideally, discharge planning for a hospitalized surgical patient should begin

a. following the surgical procedure.
b. when the patient is stable enough for discharge.
c. upon admission for surgery.
d. before admission for surgery.

39. The most effective complementary care intervention to reduce stress in preoperative pediatric patients is likely;

a. humor
b. music
c. aromatherapy
d. hypnosis

40. If using the situation, background, assessment, and recommendations (SBAR) tool for handoff of a patient to the PACU, the presence or absence of surgical complications would be discussed under the category of:

a. situation (S)
b. background (B)
c. assessment (A)
d. recommendations (I)

41. When assessing a patient for risk for difficulty with mask ventilation, which of the following increases risk?

a. Age <55
b. Long neck
c. Increased hyomental distance
d. Decreased hyomental distance

42. Which of the following surgical energy devices generates the smallest aerodynamic particle size?

a. Electrocautery
b. Laser tissue ablation
c. Ultrasonic scalpel
d. Laser tissue ablation and ultrasonic scalpel

43. A cranial bone flap has been removed and cleaned for preservation. If storage is in plastic bags, how many bags should be used to encase the specimen before it is moved from the sterile field?

a. 1
b. 2
c. 3
d. 4

44. The recommended treatment for LAST is:

a. 20% lipid emulsion
b. dexamethasone
c. phentolamine
d. blood transfusion

45. If many mistakes have occurred during the cleaning and packaging of instruments, what is the best management approach to resolving the problem?

a. Reprimand those making the mistakes.
b. Supervise the process directly.
c. Arrange for retraining for those involved.
d. Assign the task to different individuals.

46. If each surgical site infection costs $30,000 and the institution averages 10 surgical site infections a year, the product selection with the best cost-benefit is

a. a product that costs $80,000 year and reduces infections by 5 (50%).
b. a product that costs $40,000 a year and reduces infections by 2 (20%).
c. a product that costs $100,000 a year and reduces infections by 8 (80%).
d. a product that costs $20,000 and reduces infections by 1 (10%).

47. When transporting a patient who is on droplet precautions, who must wear a mask?

a. The patient only
b. The patient and the transporter
c. The transporter only
d. Neither the patient nor the transporter

48. In a single endoscopy processing room, clean areas and contaminated areas must be separated by at least:

a. 3 feet
b. 4 feet
c. 5 feet
d. 6 feet

49. According to the Health Information Management Association, the register of surgical procedures should be maintained:

a. for 5 years
b. for 10 years
c. for 15 years
d. indefinitely

50. A parent or family member may be allowed into the OR

a. during induction of a child (usually younger than 12) or mentally disabled adult.
b. upon request and permission of patient.
c. never.
d. at the physician's discretion.

51. When do most errors occur with specimen management?

a. All phases equally
b. The preanalytical phase
c. The analytical phase
d. The postanalytical phase

52. Flexible endoscopes should be stored in a cabinet with:

a. all valves open and removable parts detached
b. all valves open and removable parts attached
c. all valves closed and removable parts detached
d. all valves closed and removable parts attached

53. If there is a count discrepancy at the end of a procedure, which member(s) of the perioperative team should take immediate action?

a. All team members
b. Surgeon
c. Scrub nurse
d. Circulating nurse

54. If the bone cement methyl methacrylate (MMA) is spilled during preparation, the correct response is to ventilate the area and:

a. flood the MMA with water
b. wipe up the MMA with gauze pads
c. cover the MMA with an activated charcoal absorbent
d. spray the MMA with a fire extinguisher

55. If an audit shows that the length of the notes in the patients' EHR has increased markedly but the time spent documenting has decreased, this is probably an indication of

a. conscientious documentation.
b. more complex patient issues.
c. staff confusion regarding required documentation.
d. overuse of copy and paste.

56. The scrub nurse notes that a biomedical engineer who was called into the operating room for an equipment malfunction has stepped into the sterile field. The scrub nurse should

a. tell the engineer to step away.
b. stop the surgical procedure.
c. immediately notify the team.
d. wait for guidance from the team.

57. The use of standardized preprinted order sets:

a. increases the risk of errors
b. is prohibited by CMS regulations
c. increases the risk of civil liability
d. reduces errors and improves documentation

58. Outcomes evaluation can include all of the following EXCEPT

a. negotiating with staff.
b. monitoring treatment.
c. evaluating results.
d. replacing treatment.

59. When recommending the purchase of specific equipment, what information must the nurse disclose to avoid the appearance of commercial bias?

a. Survey results showing staff preference for the equipment.
b. Survey results showing staff preference for other equipment.
c. Personal history using the equipment in employment.
d. Having a close family member serving as a sales representative for the equipment.

60. If a patient with an active case of COVID-19 requires surgery, the surgery should be scheduled:

a. first thing in the morning
b. at any convenient time
c. midday when some staff members are on break
d. at the end of the day

61. If a patient needs hair removal for a surgical procedure, this should be done:

a. the day before in the patient's room or as an outpatient
b. within 4 hours of the surgery in the patient's room
c. in a room near the operating room immediately before surgery
d. in the operating room immediately before surgery

62. Unused materials in surgical packages used during surgery for a patient cannot be

a. donated for use in developing countries.
b. resterilized for use on other patients.
c. disposed of properly.
d. recycled.

63. After an employee has received the third hepatitis B vaccination in the series of three, when should serologic testing be carried out to determine if antibody levels are sufficient?

a. In 1–2 weeks
b. In 1–2 months
c. In 6 months
d. In 12 months

64. During laser procedures, reflective instruments should be:

a. used with caution
b. replaced with nonreflective instruments
c. used as per routine surgery
d. coated with a water-soluble lubricant

65. All of the following are elements of the 5 rights of medication administration EXCEPT

a. right reason.
b. right patient.
c. right drug.
d. right dose.

66. The wrappers used for packaging instruments for sterilization should be held at room temperature for a minimum of __________ hour(s) prior to sterilization.

a. 1
b. 2
c. 2.5
d. 3

67. In the perioperative setting, the "sterile cockpit" rule is applied:

a. at all times
b. during important tasks
c. during transport of patients
d. during scrubbing procedures

68. Which type of chemical indicator demonstrates only that a package has been exposed to the sterilization process?

a. Type 1
b. Type 2
c. Type 3
d. Type 4

69. If using binaural beats with a postoperative patient to reduce anxiety, the primary concern is:

a. hallucinations
b. hearing damage
c. delirium
d. paranoia

70. The leadership style associated with following organizational rules exactly and expecting others to do so is

a. autocratic.
b. consultative.
c. bureaucratic.
d. democratic.

71. The ethical principle that relates to the distribution of limited resources of health care benefits to the members of society is

a. autonomy.
b. justice.
c. beneficence.
d. nonmaleficence.

72. Which of the following is a violation of patient's confidentiality?

a. Password-protected computerized charting.
b. Computer screen for electronic charting facing the hallway.
c. Providing report to a minor's parents.
d. Describing patient's behavior to the patient's attending physician.

73. According to advanced cardiovascular life support guidelines, if an adult patient goes into cardiac arrest, the rate of compressions to ventilations is

a. 4:1.
b. 15:2.
c. 30:2.
d. 60:4.

74. If using multimodal complementary care to control a patient's postoperative nausea and vomiting, in addition to medication, the patient may be offered:

a. music therapy
b. aromatherapy (essential oils)
c. distraction
d. transcutaneous electrical acupoint stimulation

75. The first step in removing disposable gown and gloves following a surgical procedure is to:

a. undo the fastener at the neck
b. remove gloves
c. grasp the front of the gown and pull
d. grasp the neck of the gown and pull

76. An example of a group 1 endoscope is a:

a. bronchoscope
b. colonoscope
c. enteroscope
d. cystoscope

77. Which of the following applies to terminal clearing of an operating room?

a. The floor may be sprayed with disinfectant before mopping
b. The floor is cleaned with dry cleaning preparations only
c. The floor may be mopped or wet vacuumed
d. The floor around the equipment is mopped

78. The type of water that should be used in the final rinse when reprocessing flexible endoscopes is:

a. deionized water
b. critical water
c. utility water
d. chlorinated water

79. A patient should have a nursing diagnosis of risk for pressure ulcer if the patient's Braden Scale score is less than

a. 6.
b. 12.
c. 18.
d. 22.

80. The maximum volume of alcohol-based rub in a dispenser in a room, corridor, or area open to corridors is:

a. 500 mL
b. 750 mL
c. 1,000 mL
d. 1,200 mL

81. During the skin assessment of a patient scheduled for right knee surgery, a large pustule is found on the right posterior calf. The nurse should immediately

a. notify the surgeon.
b. describe the pustule in the patient's EHR.
c. cover the pustule with a bandage.
d. cancel the operative procedure.

82. When cleaning with disinfectant, the appropriate method is to clean:

a. from top to bottom
b. from bottom to top
c. from dirty to clean
d. in a counterclockwise direction only

83. When examining the patient's mouth as part of the assessment for moderate sedation, only the upper portion of the uvula and the soft palate are visible. This corresponds to the Mallampati classification of:

a. class I
b. class II
c. class III
d. class IV

84. The anesthesia provider can leave the patient in the postanesthesia care unit (PACU) when

a. the patient is in the PACU and monitoring has begun.
b. the oral transfer report is completed.
c. the PACU nurse accepts responsibility for the patient.
d. the documentation is complete.

85. After teaching a patient wound care, the best technique to ensure the patient understands is

a. ask the patient to give a return demonstration.
b. give the patient a brief quiz.
c. ask the patient to explain the procedure.
d. provide written directions for the patient to refer to.

86. When is a post-transplant patient at the most risk for infection?

a. In the first three days after surgery.
b. The first two weeks after the transplant.
c. The first year after the transplant.
d. One to six months post-transplant.

87. In the OR, a health care industry representative (HCIR) should not

a. enter the patient's sterile field.
b. observe patient procedures.
c. provide technical support for product use.
d. perform calibrations of equipment.

88. Which of the following may make a patient susceptible to iodism from iodine and iodophor-based antiseptics?

a. Diabetes mellitus
b. Burns
c. Cardiovascular disorders
d. Fractures

89. Which of the following is characteristic of targeted screening and decolonization for *Staphylococcus aureus*?

a. Simple medication prescription.
b. All carriers are identified.
c. Horizontal approach to treatment.
d. All patients are screened.

90. According to AORN guidelines, when lasers are not in use, they should be disabled by

a. placing them in standby mode.
b. unplugging the device from the power outlet.
c. removing the key and placing it in a secure location.
d. using beam shutters.

91. If receiving verbal orders from a physician, the nurse must:

a. double-check the dosages
b. ask the physician to repeat the orders
c. verify the orders with a second nurse
d. confirm the orders through readback

92. Under HIPAA guidelines, which of the following information can be communicated to a friend who is visiting a postoperative patient?

a. A report of general condition.
b. A detailed report of surgery.
c. Prognosis.
d. No information.

93. The area within which direct, reflected, or scattered radiation associated with laser use exceeds the maximum permissible exposure level is the:

a. nominal hazard zone
b. laser safety zone
c. laser-treatment controlled area
d. restricted zone

94. What are the acceptable upper limits of the temperature range for a decontamination room used in reprocessing instruments?

a. 66 °F to 70 °F (19 °C to 21 °C)
b. 70 °F to 74 °F (21 °C to 23.3 °C)
c. 74 °F to 76 °F (23.3 °C to 24.4 °C)
d. 72 °F to 78 °F (22 °C to 26 °C)

95. According to the American Society of Heating, Refrigerating and Air-Conditioning Engineers standards, what is the minimum number of total air exchanges per hour that should be used for operating rooms?

a. 10
b. 12
c. 16
d. 20

96. If surgical drapes become ignited during a surgical procedure, the immediate response should be to remove the drapes and:

a. extinguish the fire with water or NS
b. get a fire extinguisher to extinguish the fire
c. apply a fire blanket
d. call for help

97. According to the guidelines for the World Health Organization's Surgical Safety Checklist, every item on the checklist should be

a. optional.
b. actionable.
c. advisory.
d. static.

98. The five Hs that represent reversible causes of cardiac arrest are (1) hypovolemia, (2) hypoxia, (3) hydrogen ion (acidosis), (4) hypo-/hyperkalemia, and (5)

a. hemorrhage.
b. hypothermia.
c. hemolysis.
d. hyperthermia.

99. If a large specimen (such as an amputated leg) does not fit into a container, it can be transported by:

a. placing it inside of two sealed red hazard bags
b. placing it inside of one clear plastic bag
c. leaving it open on a cart and covered with a towel
d. leaving it open on a cart and covered with plastic

100. The most common unintentionally retained surgical items are:

a. surgical sponges
b. needles
c. guidewires
d. rectal tube caps

101. The period of time in which an activated high-level disinfectant can be used is the:

a. activation date
b. shelf-life date
c. use life
d. reuse-life date

102. When conflict arises among OR team members, the first step in conflict resolution is

a. encourage cooperation and compromise.
b. allow both sides to present their ideas.
c. utilize humor and empathy.
d. evaluate the need for formal resolution process.

103. During surgery that involves the use of a monopolar electrosurgical unit, monitoring electrodes should be placed:

a. as far from the operative site as possible
b. as near to the operative site as possible
c. parallel to the operative site
d. above the operative site

104. Immediately after receiving a local anesthetic injection, the patient becomes agitated and confused, exhibits dysarthria, and complains of numbness about the mouth and a metallic taste, as well as ringing in the ears. These symptoms are consistent with:

a. anaphylaxis
b. panic attack
c. local anesthetic systemic toxicity (LAST)
d. methemoglobinemia

105. When transporting a flexible endoscope from the procedure room to the processing room, the parts should be:

a. submerged in cleaning solution
b. dry
c. carried in an open container
d. wet or damp

106. For all chemicals such as high-level disinfectants used in a facility, the organization must create a hazard communication program. The three components that must be included are the (1) safety data sheets (SDSs), (2) specific hazards of each chemical, and (3):

a. neutralizing agents
b. antidotes
c. storage requirements
d. labeling requirements

107. The most important factor in a patient safety culture is:

a. fostering learning
b. reporting safety statistics
c. rewarding compliance
d. communicating concerns

108. Twelve hours after a total hip arthroplasty because of a fractured head of the right femur, the patient develops dyspnea with hypoxemia, tachycardia, petechial rash on the upper body, restlessness, and confusion. The nurse should suspect

a. fat embolism syndrome.
b. pulmonary embolism.
c. infection.
d. allergic reaction.

109. A patient scheduled for surgery has been assessed by the anesthesiologist and classified under the American Society of Anesthesiologists (ASA) Physical Status Classification as ASA III. What does this indicate about the patient's general condition?

a. The patient has mild systemic disease.
b. The patient is moribund.
c. The patient has severe systemic disease.
d. The patient is normal and healthy.

110. Following a procedure carried out with moderate sedation, the patient is usually ready to transfer from the PACU when the Aldrete score is:

a. 10–12
b. 8–10
c. 6–8
d. 4–6

111. According to AORN guidelines regarding hair removal at a surgical site, the hair should generally

a. be left in place.
b. be removed only along the incision line.
c. be removed in the operating room.
d. be removed with a razor.

112. Reiki reduces stress and induces relaxation through:

a. deep massage
b. breathing exercises
c. gentle touch
d. visualization

113. IV solution containers that have been spiked must be administered within:

a. 30 minutes
b. 60 minutes
c. 90 minutes
d. 2 hours

114. Which one of the following is the appropriate marking for a surgical site?

a. A line of dots.
b. A circle.
c. An X.
d. An arrow.

115. Which of the following is an essential external distraction in the operating room?

a. Nonsurgical related conversation
b. Music
c. Interruptions unrelated to the surgical procedure
d. Equipment noise

116. A patient requires nasogastric tube insertion because of paralytic ileus. After insertion, the nurse aspirates and finds that the aspirant has a pH of 6. What does this likely indicate?

a. Placement into the small intestine.
b. Placement into the stomach.
c. Placement into a bronchial tree or lung.
d. Placement into the esophagus.

117. Which of the following is sufficient for sterilization?

a. Quaternary ammonium compounds
b. 7.35% Hydrogen peroxide with 0.23% peracetic acid
c. Phenolics
d. ≥2.4% glutaraldehyde solution

118. Following surgery on a patient with a Methicillin-resistant *Staphylococcus aureus* infection, the operating room should:

a. be closed to further surgeries
b. undergo standard cleaning
c. undergo terminal cleaning
d. undergo enhanced cleaning

119. When packaging sterile instrument sets, the total weight of the sterile packaging system and contents should not exceed:

a. 15 pounds
b. 20 pounds
c. 25 pounds
d. 30 pounds

120. Which of the following laws regulates the right to privacy for operative patients?

a. Americans with Disabilities Act (ADA).
b. Patient Self-Determination Act (PSDA).
c. Patient Protection and Affordable Care Act (PPACA).
d. Health Insurance Portability and Accountability Act (HIPAA).

121. To save time during turnover cleaning between patients in the operating room, staff members have been placing all contaminated, discarded, and disposable items into the hazardous waste bags for disposal. Is this an efficient practice?

a. No, because the bags are more likely to leak or break.
b. No, because it is costly, and many of the items are recyclable.
c. Yes, because it saves time in turnover.
d. Yes, because it saves money to use one type of disposal bag.

122. Which of the following is NOT a function of the stomach?

a. Acceptance and storage of ingested substances.
b. Digestion through gastric lipase, pepsinogen, and hydrochloric acid.
c. Absorption of essential nutrients with 95% efficiency.
d. Regulate the rate of delivery of digested food to the small intestine.

123. The Perioperative Nursing Data Set (PNDS) begins with:

a. outcomes
b. nursing diagnoses
c. interventions
d. measures

124. When assessing the patient's physiological response and depth of sedation, the nurse notes that the patient has adequate ventilation and cardiovascular function without intervention and has a purposeful response to verbal or tactile stimulation. This is consistent with:

a. minimal sedation
b. moderate sedation
c. deep sedation
d. general anesthesia

125. A patient with an Aldrete score of 7 in the PACU will generally be

a. transferred out of the PACU to the surgical unit.
b. transferred out of the PACU into the ICU.
c. returned to the OR.
d. retained in the PACU until condition improves.

126. If a patient's surgery is delayed because the bariatric surgical bed that the patient needs is not ready yet, the most appropriate way to communicate this information to the patient is:

a. "We have only one surgical bed for obese patients, and it's still in use."
b. "The operating room is not ready for you yet."
c. "You are too big for standard operating beds, so we have to wait until the large bed is available."
d. "We are waiting for the appropriate bed for your procedure."

127. A patient is scheduled for laser perineal surgery. What precaution is necessary to decrease risk of fire?

a. Coat the entire perineal area with a water-soluble lubricant
b. Have moistened radiopaque sponges readily available
c. Use moistened radiopaque sponges as rectal packing
d. Increase the relative humidity of the room

128. The relative humidity in operating rooms should be maintained between:

a. 10% and 30%
b. 20% and 40%
c. 20% and 60%
d. 40% and 70%

129. If a patient has a cochlear implant, use of monopolar electrosurgery should be limited to below the:

a. clavicles
b. umbilicus
c. thyroid notch
d. xiphoid process

130. When removing chemical indicator tape from a sterilized pack with a reusable wrapping, the correct procedure is to

a. tear the tape and remove it completely.
b. remove the intact tape completely.
c. tear the tape and leave it on the wrap.
d. loosen the tape from one end, leaving it attached at the other end.

131. In perioperative care, methods to prevent or treat hypothermia should be used for:

a. all patients
b. patients at risk
c. patients with a low baseline temperature
d. patients undergoing prolonged procedures

132. The radiation that emanates from the x-ray equipment/housing is referred to as:

a. primary radiation
b. scatter radiation
c. incidental radiation
d. leakage radiation

133. If a patient experiences symptomatic bradycardia with a pulse rate varying from 30 to 42 beats per minute, the patient is hypotensive, dyspneic, slightly confused, and complains of chest discomfort, the initial emergent treatment is typically

a. epinephrine.
b. amiodarone.
c. atropine.
d. dopamine.

134. When labeling an autograft package, if the specimen has not been tested for infectious diseases, the labeling should state:

a. "Test for infectious substances before use."
b. "Beware, hazardous material."
c. "Possible contagions in specimen."
d. "Not evaluated for infectious substances."

135. A patient who identifies as a Jehovah's Witness has severe internal bleeding after a traumatic injury, but the patient refuses transfusions of donated blood. What is likely the best solution?

a. Cell salvage.
b. IV colloids.
c. Tranexamic acid.
d. IV crystalloids.

136. According to the Nuclear Regulatory Commission and the Code of Federal Regulations Standards for Protection Against Radiation, the total effective dose equivalent for the whole body for radiation workers is:

a. 0.1 rem
b. 0.5 rem
c. 5 rem
d. 50 rem

137. When an injury to a patient occurs during surgery because of procedure violation, under the Reason Model for determining culpability, the first step is to

a. determine whether substance abuse is involved.
b. do a substitution test.
c. establish intent.
d. examine mitigating circumstances.

138. If a near-miss situation regarding patient safety has occurred and the perioperative team is conducting a brief safety huddle, an appropriate first question is:

a. "Who is responsible for this safety issue?"
b. "What happened to threaten patient safety?"
c. "Why did this safety problem happen?"
d. "What should have happened to prevent this near miss?"

139. Before access to the OR, a health care industry representative (HCIR) must have training/certification in all of the following EXCEPT

a. bloodborne pathogens.
b. CPR.
c. OR protocol.
d. HIPAA.

140. When eschar builds up on the nonstick-coated tip of an electrosurgical unit, it should be cleaned with a(n):

a. sterile sponge moistened with sterile water
b. antiseptic wipe
c. abrasive electrode cleaning pad
d. squeeze bottle with sterile water

141. If a nurse keeps notes about patients on a personal smartphone and then transcribes the information onto patients' EHRs when the unit is less busy, this is

a. a time-saving method.
b. an inefficient method.
c. a HIPAA violation
d. an act of malpractice.

142. Following implantation of a Watchman device, a patient is at risk for reduced cardiac output. The patient's cardiac monitoring shows the following:

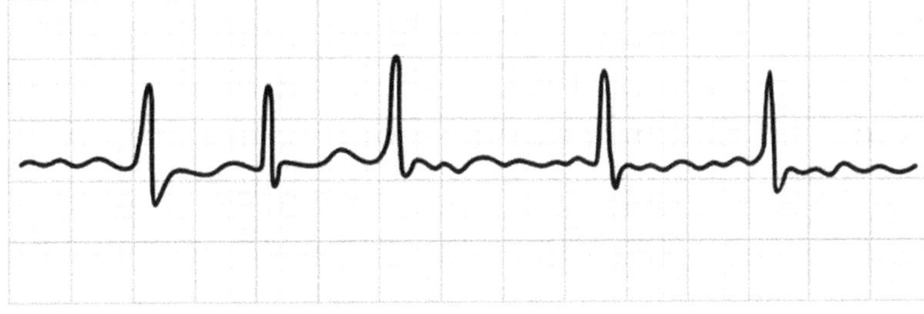

What dysrhythmia does this represent?

a. Atrial tachycardia with variable block.
b. Wandering atrial pacemaker.
c. Atrial flutter.
d. Atrial fibrillation.

143. Which peripheral temperature measurement site has proven inaccurate in measuring the core temperature of perioperative patients?

a. Oral with a thermometer
b. Temporal artery with thermometer
c. Bladder catheter with thermometer
d. Tympanic membrane with infrared sensor

144. If, during an operative procedure, a specimen containing a radioactive seed is excised, the location of the seed should be verified by a:

a. handheld radiation detection device
b. surgeon's report and a radiograph
c. handheld radiation detection device and a radiograph
d. surgeon's report and a handheld radiation detection device

145. If reusable surgical attire is contaminated with blood or other body fluids, it must be:

a. rinsed and then bagged
b. sorted and then bagged
c. bagged
d. pretreated with disinfectant and then bagged

146. Critical water should have a pH in the range of:

a. 4–5
b. 5–7
c. 6–9
d. 9–10

147. Approximately 90 minutes after exposure to local anesthesia, a patient develops headache, tachypnea, tachycardia, lightheadedness, decreasing oxygen saturation, and cyanosis. What medication should the nurse anticipate that the physician will order?

a. Methylene blue
b. Epinephrine
c. Phentolamine
d. Dexamethasone

148. When using a brush in the decontamination area to clean soiled surgical instruments, it is necessary to brush:

a. above the water
b. under cool water
c. under running water
d. under hot water

149. With a hysteroscopy, the use of Dextran as an irrigating or distension media should be limited to a volume that does not exceed:

a. 200 mL
b. 500 mL
c. 700 mL
d. 1,000 mL

150. When disposing of bodily waste with low levels of radioactivity, the appropriate method is to:

a. dilute and disperse
b. delay and decay
c. concentrate and contain
d. incinerate

151. When reviewing a patient's history, which finding should alert the nurse to a risk of the development of postoperative nausea and vomiting?

a. Male gender
b. History of migraines
c. History of smoking
d. History of constipation

152. What is the primary purpose of checking the load control label on sterile packs?

a. To ensure that the pack is sterile.
b. To determine who was responsible for sterilization.
c. To track problems in sterilization or packaging.
d. To check the sterilization and expiration dates.

153. If using the Richmond Agitation-Sedation Scale (RASS) to assess a patient's level of sedation and readiness for transfer, what score indicates that the patient is alert and calm?

a. 0.
b. +4.
c. +1.
d. –2.

154. A community resource that can provide nursing and personal care in the home is

a. public health department.
b. Visiting Nurse Association.
c. Social Services.
d. Senior Citizens' organization.

155. Which of the following anatomical structures pose the greatest risk of fire?

a. Heart and coronary arteries
b. Uterus and ovaries
c. Bowels and trachea
d. Kidneys and bladder

156. If a patient is to have open reduction and internal fixation surgery of a fracture of the femoral shaft, skin prep should extend from:

a. below the umbilicus to the foot
b. the femoral region to the foot
c. the umbilicus to below the knee
d. the femoral area to below the knee

157. Screening is an especially important aspect of which type of perioperative decolonization?

a. Horizontal
b. Vertical
c. Blended
d. Standard

158. If the surgeon has employed a scribe to assist with documentation, the scribe's responsibilities include

a. documenting information from all members of the surgical team.
b. communicating orders for patient care.
c. recording independent notes.
d. documenting the dictated patient information.

159. A parent is to accompany a small child into the operating room and remain during induction. What is the primary role of the operating room nurse?

a. Educate the parent about the operating room, the induction process, and the parent's role.
b. Talk though the induction process while it is occurring.
c. Monitor the parent's well-being.
d. Provide emotional support for the parent.

160. The cost containment method that uses average cost of an event and the cost of intervention to demonstrate savings is

a. cost-utility analysis.
b. efficacy study.
c. cost-effective analysis.
d. cost-benefit analysis.

161. The five Ps handoff procedure includes

a. patient, plan, purpose, problems, and precautions.
b. patient, performance, pathology, plan, and patterns.
c. person, parameters, pathology, problems, and progression.
d. patient, pathology, plan, problems, and precautions.

162. Which of the following operating room temperatures most likely will need to be corrected to meet recommendations prior to operating room use?

a. 68 °F (20 °C)
b. 70 °F (21.1 °C)
c. 66 °F (18.9 °C)
d. 75 °F (24 °C)

163. Which type of surgical glove provides the best protection for glove punctures?

a. Natural rubber latex
b. Nitrile
c. Thermoplastic elastomer
d. Neoprene

164. After steam sterilization and removal of the sterilization rack from the chamber, sterilized items can be removed:

a. at any time
b. after 30 minutes
c. when cooled to a mildly hot temperature
d. when cooled to room temperature

165. An appropriate site for measuring core temperature before, during, and after surgery is

a. rectal.
b. axillary.
c. the nasopharynx.
d. the bladder.

166. If a formula-fed infant is scheduled for surgery, the minimal nothing-by-mouth fasting guideline for infant formula is:

a. 1 hour
b. 2 hours
c. 4 hours
d. 6 hours

167. If using charting by exception, it is critically important to:

a. accurately record baseline data
b. record all observations
c. always use narrative descriptions
d. use check marks only and no narratives

168. Which of the following should trigger an evaluation for latex allergy?

a. A patient works in a clothing store selling men's clothing
b. A patient reports being allergic to bee stings and dust mites
c. A patient developed an unexplained anaphylactic reaction while receiving treatment in the emergency department for the flu
d. A patient has a history of one previous surgery without incident

169. If, during administration of local anesthesia, vasoconstrictor-induced ischemia occurs, the emergent treatment is:

a. epinephrine
b. atropine
c. dexamethasone
d. phentolamine

170. When carrying out hand hygiene with soap and water, after wetting the hands and applying soap, the hands must be rubbed together vigorously for at least:

a. 5 seconds
b. 15 seconds
c. 30 seconds
d. 40 seconds

171. When preparing a patient for surgery on the right hand, the nurse notes that there is no marking on the site even though this is required by protocol. The most appropriate response is to:

a. continue with the prep
b. check the consent form before proceeding
c. continue with the prep but verify with the physician before surgery begins
d. hold the procedure until the surgeon verifies the correct site

172. During the presurgical neurological assessment, there is dysfunction of cranial nerves IX and X. This could place the patient at risk for

a. abnormal eye movements.
b. aspiration.
c. corneal injury.
d. complicated intubation.

173. The bispectral index system (BIS) is used with a patient to monitor the sedation level. What index level is considered optimal anesthesia?

a. 20–40
b. 40–60
c. 60–80
d. 80–100

174. The medication most commonly used for nasal decolonization is:

a. nasal povidone-iodine
b. topical mupirocin 2%
c. an alcohol-based nasal antiseptic
d. nasal erythromycin

175. Reservoirs of critical water used in the cleaning and reprocessing of instruments should be cleaned every:

a. 7 days
b. 2 weeks
c. 1 month
d. 2 months

176. If graduated compression stockings are applied to a patient and a reverse gradient occurs, this means that:

a. the distal pressure is higher than the proximal pressure
b. the proximal pressure is higher than the distal pressure
c. neither the proximal nor the distal pressure is adequate
d. the distal pressure and the proximal pressure are the same

177. If a patient scheduled for moderate sedation has a history of sleep apnea, what precaution is necessary?

a. Prepare for possible noninvasive positive pressure ventilation
b. Avoid the use of opioids or nonopioid analgesia
c. Position the patient with the head elevated
d. Apply a neck brace prior to induction

178. When the circulating nurse transfers a medication to the sterile field, the person receiving the medication must:

a. acknowledge receiving the medication by name
b. concurrently verify the name, strength, dosage, and expiration date
c. ask the circulating nurse to pour a liquid medication into a secondary container on the sterile field
d. ensure that all medications are delivered at the beginning of the procedure

179. During the preoperative assessment, the patient reports taking routine morning medications before coming to the ambulatory surgery center. Which medication may be cause for concern?

a. One-quarter the usual dosage of insulin
b. Metoprolol
c. Ibuprofen
d. Docusate sodium

180. Prior to transfer from the postanesthesia care unit, the AVPU scale may be used to

a. assess the patient's level of consciousness.
b. quantify the patient's level of consciousness.
c. asses the patient's level of pain.
d. monitor trends over time.

181. A patient with multiple body piercings is scheduled for general anesthesia and states that all jewelry has been removed. The nurse should

a. document that all jewelry has been removed.
b. verify removal and document sites of piercings.
c. ask patient to list piercing sites and document.
d. verify removal and document that all jewelry has been removed.

182. If a patient with a traumatic brain injury exhibits Cushing's triad (i.e., bradycardia, hypertension with widened pulse pressure, and irregular respirations), this is likely an indication of

a. hydrocephalus.
b. cerebral ischemia.
c. meningitis.
d. brain stem herniation.

183. If a solution is used to irrigate a surgical wound during an operative procedure, the maximum temperature of the solution should be no more than:

a. 68 °F (19.3 °C)
b. 98 °F (36.7 °C)
c. 104 °F (40 °C)
d. 112 °F (44.4 °C)

184. If during the initial count, a standard 10-pack of surgical sponges is found to contain only 9 sponges, the correct response is to:

a. include the 9 sponges in the count
b. add a sponge from another pack to bring the total to 10
c. exclude the pack from the count and remove it from the field
d. remove 4 sponges and count it as a standard 5 pack

185. The individual who has primary responsibility for initiating the counting process of surgical items before a surgical procedure is the:

a. surgeon
b. anesthetist
c. scrub nurse
d. circulating nurse

186. The dispersive electrode for an electrosurgical unit should be placed:

a. as far as possible from the operative site
b. on the opposite side of the operative site
c. over a bony prominence
d. over a large perfused muscle mass

187. Documentation regarding exposure incidents have to be maintained for the duration of the employee's employment and an additional:

a. 5 years
b. 7 years
c. 20 years
d. 30 years

188. When preparing a 5-year-old child for a surgical procedure, which explanation to the child is the most appropriate?

a. "Don't worry; you will be asleep and won't feel anything."
b. "While you are sleeping, the doctor will make a small opening to remove that lump."
c. "The doctor is going to cut that tumor out of you."
d. "You will wake up after surgery and feel just fine."

189. A 30-year-old male postsurgical patient has a history of drug abuse and is found using heroin while hospitalized, stating that he uses drugs when he is anxious. What is an appropriate nursing diagnosis for this situation?

a. Ineffective health maintenance.
b. Ineffective coping.
c. Risk for injury.
d. Risk for poisoning.

190. If a patient with upper GI tract bleeding scores 5 on the Rockall Risk Scoring System after an episode of upper GI bleeding, the risk for rebleeding is approximately

a. 5%.
b. 11%.
c. 24%.
d. 33%.

191. If a large amount of blood has spilled on the floor, the first step is to:

a. apply absorbent material to the spill
b. wipe up the blood with absorbent pads
c. apply an appropriate Environmental Protection Agency (EPA)-registered disinfectant
d. suction the blood from the floor surface

192. Following cardiac surgery, a patient receives low-molecular-weight heparin. On postoperative day 6, the patient has a sudden drop of platelets from 158,000 to 64,000; erythema at the heparin injection sites; and signs of deep vein thrombosis. The most likely cause is

a. disseminated intravascular coagulation.
b. heparin-induced thrombocytopenia.
c. allergic reaction.
d. sepsis.

193. Flammable wet antiseptic materials used in skin prep need to be disposed of outside the vicinity of care in the operating room. The vicinity of care extends how far beyond the usual position of the operating bed?

a. 3 feet
b. 4 feet
c. 6 feet
d. 8 feet

194. Which of the following classes of lasers pose the greatest risk of materials burn hazard?

a. 1M
b. 2
c. 3R
d. 4

195. The relevant factors for deep vein thrombosis (DVT) that the perioperative nurse must identify when reviewing a patient's medical record include all of the following EXCEPT

a. age older than 50.
b. history of varicose veins.
c. history of heart disease.
d. history of ovarian cysts.

196. When assessing the underlying causes of perioperative cardiac arrest by applying the five Ts, the Ts stand for (1) cardiac tamponade, (2) tension pneumothorax, (3) toxins, (4) pulmonary thrombosis, and (5)

a. coronary thrombosis.
b. torsades de pointes.
c. temperature extremes.
d. physical trauma.

197. A medical student who observed a surgery asked many questions and made numerous comments during the procedure and is now scheduled to observe another surgery. How should the nurse manage this medical student?

a. Encourage the student to continue to ask questions.
b. Tell the student that asking questions is inappropriate.
c. Ask the student to remain quiet during the surgery and to make a list of questions to ask after the procedure.
d. Tell the student's instructor that the student is being disruptive.

198. Tissue vaporizes, producing surgical smoke, when surgical energy devices raise the intracellular temperature of the tissue to:

a. ≥239 °F (115 °C)
b. ≥212 °F (100 °C)
c. ≥194 °F (90 °C)
d. ≥185 °F (85 °C)

199. For a patient with a nursing diagnosis of impaired swallowing, which stage of swallowing is within the patient's voluntary control?

a. Oral stage.
b. Pharyngeal stage.
c. Esophageal stage.
d. No stage is within the patient's control.

200. The best procedure for dealing with a piece of equipment with an electrical cord too short to reach the operating table is to

a. attach an extension cord and tape cord flat.
b. change cord to one of a longer length.
c. move the operating table closer to the outlet.
d. replace the equipment.

Answer Key and Explanations for Test #1

1. B: If an operating room is frequently flooded during procedures with the patient present, the room should be designated as a wet location. The room must have an isolated power system or ground fault circuit interrupters to prevent inadvertent shocks. The wet location designation is applied if a room often has standing fluids or splashing of fluids. Operating rooms are generally considered wet locations unless the governing body of the facility carries out a risk assessment showing that an operating room is not a wet location.

2. A: Visualization and various types of relaxation exercises can be used as complementary care for patients without having formal training, education, or licensure. Some types of complementary therapy cannot be used unless a practitioner is trained and licensed; these include massage therapy, acupuncture, biofield interventions, and hypnosis. In the perioperative setting, use of complementary care should be standardized so that staff use the same intervention techniques and document outcome-specific assessments.

3. C: Sickle cell disease is a systemic contraindication to the use of a pneumatic tourniquet because it may result in increased sickling. Other systemic contraindications include the presence of an arteriovenous graft or fistula, peripheral vascular disease, history of revascularization, diabetic neuropathy, severe infection, and the presence or history of venous thromboembolism (VTE). Pneumatic tourniquets should also be used with caution in older adults (age >60) because of the increased risk of delayed functional recovery, increased atrophy and risk of pulmonary embolism, and increased risk of neurological complications.

4. A: If a patient has been admitted to the postanesthesia care unit (PACU) after surgery and has a persistent Aldrete score that is 3 points less than the baseline, this indicates that the patient should be maintained on one-to-one nursing and should have vital signs checked every 5 minutes. The Aldrete score is based on five parameters—activity, respirations, circulation, consciousness, and oxygen saturation—scored 0 to 2 (with 2 being optimal). The patient is usually scored on admission to the PACU and at least every 30 minutes during the stay and again on discharge, depending on the response. If the patient is 2 points less than the baseline, he or she should be checked every 15 minutes; if the patient is 1 point below the baseline, then checking occurs every 15–30 minutes.

5. C: Some patients with complex medical needs are transferred directly from the operating room to the intensive care unit (ICU). The ICU staff should be notified before the patient leaves the operating room so that they can prepare. During this notification, the staff should be advised of ventilator settings, drainage requirements, and any necessary monitoring or isolation procedures. A summary data sheet (written or digital) should accompany the patient. The transferring nurse should ask for a safety pause at the beginning of handover and should assist with patient care tasks, such as connecting the patient's breathing circuit to the ICU ventilator.

6. D: Hypothermia can result in a number of adverse effects: decreased blood clotting (i.e., a 10% decrease in clotting factors for every 1 °C [1.8 °F] decrease), vasoconstriction resulting from increased levels of epinephrine and norepinephrine, increased oxygen consumption by up to 400% resulting from shivering, decreased heart rate, and decreased BP. Additionally, if the hypothermia is not adequately treated, the patient may develop cardiac arrhythmias that can progress to ventricular fibrillation.

7. A: If a patient with tuberculosis is hospitalized in an airborne infection isolation room (AIIR) but needs surgery, when transporting the patient to the surgical area, the patient should be taken directly to the operating room rather than to the preoperative area in order to keep exposure to a minimum. Following surgery, the patient should be immediately returned to the AIIR under appropriate postoperative care rather than transferred to the PACU.

8. C: On all sides of an operating bed or procedure chair, the sterile field clear area is 3 feet (0.91 m). Standard-size operating beds measure 3 × 7 feet. The circulation pathway measures 3 feet at the head and sides of an operating bed or procedure chair but only 2 feet at the foot. The movable equipment zone for a 400 square foot room extends 2.5 feet on three sides and 2 feet at the foot. For smaller rooms, the circulation pathway and mobile equipment zones are combined into just the circulation pathway. The anesthesia zone extends 6 × 8 feet at the head of the bed.

9. B: When handling hazardous medications, such as chemotherapeutic agents, gloves must be changed every 30 minutes. Two pairs of powder-free chemotherapy gloves should be worn because chemotherapeutic agents may permeate a single glove. In addition, PPE should include a single-use chemotherapy gown and goggles with full face shields. If there is a risk of airborne powder or aerosolization, then an N95 or a more protective respirator must be worn.

10. D: If a patient has an implantable electronic device (IED), the surgical device that poses the most risk to the patient is monopolar electrosurgery. Therefore, whenever possible, alternate technology (electrocautery, bipolar forceps) should be used. The IED and its leads must be as far away as possible from the electrosurgical device and lead, and they must not be between the active and dispersive electrodes. If possible, the IED should be inactivated or reprogrammed during the surgical procedure.

11. D: Unless otherwise specified (such as by the manufacturer), the beyond-use date of a multi-dose vial after first use is 28 days. At the time of first use, the vial must be clearly labeled with the beyond-use date. The date should be verified before each subsequent use of the medication, and the medication should be disposed of when the beyond-use date is met. A multidose vial should be used for one patient only and stored outside of the immediate patient treatment area if possible.

12. B: The most common signs of pulmonary embolism are tachypnea and tachycardia; other signs and symptoms include apprehension or anxiety, dyspnea, chest pain, hemoptysis, and elevated temperature. Typical arterial blood gas findings include decreased PaO_2 (hypoxemia), decreased $PaCO_2$ (hypocarbia), and increased pH (acidic), resulting in respiratory alkalosis. Chest x-rays may appear normal, so they should not be used for diagnostic purposes. Computed tomography and pulmonary angiography are used for diagnosis.

13. D: Although all of these are important, a key element in product evaluation and selection is the financial impact analysis, which should consider:

- Direct costs: Cost of the product and other necessary equipment
- Indirect costs: Utilities, education, storage, energy use
- Reimbursement: CMS value-based purchasing
- Group purchasing options: If applicable

14. D: The nurse should always check the date upon which a surgical pack was sterilized before accepting the pack onto the surgical field. If the sterilization date on the pack is smudged and unreadable, the pack should be rejected and replaced with another pack. The supervisor should be advised of the unreadable label, and the incident should be documented. A smudged and unreadable label can indicate that an incorrect pen was used for marking it or that the pack was contaminated, such as by contact with liquid.

15. D: If a patient is to receive a benzodiazepine as part of moderate sedation/analgesia, flumazenil must be readily available. Naloxone is the reversal agent for opioids, such as morphine and fentanyl. Sugammadex and neostigmine can both be used to reverse neuromuscular blockade. Sugammadex, for example, is used for rocuronium. Neostigmine should be given with an anticholinergic drug because it can cause increased salivation and nausea.

16. B: The maximum duration of time that a pneumatic tourniquet should generally stay inflated on a lower extremity (adult) is 2 hours. Generally, there is little risk of permanent injury within this time frame. In some cases, to further decrease risk of complications, tourniquets are released every hour for 10 minutes, the limb is cooled, or alternating dual cuffs are used in order to decrease the risk of complications for restricted blood flow.

17. A: If using the 3-bucket venous thromboembolism (VTE) risk assessment model, no prophylaxis is recommended for a fully ambulatory patient undergoing minor surgical procedures or observation patients whose hospital stay is expected to be less than 48 hours. Patients should be encouraged to ambulate and should be periodically reassessed, but no other pharmacologic prophylaxis is needed. Risk levels are as follows:

- Low risk: As above.
- Moderate risk: Open, thoracic, gynecologic, or GU surgeries and patients who have impaired mobility (from baseline) and/or have an acute illness. Prophylaxis is unfractionated heparin or low-molecular-weight heparin.
- High risk: Hip or knee arthroplasty, hip fracture repair, multiple major traumas, spinal cord injury or other major spinal procedure, and abdominal-pelvic operations for cancer. Prophylaxis includes intermittent pneumatic compression device AND low molecular weight heparin or another anticoagulant.

18. A: Shivering increases cardiac demand and may lead to cardiac ischemia and arrest in this vascular surgery patient, especially due to her already-compromised cardiac status.

19. B: Although blankets and warm IV fluids are helpful in warming a patient, the use of forced-air warming blankets have been shown to be the most effective in warming hypothermic patients. These devices have been found to be useful in pre-, intra-, and postoperative areas.

20. C: Any vascular surgery that requires catheter placement, such as a pacemaker, may need a chest x ray postoperatively to verify proper placement. This is usually done in the PACU area. Although this patient might require additional lines or a blood transfusion due to her overall disease process, it would not be a routine order for a pacemaker placement patient.

21. D: If a perioperative team prepares the wrong site for surgery, resulting in a delay while the patient is prepped correctly, in a just culture, the initial response should be to investigate the root cause. A just culture considers the need to change the system rather than the individual and differentiates among the following:

- Human error: Inadvertent actions, mistakes, or lapses in proper procedure, requiring consolation and training or changes in processes/procedures
- At-risk behavior: Unjustified risk, choice, requiring incentives/disincentives and coaching
- Reckless behavior: Conscious disregard for proper procedures, requiring remedial action and/or punitive action

22. C: Perioperative personnel who may experience radiation exposure must receive education regarding radiation safety and verify competency upon hiring and annually. Education about radiation must include:

- Exposure risks
- Biological effects
- Principles of protection
- Dosimetry
- Safe operation of equipment
- Regulatory requirements

23. B: When conducting leak testing for a flexible endoscope and the endoscope is pressurized with an automatic or manual pressure tester, the pressure should be maintained for a minimum of 30 seconds. The manufacturer's pressure recommendations must be followed because if the pressure is too low, leaks may go undetected; alternately, if the pressure is too high, this may damage the endoscope. A handheld pressure tester allows a leak to be detected before the instrument is submerged because the pressure falls as the air escapes.

24. D: If a patient is scheduled for an outpatient procedure, but during the preoperative assessment, the nurse notes what appears to be needle tracks on both arms despite the patient denying any recent drug use, the appropriate response is to notify the surgeon and the anesthesiologist of the observation. Patients who are current substance abusers are not good candidates for ambulatory surgery. A history of substance abuse may also preclude ambulatory surgery depending on the length of time since abstinence.

25. D: Unless otherwise mandated by state law, under federal regulations, verbal orders must be authenticated by a responsible physician within 48 hours. Verbal orders are expected to be carried out immediately and must be carefully documented to include the date and time the orders were received. If orders are entered into the record by a documentation assistant, these orders are not considered verbal orders because the physician or other licensed independent practitioner is present and should verify that the orders are correct.

26. B: The fuel source that is most often associated with surgical fires is surgical drapes. In fact, >80% of surgical fires involve surgical drapes. Flammable skin antiseptic agents (such as isopropyl alcohol) must dry completely before surgical drapes are applied in order to prevent pooling of volatile fumes. Other sources of fuel include tissue, the patient's hair, and GI tract gases. Drapes placed over the patient's head must allow oxygen to flow freely and not pool under the drapes.

27. C: For the Mohs procedure, to ensure that the correct site is excised after the biopsy site has healed, the safest method is to rely on a high-quality photo of the lesion and surrounding site (taken before the biopsy). Relying on recollection or notes without photographs may result in surgery on the wrong site, and there may be no obvious scarring from a biopsy. The photo may include a ruler indicating distances of landmarks, such as eyebrows. Different views, such as close-up and distant shots, may be indicated as well as circling the lesion with a surgical skin marker to ensure that the correct lesion is identified later.

28. C: Class III. Modified Mallampati classification:

- 0: All parts of the epiglottis are visible.
- I: The entire uvula, soft palate, and tonsillar pillars are visible.
- II: The upper portion of the uvula and the soft palate are visible.

- III: Only the soft palate and base of the uvula are visible.
- IV: The uvula and soft palate are not visible at all.

The patient should be assessed while sitting upright with the mouth open and the tongue protruding. Studies have indicated that the Mallampati classification is often inaccurate when used to identify difficult airways; however, it is a good predictor of obstructive sleep apnea.

29. D: Pulse oximetry measures oxygenation but not ventilation. Patients who have 100% oxygenation could have respiratory acidosis from inadequate ventilation. Readings under 90% indicate significant hypoxemia. Bright lights interfere with the accuracy of the pulse oximeter, so cover the patient's hand bearing the oximeter with a drape or blanket. Methylene blue and other IV dyes may interfere with the performance of the pulse oximeter.

30. D: Gingko biloba may increase the risk of postoperative bleeding because it slows blood clotting, especially if combined with aspirin or other nonsteroidal anti-inflammatory drugs (NSAIDs). Most patients do not consider herbal supplements as medications and tend not to list nonprescribed drugs on their medication lists, so patients should always be asked specifically about their use of herbal supplements and over-the-counter drugs. People with or fearful of mild cognitive impairment often take gingko biloba because it is purported to boost memory.

31. C: The label for a specimen container must include two patient identifiers (such as name, record number, and birthdate), the specimen name, the specimen site (including right or left to indicate laterality), and the date of excision. Containers should not be prelabeled, and only one specimen should be labeled at a time. Dark indelible ink should be used for labeling so that it does not smudge.

32. A: Chills, headache, fever, and muscle ache are consistent with febrile nonhemolytic reaction, which usually occurs within 2 hours of initiation of a transfusion. The correct response is to stop the transfusion until the physician orders it to be restarted, although the patient should be monitored carefully for signs of infection or acute hemolytic reaction. Febrile nonhemolytic reaction occurs because packed red blood cells (PRBCs) may contain small amounts of WBCs, to which a person's antibodies react. Treatment is with acetaminophen or a nonsteroidal anti-inflammatory drug such as ibuprofen.

33. A: Precleaning processes for flexible endoscopes should be carried out in the procedure room (point of use) immediately after the procedure is completed in order to prevent the development of biofilms. The instrument should be wiped of any soil so that it does not dry on the device, and the recommended cleaning solution is suctioned through the suction and biopsy channels. Additionally, air and solution should be alternately flushed through the channels, ending with air. Further cleaning should then be carried out in a special endoscopy processing room, which is reserved for only this purpose.

34. D: A disinfectant that is appropriate to use for reprocessing flexible endoscopes is 2–2.4% glutaraldehyde. Peracetic acid (type III) has also been shown to be effective. Skin antiseptics, such as chlorhexidine gluconate, povidone-iodine, and alcohol, are not appropriate to use for disinfection. Hypochlorites may become inactivated by organic material and are corrosive to the materials in endoscopes. Phenolics may be irritating to the tissue if residue remains.

35. A: If using enzymes to target soil, the type of enzyme that is effective for organic material is proteases. Amylases are effective for carbohydrates, starches, and sugars; lipases, for fats and oils; and celluloses, for cellulose. Many concentrated enzymatic cleaners used to clean and reprocess surgical instruments contain a combination of different enzymes. For example, NOSOZYM contains protease, lipase, and amylase.

36. D: Nonshockable rhythms include asystole and pulseless electrical activity. With these conditions, defibrillation is ineffective. The patient should immediately receive cardiopulmonary resuscitation (CPR), and epinephrine is administered as soon as possible at 1 mg by IV (preferred) or intraosseously, repeated every 3–5 minutes as needed. CPR should be continued for cycles of 2 minutes; then perform rhythm checks for 10 seconds. An advanced airway and capnography should be considered. With the airway in place, breaths are administered every 6 seconds. Treatment is continued until the return of spontaneous circulation or upon the determination of death.

37. C: An ankle-brachial value of <0.9 is consistent with a diagnosis of peripheral arterial disease and supports the nursing diagnosis of ineffective peripheral tissue perfusion.

>1.4	Calcified, noncompressible vessel
1.0–1.39	Normal range
0.9–0.99	Acceptable range
0.8–0.89	Mild arterial disease (treat the risk factors)
0.5–0.79	Moderate arterial disease
<0.5	Severe arterial disease

With mild arterial disease, risk factors such as smoking, hypertension, diabetes, and high cholesterol should be addressed. With moderate to severe arterial disease, lifestyle changes, medications, and surgical procedures (such as angioplasty with stent placement or bypass surgery) may be indicated.

38. D: Ideally, if a surgical patient is hospitalized, discharge planning should begin before the patient is admitted in order to explore the patient's needs and the ability of the family to assist in care if necessary or to find available community resources, such as home health care and home meal programs. Early discharge planning can enhance coordination between different healthcare providers, such as occupational and physical therapists. In some cases, educating the patient and family about postoperative care and medication management should begin prior to admission, especially for patients with complex medical needs.

39. A: The most effective complementary care intervention to reduce stress in preoperative pediatric patients is likely humor. Young children especially respond well to humor, which may occur in face-to-face interactions or video presentations about the child's procedure. Clown humor interventions can also be used, although it is important to ascertain whether the child has a fear of or aversion to clowns before the clown appears. When the child is more relaxed, the child's parent or caregiver is often also more relaxed.

40. C: If using the situation, background, assessment, and recommendations (SBAR) tool for handoff of a patient to the PACU, the presence or absence of surgical complications would be discussed under the category of assessment (A). SBAR stands for:

- Situation (S): Name, birthdate, surgeon, operative site, procedures performed
- Background (B): Type of anesthesia, anesthesia provider, intraoperative medications, IV fluids, estimated blood loss, wound information (drains, packing, tubing), significant operative events

- Assessment (A): Hemodynamic stability, airway status, thermal status, urinary output, surgical complications, level of pain, pain management
- Recommendations (R): Review postoperative orders, discharge protocol, questions/answers

41. D: When assessing a patient for risk for difficulty with mask ventilation, a decreased hyomental distance (smaller than three finger widths) increases risk. Other risk factors include age >55, obesity, dental problems, snoring, stridor, sleep apnea, facial hair, short neck, neck mass, limited neck extension, cervical spine abnormality, facial dysmorphia, mouth opening <3 cm (adult), large tongue, high arched palate, jaw abnormalities, rheumatoid arthritis, genetic chromosomal disorders, and a Mallampati classification of III or IV.

42. A: The surgical energy device that generates the smallest aerodynamic particle size is electrocautery. Particle sizes that are generated by different surgical devices include:

- Electrocautery: 0.07-0.1 µm
- Laser tissue ablation: 0.31 µm
- Ultrasonic scalpel: 0.35-6.5 µm

Particles that are 5 µm or greater may settle in the nasopharynx, but those that are smaller than 5 µm may damage the lungs. Particles that are 2.0-5.0 µm may settle in the trachea or bronchus, and those that are 0.8-3.0 µm may settle in the alveoli.

43. C: If a cranial bone flap has been removed and cleaned for preservation and is to be stored in plastic bags, then the specimen must be sealed into three sterile bags, one after the other, before it can be removed from the sterile field. Preparation includes removal of blood and excess soft tissue, irrigating or immersing the cranial bone flap in normal saline (NS) and antibiotic or povidone-iodine, drying, and wrapping it in sterile gauze. Cranial bone flaps are typically stored under cryopreservation if they are not placed in a subcutaneous pocket.

44. A: The recommended treatment for LAST is 20% lipid emulsion (1 L total), administered intravenously. Other emergent treatment includes discontinuing the anesthesia, calling for help and retrieving the rescue kit (which should contain the lipid emulsion), maintaining the airway, ventilating with 100% oxygen, establishing IV access, and carrying out advanced cardiac life support as needed. LAST most often occurs as the result of inadvertent intravenous (IV) administration of the anesthesia.

45. C: Retraining is sometimes needed when repeated mistakes are occurring, usually indicating that personnel are taking shortcuts or are confused about the correct procedures. When planning for retraining, it is important to assess the type of mistakes that are occurring and where in the procedure they occur because sometimes the procedure itself needs to be corrected in some way, especially if it is confusing or ambiguous. The nurse should avoid reprimanding individuals unless the mistakes are clearly related to negligence, although all of the staff members involved should be made aware of the problems.

46. C: The current cost of infections is $300,000 a year (10 x $30,000), so the most cost-effective solution is a product that costs $100,000 a year and reduces infections by 8 (leaving a cost of $60,000 for infections): $100,000 plus $60,000 = $160,000, a savings of $140,000. When determining the cost-benefit analysis, both the cost and the savings must be calculated because sometimes the least expensive product does not provide the best savings. For example, the product that costs $20,000 and reduces infections by only 1 (10%) costs $20,000 plus $270,000 ($30,000 x 9) for a total cost of $290,000 and a savings of only $10,000.

47. A: When transporting a patient who is on droplet precautions, the patient is required to wear a mask but not the transporter. The patient should be advised to practice appropriate cough etiquette and respiratory hygiene. Ideally, the patient should have a private room, but if rooming with other patients, a distance of at least 3 feet should be maintained and a privacy curtain should be drawn between the beds to minimize contact.

48. A: In a single endoscopy processing room, clean areas and contaminated areas must be separated by at least 3 feet. Additionally, a wall or barrier must separate the areas and extend at least 4 feet (1.2 m) above the level of the sink. Contaminated droplets can travel about 1 meter, so separation is necessary to prevent contamination of the clean area. The room should be designed so there is a unidirectional workflow.

49. D: According to the Health Information Management Association, the register of surgical procedures should be maintained indefinitely. Most other health records must be kept for a minimum number of years after the last date of service or after a patient's death. The number of years varies, but most range between 5 and 10. Medical records for minors are usually kept for a minimum number of years after the child reaches the age of majority. For example, in California, adult records are kept for 7 years after the patient is discharged and 7 years after a minor is discharged or 1 year after the child reaches the age of majority or turns 19.

50. A: A parent or family member may be allowed into the OR for a child (usually younger than 12 years) or a mentally disabled adult during the induction phase of anesthesia only and then should be escorted to the waiting area. Visitors should be strictly limited to only those authorized, such as medical students, interns, and health care industry representatives. Law enforcement officers may, in some instances, be allowed to accompany and stay with a patient but should be in surgical attire and provided clear instructions. In some cases, the officer may remain outside the OR door.

51. B: With specimen management, most errors occur in the preanalytical phase. Because these errors occur before the specimen is analyzed, they can lead to further errors as the specimen is processed. Preanalytical errors can encompass ordering, collecting, handling, containing, labeling, storing, and transporting. Preanalytical management is generally under the purview of perioperative nurses, so careful adherence to evidence-based guidelines can prevent further errors.

52. A: Flexible endoscopes should be stored in a cabinet with all valves open and removable parts detached because this facilitates complete drying and inhibits microbial growth and development of biofilms. Before using a stored endoscope, it should be visually inspected to ensure there is no sign of soil, moisture, or odor (fecal), which would indicate the need for reprocessing. If one endoscope in a cabinet is found to be contaminated, the others may also be contaminated.

53. A: If there is a count discrepancy at the end of a procedure, all members of the perioperative team should take immediate action:

- Surgeon and first assistant: Suspend closure of the wound and examine the wound, participate in imaging if necessary and remain with the patient until the missing item is found.
- Circulating nurse: Notify the team, call for assistance, search the room, and recount with the scrub person.
- Scrub person: Organize and search the sterile field and recount with the circulating nurse.

54. C: If the bone cement methyl methacrylate (MMA) is spilled during preparation, the correct response is to ventilate the area and cover the MMA with an activated charcoal absorbent. All sources of ignition should be removed from near the MMA, and personal protective equipment (PPE) should be worn during cleanup. A closed system should be used to mix the powder and solution to form the cement in order to minimize risks, and the cement should not be handled with gloved hands until it has reached the dough stage because MMA can penetrate plastic and latex gloves.

55. D: The copy and paste function in EHRs is often overused, resulting in bloated records with duplications and propagation of errors since they may be copied and pasted repeatedly. Additionally, copying and pasting may result in notes that do not accurately reflect the patient's condition, which can impact the patient's plan of care. Although copying and pasting can make documenting more efficient, this function should be reserved for information that is unlikely to change, such as a patient's health history, and the accuracy of that information should be verified.

56. C: If the scrub nurse notes that a person who is non-operating room personnel, such as a biomedical engineer, has stepped into the sterile field, the scrub nurse must immediately notify the team (e.g., by saying "Sterile field breach") and indicate where the breach occurred and what appears to have been contaminated. The nurse should remain calm and professional. Upon notification, the team leader, who may be the circulating nurse or the surgeon, and the rest of the team will apprise the situation and determine what steps need to be taken to ensure that the sterile field is intact.

57. D: The use of standardized preprinted order sets reduces errors and improves documentation; however, the order sets must be current, updated, and free from problematic entries, such as the use of unacceptable abbreviations (cc, BT, OD, D/C) and the use of trailing zeros in medication dosages (3.0 mL). The order sets should use standardized terminology for treatments and interventions and should be reviewed by the attending physician to make sure they are accurate.

58. A: Negotiating with staff is not part of outcomes evaluation, which includes:

- Monitoring over the course of treatment involves careful observation and record keeping that notes progress, with supporting laboratory and radiographic evidence as indicated by condition and treatment.
- Evaluating results includes reviewing records as well as current research to determine if outcomes are within acceptable parameters.
- Sustaining involves continuing treatment, but continuing to monitor and evaluate.
- Improving means to continue the treatment but with additions or modifications in order to improve outcomes.
- Replacing the treatment with a different treatment must be done if outcomes evaluation indicates that current treatment is ineffective.

59. D: Commercial bias is showing preference for one commercial product or company over another because of personal feelings or personal benefit rather than evidence of quality. Commercial bias may also be an issue if a close family member has an interest in a supplier company. The nurse should avoid promoting a particular product or service and should make full disclosure if a conflict of interest, such as a financial interest in a company, occurs. Disclosure should include any financial incentive/payment, the name of the company, and the person's relationship to the company. Recommendations should be based on evidence-based research, quality, and cost-effectiveness.

60. D: If a patient with an active case of COVID-19 requires surgery, the surgery should be scheduled at the end of the day when the number of staff present is minimal and few other patients are in the operating rooms. COVID-19 is an airborne disease, so airborne precautions must be used. If possible, surgery should be postponed until the patient tests negative and is no longer infectious. This is true for all patients with suspected or confirmed airborne infections.

61. C: If a patient needs hair removal for a surgical procedure, this should be done in a room near the operating room immediately before surgery. Hair removal should not be carried out in the operating room because of the risk of hair contamination of the equipment and the operative site. Hair removal should be done only if absolutely necessary. Clipping is preferable to any type of shaving, and razors should not be used because of the risk of small cuts to the skin.

62. B: Unused materials in surgical packages cannot be resterilized for use on other patients but must be disposed of properly. Some materials may be recycled in accordance with institution policies. Some charitable organizations, such as the REMEDY program (established at Yale-New Haven hospital), collect opened but still clean or sterile supplies for use in developing countries where access to medical supplies is limited. Some other types of supplies and equipment (such as older equipment and excess supplies) may also be donated for use.

63. B: After an employee has received the third hepatitis B vaccination in the series of three, serologic testing should be carried out to determine if antibody levels are sufficient in 1–2 months. If the antibody level is <10 mIU/mL, then the person should be revaccinated and tested again when the series is completed. The Occupational Safety and Health Administration (OSHA) requires that organizations make hepatitis B vaccinations available to all perioperative employees.

64. B: During laser procedures, reflective instruments should be replaced with nonreflective (matte, dull) or ebonized (black-coated) instruments to eliminate glare because laser beams may reflect off of reflective surfaces and cause a fire. Ebonized coatings are designed to absorb energy. If reflective instruments must be used, they must be covered with nonreflective material, such as saline-saturated radiopaque sponges. If instruments are ebonized, they must be carefully examined for damage to the coating before use.

65. A: The "right reason" is not part of the 5 rights of medication administration although it is certainly an important consideration. The 5 rights include:

- Right patient: Verified by at least 2 identifiers, such as name and birth date.
- Right drug: Checked against physician order and patient diagnosis.
- Right dose: Evaluated in terms of usual dose for age and size patient.
- Right route: Double-checked for parenteral medications to ensure IM and IV are not confused.
- Right time: Verified by checking order and previous administration.

66. B: The wrappers used for packaging of surgical instruments should be held at room temperature for a minimum of 2 hours prior to sterilization. This is especially important for moisture-permeable wrappers. If wrappers are cold, they may form condensation in the warmer environment of the sterilizer, and this can compromise the instruments' sterility. Additionally, some wrapping material is less flexible when cold. Waiting for 2 hours allows the materials to acclimate to the ambient temperature. The handling of wrappers may vary somewhat depending on the type of sterilization process used.

67. B: In the perioperative setting, the sterile cockpit rule is applied during important tasks such as the sponge and instrument count and during induction of anesthesia. The sterile cockpit rule requires that no nonessential activities or distractions take place during the task to prevent errors. The sterile cockpit rule is borrowed from aeronautics and is used in aircraft to prohibit crew members from engaging in nonessential activities during taxiing, take-off, and landing.

68. A: Type 1 chemical indicators demonstrate only that a package has been exposed to the sterilization process. This helps to distinguish between packages that have been processed and those that have not. Type 2 chemical indicators are used for a specific purpose, type 3 is a single-parameter indicator, type 4 is a multiparameter indicator, type 5 is an integrating indicator, and type 6 an emulating indicator. Chemical indicators are used to monitor exposure to various sterilization parameters.

69. B: If using binaural beats with a postoperative patient to reduce anxiety, the primary concern is hearing damage. With binaural beats, the patient listens to different tones in each ear through headphones for 30–60 minutes, so it is important that the volume stay below 7 decibels because prolonged exposure to high decibels can result in hearing impairment. Binaural beats can be adjusted to promote different types of brain waves; for example, the alpha pattern (7–13 Hz) promotes relaxation, and the beta pattern (13–30 Hz) promotes alertness.

70. C: Bureaucratic leaders follow organizational rules exactly and expect others to do so. Autocratic leaders make decisions independently and strictly enforce rules. Consultative leaders present a decision and welcome input and questions, although decisions rarely change. Democratic leaders present a problem and ask staff or teams to arrive at a solution; however, the leader usually makes the final decision. Charismatic leaders depend on personal charisma to influence people. Participatory leaders present a potential decision and make a final decision based on input from others. Laissez-faire leaders exert little direct control and allow others to make decisions with little interference.

71. B: Justice is the ethical principle that relates to the distribution of the limited resources of health care benefits to the members of society. These resources must be distributed fairly. Autonomy is the ethical principle that the individual has the right to make decisions about his or her own care. Beneficence is the ethical principle that involves performing actions that are for the purpose of benefitting another person, so medical treatment should benefit the patient. Nonmaleficence is the ethical principle that indicates health care workers should provide care in a manner that does not cause direct, intentional harm to the patient.

72. B: Charting electronically with a computer screen open to view, such as a hallway, is a violation of patient's confidentiality because unauthorized personnel and visitors may be able to read the records. Computerized record keeping should always be password protected. Parents have a legal right to information about their child unless their child is legally emancipated. Patients have a right to expect that when they divulge personal information to a nurse that only those with a need to know (such as the physician and other nurses) will be provided this information.

73. C: According to advanced cardiovascular life support guidelines, cardiac compressions should be administered at the rate of 30 compressions to two ventilations at a 2-inch depth and a rate of 100–120 compressions per minute. If an airway is already established, oxygen should be administered at 100% and a monitor/defibrillator is attached to determine if the rate is shockable or nonshockable. Shockable rhythms include ventricular fibrillation and pulseless ventricular tachycardia. Nonshockable rhythms include asystole and pulseless electrical activity.

74. B: If using multimodal complementary care to control a patient's postoperative nausea and vomiting, in addition to medication, the patient may be offered aromatherapy with essential oils. Oil of ginger (a combination of ginger, spearmint or peppermint, and cardamom), lavender oil, and fennel oil have been shown to reduce the intensity of nausea and vomiting and the need for antiemetics. Essential oils should generally be infused rather than applied to the skin. Aromatherapy with isopropyl alcohol has also been shown to be effective.

75. C: The first step in removing disposable gown and gloves following a surgical procedure is to grasp the front of the gown and pull it away from the body. The fasteners will pull apart and break. The gown and glove doffing steps are as follows:

6. While pulling the gown away from the body, roll it inside out because the outside is contaminated, touching only the outside with gloved hands.
7. Peel away the glove while removing the gown, touching only the inside of the gloves.
8. Use bare hands only when touching the inside of gloves or the inside of the gown.
9. Discard in an appropriate container.

76. B: An example of a group 1 endoscope is a colonoscope. Flexible endoscopes are classified as group 1, 2, or 3 depending on the purpose and structure:

- Group 1: GI endoscopes include gastroscopes, colonoscopes, and duodenoscopes (with an encapsulated elevator channel).
- Group 2: GI endoscopes with air/water and instrument/channel and sometimes additional channels include duodenoscopes (with an open elevator channel), echoendoscopes, and enteroscopes.
- Group 3: Other types of endoscopes with only one channel system or with no channel system include bronchoscopes, cystoscopes, laryngoscopes, and nasendoscopes.

77. C: With terminal clearing of an operating room, the floor may be mopped or wet vacuumed. Dry cleaning preparations and spraying should be avoided. Cleaning the floor around equipment is insufficient; the equipment, including the operating bed, must be moved so the floor underneath can be cleaned. In addition, all exposed surfaces in the room must be cleaned and disinfected, including all furniture and equipment in the room (including the anesthesia cart) as well as wheels and casters, positioning devices, and transfer devices.

78. B: The type of water that should be used in the final rinse when reprocessing flexible endoscopes is critical water, which has low levels of minerals. Critical water composition is as follows:

- <1 mg/L calcium carbonate
- 5–7 pH
- <1 mg/L chloride
- <10 colony forming units (CFU)/mL bacteria
- <10 endotoxin units/mL

79. C: A Braden Scale score of less than 18 indicates that the patient is at risk for pressure ulcer. The Braden Scale scores six different areas with 1–4 points: sensory perception, moisture, activity, mobility, usual nutrition pattern, and friction and shear. Scores can range from 6 (worst) to 23 (best):

- 23: Excellent prognosis, very minimal risk.
- ≤16–18: Breakpoint for risk of pressure ulcer (will vary somewhat for different populations).
- 6: The prognosis is very poor; there is a strong likelihood of developing pressure ulcers.

Other risk factors include cognitive impairment, impaired sensorium, anemia, cardiovascular disease and an American Society of Anesthesiologists Physical Status Classification score ≥2.

80. D: The maximum volume of alcohol-based rub in a dispenser in a room, corridor, or area open to corridors is 1,200 mL. Precautions are necessary because alcohol-based rubs are flammable. Dispensers must be at least 4 feet apart and must not be placed above or within 1 inch of light switches, electrical outlets, or other ignition sources. Alcohol-based hand rubs contain ethyl alcohol and can evaporate and form a vapor that can ignite.

81. A: If any type of skin lesion, such as a pustule, is found in close proximity to an operative site or elsewhere on the body, the surgeon should be notified immediately to determine whether the surgical procedure should be postponed. The pustule should be examined carefully, noting its size, its appearance, and the existence of any erythema and swelling that might indicate an active infection. Information about the lesion should be entered into the EHR. If facility policy permits, a photograph may also be entered into the record.

82. A: When cleaning with disinfectant, the appropriate method is to clean from top to bottom and from clean to dirty in order to avoid spreading contamination from the dirty area to the clean. If cleaning is done from bottom to top, some dust or debris may fall on the already cleaned lower surface. Cleaning may be done in a clockwise or counterclockwise direction, but the direction should be consistent.

83. B: Finding only the upper portion of the uvula and the soft palate visible when examining the patient's mouth as part of the assessment for moderate sedation corresponds to class II of the Mallampati classification. Classifications are as follows:

- I: The entire uvula, soft palate, and tonsillar pillars are visible.
- II: The upper portion of the uvula and soft palate are visible.
- III: Only the base of the uvula is visible.
- IV: The uvula and soft palate are not visible at all.

84. C: The anesthesia provider must accompany the patient from the surgical suite to the PACU and remain with the patient until the PACU nurse accepts responsibility for the patient. Before accepting responsibility, the PACU nurse assesses the airway and circulation (ABCs) and connects the patient to monitoring devices, such as an oximeter and cardiac monitor. The hand-off reports from both the anesthesia provider and the perioperative nurse must be completed and include time for questions and answers.

85. A: A return demonstration is given by patients to show mastery of a procedure. This may be done for each step during initial instruction but should eventually include a demonstration of the entire procedure:

- The nurse should ask if the patient has any questions before the demonstration.
- The patient should gather all necessary equipment, using a checklist to ensure that nothing is forgotten.
- The patient should explain the steps
- The nurse should provide positive feedback occasionally during the procedure: "You've placed the equipment exactly right," and may remind the patient to look at the checklist.

86. D: The first to sixth months have the highest risk for infections because the immunosuppression therapy is still at a high dose, putting the patient at risk for all types of infections.

87. A: The HCIR should not enter the patient's sterile field, scrub in, or assist in direct patient care. The HCIR may observe patient procedures in accordance with policies (institutional, state, and federal) and may provide technical support concerning the use of the product as well as calibrations of equipment (such as lasers, radiofrequency devices, and implantable devices) under the direct supervision of a physician. The HCIR must wear appropriate surgical attire and wear an identifying badge, and the patient should provide informed consent prior to surgery.

88. B: Burns may make a patient susceptible to iodism from iodine and iodophor-based antiseptics because the antiseptics may be easily absorbed. Other disorders or conditions that increase susceptibility include thyroid disorders, pregnancy, and lactation. Iodism is a toxic reaction to iodine or its compound. With burns, iodism occurs when iodine is absorbed, most often after repeated exposures, and this results in hyperthyroidism or metabolic acidosis.

89. D: A characteristic of targeted screening and decolonization for *Staphylococcus aureus* is that all patients are screened, and only those identified as carriers are treated with mupirocin and other medications. The logistics of targeted screening and decolonization tend to be more complex than universal screening, and some carriers may be missed because tests are not 100% sensitive and some are non-nasal carriers. With universal decolonization, all patients are treated as though they are carriers and no screening is necessary.

90. C: The key switch for laser devices is usually located on the front or a side panel and is an opening into which a metal key is inserted. Because the key needs to be inserted before the laser device can be activated, this prevents inadvertent activation. When disabling the device, the key is turned to the off position and the key is removed. The key should be stored in a secure place and not attached to the laser device because it must only be accessible to authorized personnel.

91. D: If receiving verbal orders from a physician, the nurse must confirm orders through readback. Verbal orders are more prone to error than written orders because of misunderstanding what is said, background noises, or accents. For example, 15 mg and 50 mg may sound similar. Protocol for readback requires that after receiving the orders, the receiver reads back the orders word by word and digit by digit, spelling out words for clarity if necessary for confirmation before acting on the orders.

92. D: No information can be provided without explicit permission of the patient. HIPAA regulations are designed to protect the rights of individuals regarding the privacy of their health information. The nurse must not release any information or documentation about a patient's condition or treatment without consent, as the individual has the right to determine who has access to personal information. Personal information about the patient is considered protected health information (PHI) and consists of any identifying or personal information about the patient, such as health history, condition, or treatments in any form, and any documentation.

93. A: The area within which direct, reflected, or scattered radiation associated with laser use exceeds the maximum permissible exposure level is the nominal hazard zone. The nominal hazard zone may vary from one class of lasers to another. This zone often exceeds the size of the laser procedure room, so precautions must be taken to prevent exposure outside of the procedure room, such as through closed doors, controlled entry, covered windows, and screening. Appropriate eye protection must be used in the nominal hazard zone.

94. D: The acceptable upper limits for the temperature range for a decontamination room used in reprocessing instruments ranges from 72-78 °F (22-26 °C). The temperature may be adjusted to cooler than 72 °F (22 °C) for the comfort of staff, who may become too hot because of wearing PPE, but it should not be adjusted to warmer than 78 °F (26 °C). Any variance in temperature (higher or lower that the acceptable range) should be reported and resolved.

95. D: According to the American Society of Heating, Refrigerating and Air-Conditioning Engineers standards, the minimum number of total air exchanges per hour that should be used for operating rooms is 20 in order to ensure proper ventilation. It is currently common for hospitals to use 20-25 or more air exchanges per hour to decrease the risk of infection. Air exchanges of outdoor air must be done at least 4 times per hour. Fresh air intakes must be located at least 25 feet from contaminated air outlets or any structures that emit dust, fumes, or exhaust.

96. A: If surgical drapes become ignited during a surgical procedure, the immediate response should be to remove the drapes and extinguish the fire with water, NS, or another noncombustible, nonflammable solution from the back table because this is usually more easily accessible than fire extinguishers, which are not the first line of fire defense. Fire blankets should not be used in the operating rooms because they may trap a fire and may burn in some cases.

97. B: According to the World Health Organization's Surgical Safety Checklist, every item on the checklist must be actionable, that is, tied to a specific action. There are three sections of the checklist:

- Before anesthetic induction: Patient identification is confirmed, site is marked, anesthesia/medication check, pulse oximeter is in place and is functioning, known allergies, difficult airway/aspiration risk, risk of >500 mL blood loss (7 mL/kg for pediatric patients).
- Before skin incision: All team members are introduced; confirm the patient's identification, procedure, and incision site; antibiotic prophylaxis and anticipated critical events; imaging is displayed.
- Before leaving the operating room: Verbal confirmation of procedure, counts, specimens and labeling, equipment problems, and concerns for recovery.

98. B: The five Hs of reversible causes for cardiac arrest include the following:

- Hypovolemia: Decreased cardiac output and inadequate perfusion.
- Hypoxia: Tissue ischemia, myocardial dysfunction.
- Hydrogen ion (acidosis): Especially metabolic acidosis from ketoacidosis, renal failure, sepsis. Impairs myocardial contractility.

- Hypo-/Hyperkalemia: Hypokalemia impairs myocardial contractility and causes arrhythmias. Hyperkalemia leads to arrythmias and cardiac arrest.
- Hypothermia: A body temperature of less than 35 °C (95 °F) impairs cardiac function.

The five Ts are usually considered with the five Hs. The five Ts include **t**ension pneumothorax, cardiac **t**amponade, **t**oxins, pulmonary **t**hrombosis, and coronary **t**hrombosis.

99. A: If a large specimen (such as an amputated leg) does not fit into a container, it can be transported by placing it inside of two sealed red hazard bags. The first bag is securely sealed and placed inside the second bag, which is then securely sealed. Thus, if the first bag leaks, the biological contaminants will be contained by the second bag. A cart is then used to transport the specimen. Any specimen must be contained and labeled immediately after receiving it from the sterile field.

100. A: The most common unintentionally retained surgical items are surgical sponges. The most common counting discrepancies are associated with needles. Most retained items are found in the abdomen or pelvis, although they can migrate to adjacent areas over time. Retained surgical items can occur with open surgical procedures as well as minimally invasive and endoscopic procedures. Retained surgical items are considered never events, and healthcare organizations are not reimbursed by the Centers for Medicare & Medicaid Services (CMS) for treatment needed because of a retained item.

101. D: The period of time in which an activated high-level disinfectant can be used is the reuse-life date. The activation date is the date on which the chemical became active by being mixed with another chemical. The shelf-life date is the period of time during which a stored product (before activation) remains effective. When recording high-level disinfection, the activation date, reuse-life date, and shelf life of the chemical must be recorded.

102. B: The perioperative nurse should begin conflict resolution by allowing both sides to present their side of the issue without bias, keeping the focus on the issue rather than individuals. Additional steps include encouraging cooperation and compromise while maintaining focus and avoiding arguments, evaluating the need for formal resolution or third-party negotiations, summarizing issues, and utilizing humor and empathy to help diffuse tension. The nurse should avoid forcing a resolution if possible.

103. A: During surgery that involves the use of an electrosurgical unit, monitoring electrodes, such as used for heart monitoring or oximetry, should be placed as far away from the operative site as possible to avoid burns. With electrosurgical units, the electrical current enters the patient's body. The current pathway is from the active electrode in the handpiece of the device, through the patient, and out the dispersive electrode to the generator. Monitoring electrodes should avoid this pathway.

104. C: If, immediately after receiving a local anesthetic injection, the patient becomes agitated and confused, exhibits dysarthria, and complains of numbness about the mouth and a metallic taste as well as ringing in the ears, these symptoms are consistent with local anesthetic systemic toxicity (LAST). Approximately 50% of LAST events occur within less than a minute, and 75% within 5 minutes. Patients may develop seizures and cardiovascular collapse, so rapid recognition and intervention are critical.

105. D: When transporting a flexible endoscope from the procedure room to the processing room, the parts should be wet or damp, but not submerged in cleaning solution because this could increase the risk of spillage and contamination. The parts should not be allowed to dry after precleaning because that will make the cleaning process more difficult. The parts must be transported in a closed container or transport cart that is leakproof, puncture resistant, and large enough to contain all of the parts.

106. D: For all chemicals, such as high-level disinfectants, used in a facility, the organization must write a hazard communication program. The three components that must be included are the (1) safety data sheets (SDSs), (2) specific hazards of each chemical, and (3) labeling requirements. The organization must also develop a chemical spill control and cleanup plan.

107. D: The most important factor in a patient safety culture is communicating concerns. All members of the perioperative team should be encouraged to express their concerns and report any issues of safety without reprisals. All team members should be treated with respect and encouraged to be honest, while still being held responsible for their behavior. They must also be provided with incredible supportive leadership and opportunities for shared decision making.

108. A: Fat embolism syndrome is a life-threatening complication that can occur when fat droplets are released into the blood vessels. These droplets can then become lodged in the lungs (resulting in respiratory distress), the brain (resulting in altered mental status), and the small vessels of the skin (resulting in a petechial rash). Fat embolism syndrome usually results from orthopedic trauma, especially of the long bones such as the femur, and can occur because of manipulation during the surgical procedure. Onset of symptoms is usually evident from 12 hours to 14 days after the event.

109. C: If a patient scheduled for surgery has been assessed by the anesthesiologist and classified under the American Society of Anesthesiologists (ASA) Physical Status Classification as ASA III, this indicates that the patient has severe systemic disease with considerable functional limitations. Patients who fit into this classification may have poorly controlled chronic obstructive pulmonary disease, diabetes mellitus, hypertension, active hepatitis, morbid obesity (≥40 body mass index [BMI]), substance abuse, end-stage renal disease with dialysis, or recent history of myocardial infarction (MI), cerebrovascular accident (CVA), transient ischemic attack (TIA), or coronary artery disease (CAD)/stents.

110. B: Following a procedure carried out with moderate sedation, the patient is usually ready to transfer from the PACU when the Aldrete score is 8–10. The score is based on five parameters—activity, respiration, circulation, consciousness, and oxygen saturation—scored from 0 to 2 (optimal). The patient is scored on admission to the PACU and at least every 30 minutes during the stay and again on discharge. Those three points below baseline are usually maintained with one-on-one nursing care with vital signs being checked every 5 minutes, 2 points below baseline checked every 15 minutes, and 1 point below baseline checked every 15–30 minutes.

111. A: AORN recommendations are that hair should generally be left in place during surgical procedures because shaving increases the risk of infection. However, in some cases, such as with a very hirsute individual, hair removal may be needed. In that case, the hair should be removed as close as possible to the time of surgery but not in the operating room. Clipping or the use of depilatory methods is preferred; razors should be avoided. The amount of hair removed should be kept to a minimum.

112. C: Reiki reduces stress and induces relaxation through gentle touch. The practitioner gently places the hands, without pressure, on different areas of the face and torso (front and back), holding them in place for a few minutes at each position. Touch may be applied to the limbs as well, especially if there is an injury or pain. Some practitioners hold their hands close to but not touching the skin. Typically, the patient is lying down or sitting in a chair during the therapy.

113. B: IV solution containers that have been spiked must be administered within 60 minutes in order to reduce the risk of infection, although studies have shown no bacterial growth for up to 8 hours. Any IV solution that remains at the end of a procedure and is not required for use must be discarded. No IV or irrigating solutions that are unused or opened can be reused for another patient. After an IV container has been spiked, according to the CDC, the fluids remain stable for 24 hours.

114. C: The purpose of surgical site marking is to ensure that the surgical procedure is carried out in the appropriate location. This is especially important with procedures that could be done on either side, such as a mastectomy. The marking should be done by the surgeon or an authorized member of the surgical team, and it should not be ambiguous. Dots, circles, lines, and arrows should be avoided. An X over the site is an appropriate marking, and the professional marking the site should always include his or her initials.

115. D: Because equipment noise is necessary to ensure that the equipment is functioning properly, it is an essential external distraction in the operating room. Distractions may be essential or nonessential. Other essential external distractions include alarms, timers, telephones, and pagers. Nonessential external distractions include music, non–surgical-related conversation, and interruptions unrelated to the surgical procedure or the needs/concerns of the perioperative team members.

116. A: Different parts of the GI tract tend to have different pH levels:

- Gastric placement: The pH ranges from 1 to 5.5.
- Intestinal placement: The pH ranges from 6 to 8; therefore, a pH of 6 indicates that the nasogastric tube is likely positioned in the small intestine.
- Respiratory placement: The pH is usually greater than 7.

Note that a gastric acid inhibitor may increase the pH to greater than 5.5 even though the nasogastric tube is correctly placed in the stomach, and a false-positive result may occur if placement is in the esophagus, where the pH is typically less than 5.5.

117. D: A chemical sterilant is ≥2.4% glutaraldehyde solution. Sterilants must destroy all microorganisms, including bacterial spores. Methods of sterilization include:

- High temperature: Steam (40 minutes), dry heat (1–6 hours)
- Low temperature: Ethylene oxide gas, hydrogen peroxide gas plasma, ozone, hydrogen peroxide vapor
- Liquid immersion (chemical): As above, 1.12% glutaraldehyde with 1.93% phenol, 7.35% hydrogen peroxide with 0.23% peracetic acid, and multiple other solutions

118. D: Following surgery on a patient with a methicillin-resistant *Staphylococcus aureus* infection, the operating room should undergo enhanced cleaning. This means that in addition to the routine cleaning done after every surgery, all high-touch areas and items in the room must be cleaned. This includes push plates, door handles, light switches, communication devices, computer accessories, privacy curtains, trash receptacles, linen receptacles, furniture, stools, supply charts, chairs, and storage cabinets.

119. C: When packaging sterile instrument sets, the total weight of the sterile packaging system and contents should not exceed 25 pounds. Packages greater than 25 pounds are difficult to adequately dry, and heavy weights pose ergonomic concerns. Additionally, large sterile packages are more difficult to store and more likely to be dropped, resulting in the need for resterilization.

120. D: HIPAA (1996) addresses the rights of the individual related to privacy of health information. ADA (1992) is civil rights legislation that provides the disabled, including those with mental impairment, access to employment and the community. The PSDA (1991) gives patients the rights to make their own medical decisions, refuse treatment, and create an advance medical directive. The PPACA (2010) reforms health insurance laws and extends coverage to those with preexisting conditions and expands drug coverage.

121. B: Placing all of the contaminated, discarded, and disposable items in the hazardous waste bags for disposal is a wasteful and costly practice. Hazardous waste bags are of thicker material than other waste bags, so they are more expensive, but they also require different handling, storage, transport, and disposal methods that must meet regulatory requirements. All of these things add to the cost. Additionally, many discarded items, such as solution bottles, in the surgical area can be recycled, improving environmental stewardship.

122. C: The functions of the stomach include the receipt and storage of ingested materials. The stomach digests these substances using gastric lipase, pepsinogen, hydrochloric acid, gastrin, and intrinsic factor, which aids in the absorption of vitamin B_{12}. Alcohol is absorbed in the stomach, but *most* other ingested substances are absorbed in the small intestine. Peristalsis mixes and moves the stomach contents, or *chyme*, into the duodenum at a controlled rate.

123. A: The Perioperative Nursing Data Set (PNDS) begins with outcomes, which are then defined and interpreted, and criteria are provided to measure the outcomes. Nursing interventions and actions are noted as well. The PNDS is a structured vocabulary specifically developed for perioperative nursing care. PNDS presents a controlled method of collecting and documenting information about patients so there is standardization, consistency, and clarity, thereby reducing the risk of errors.

124. B: When assessing the patient's physiological response and depth of sedation, the nurse notes that the patient has adequate ventilation and cardiovascular function without intervention and has a purposeful response to verbal or tactile stimulation; this is consistent with moderate sedation. Depths of sedation/analgesia are as follows:

- Minimal: Normal responses.
- Moderate: As above.
- Deep: Purposeful response after repeated/painful stimulation. The airway, ventilation, and cardiovascular function may need support.
- General anesthesia: Not able to be aroused; the respiratory and cardiovascular systems may need support.

125. D: A patient with an Aldrete score of 7 will usually remain in the PACU until the score is 8-20. The Aldrete score, commonly used in PACUs, is based on 5 parameters—activity, respiration, circulation, consciousness, and oxygen saturation—scored 0-2 (optimal). The patient is usually scored on admission to the PACU and at least every 30 minutes during the stay and again on discharge. Those 3 points below baseline are usually maintained with one-on-one nursing care with vital signs checked every 5 minutes, 2 points below baseline checked every 15 minutes, and 1 point below baseline checked every 15-30 minutes.

126. B: If a patient's surgery is delayed because the bariatric surgical bed that the patient needs is not ready yet, the most appropriate way to communicate this information to the patient is, "The operating room is not ready for you yet." It is important to treat patients with respect and to support their privacy. If the patient is in a waiting area with other people present, then comments about the patient's size are not only insensitive but may be overheard by other people. Additionally, pointing out that a patient is overweight serves no purpose.

127. C: If a patient is scheduled for laser perineal surgery, the precaution that is necessary to decrease the risk of fire is to use moistened radiopaque sponges as a rectal packing (or an anal covering) to prevent the escape of methane gas, which is flammable and can ignite when exposed to a laser beam. Water-soluble lubricant should be used on the skin near the surgical site, and moistened (and periodically remoistened) material should be used around the surgical site as well.

128. C: The relative humidity in the operating rooms should be maintained between 20-60% with a maximum of 60% in sterile storage rooms. However, it may be difficult to maintain this range in some geographic areas when humidity is very high or very low. Maintaining humidity at the appropriate range is necessary to prevent growth of microorganisms, provide comfort to the operating room staff, and prevent electrostatic discharge.

129. A: If a patient has a cochlear implant, use of monopolar electrosurgery should be limited to below the clavicles, and the dispersive electrode must also be placed below the clavicles. Before surgery begins, all external components must be removed and no electrosurgical device (including bipolar devices, which can be used above the clavicles) can be used within 1–2 cm of the implant generator electrodes.

130. A: The correct procedure for removing chemical indicator tape from a sterilized pack is to tear the tape into two pieces to ensure that the package cannot be retaped. Then, the pieces of tape should be completely removed from the reusable wrappings so they are not inadvertently left on during laundering, which can interfere with sterilization processes. The tape can be left in place on disposable wrappings. The chemical indicator tape should always be the first tape torn so it is clear that the pack has been breached.

131. A: In perioperative care, methods to prevent or treat hypothermia should be used for all patients during all phases of care because all patients are at risk. The method chosen to maintain normothermia depends on various factors (age, gender, cardiovascular condition, body surface area, preexisting medical conditions, type of surgery and anesthesia, positioning, use of a pneumatic tourniquet) but may include active or passive warming or insulation.

132. D: The radiation that emanates from the x-ray equipment/housing is referred to as leakage radiation. This radiation may leak through the shielding that is provided. Other types of radiation include:

- Primary radiation: This is the radiation that emanates directly from the equipment, such as when an x-ray is performed.
- Scatter radiation: This is the radiation that reflects off of other surfaces, including the patient's body.

133. C: Symptomatic bradycardia can lead to serious arrhythmias, heart failure, and cardiac arrest. The initial emergent treatment is with atropine, administering a 1 mg bolus repeated every 3–5 minutes to a maximum dosage of 3 mg. If atropine is ineffective in increasing the heart rate, then a dopamine infusion of 5–20 mcg/kg per minute is administered, titrated, and tapered. Epinephrine is given per infusion at 2–10 mcg per minute and titrated to the patient's response.

134. D: When labeling an autograft package, if the specimen has not been tested for infectious diseases, the labeling should state, "Not evaluated for infectious substances." If testing was carried out and the findings were positive, then the labeling should contain a biohazard symbol and state, "Warning: Reactive test results for [pathogenic agent]." The package should also state, "For autologous use only" and be labeled with the patient's name and medical record number and the type of tissue.

135. A: Cell salvage, which allows for the patient's own blood to be collected and reinfused, is acceptable to some Jehovah's Witnesses because it is considered an extension of the patient's own circulatory system; however, many patients will refuse a transfusion if blood is saved for future use, such as in preparation for surgery. In lieu of transfusions, volume expanders, such as crystalloids and colloids, and hemostatic agents, such as tranexamic acid, may be used.

136. C: According to the NRC and the Code of Federal Regulations Standards for Protection Against Radiation, the total effective dose equivalent for the whole body for radiation workers is 5 rem. A rem (roentgen equivalent man) is the unit used to measure radiation applied to human beings, such as when receiving x-rays. Dosages that exceed 100 rem over a short duration will cause acute radiation syndrome.

137. C: The Reason Model has 6 steps and is designed to determine if an individual responsible for an untoward event, such as injury to a patient, is culpable for the incident.

10. Establish intent: Was action deliberate?
11. Determine whether substance abuse is involved.
12. Determine if the person knowingly violated procedures: Includes assessment as to whether violation of the procedure is common.
13. Do a substitution test: Ask peers if they would have done the same. If so, the error is systems-induced.
14. Determine history of unsafe actions.
15. Examine mitigating circumstances.

138. B: If a near-miss situation regarding patient safety has occurred and the perioperative team is conducting a brief safety huddle, an appropriate first question is, "What happened to threaten patient safety?" It is important that all members of the team have a clear idea of the problem. Follow-up questions include asking what should have happened, what accounted for the difference in what did happen and what should have happened, what corrective actions to take, how to avoid a similar situation in the future, what the follow-up plan is, and who will implement the follow-up plan.

139. B: HCIRs are not required to have CPR training but must demonstrate training and certification in the following areas:

- Product: Must be familiar with all aspects of the product and able to instruct others in use, demonstrate, and supervise.
- Bloodborne pathogens: Must understand and use universal, standard, and contact precautions as indicated, including the use of PPE.

- HIPAA: Must understand the regulations regarding patient privacy and confidentiality.
- OR protocol: Must understand standard protocols for different types of procedures, responsibilities of sterile and nonsterile teams, waste disposal, and infection control.

140. A: When eschar builds up on the nonstick-coated tip of an electrosurgical unit, it should be cleaned with a sterile sponge moistened with sterile water or an instrument wipe. Abrasive pads should be avoided with nonstick surfaces because they may cause grooves, resulting in increased eschar buildup. The tips should be cleaned frequently because the eschar increases electrical impedance and may result in a spark that ignites the eschar.

141. C: Because personal smartphones lack the security and encryption necessary to comply with HIPAA regulations, they should never be used to record information about patients, even temporarily. Doing so could result in a breach of privacy and confidentiality and is noncompliant with HIPAA regulations. Additionally, transcribing information from one device to another may result in increased potential for errors. Documentation should be done in the health record (paper or electronic) as soon as a treatment or observations are completed whenever possible.

142. D: This cardiac monitoring tracing indicates atrial fibrillation. The Watchman device is implanted into the left atrial appendage to control atrial fibrillation; however, in the early postoperative period, ECG abnormalities are common. These abnormalities include atrial fibrillation, atrial flutter, premature atrial contractions, ST-T wave changes, and ventricular and supraventricular arrhythmias. These dysrhythmias are typically temporary and resolve as the heart recovers from the procedure. If dysrhythmias are persistent, they can reduce cardiac output and may require intervention.

143. D: Although checking the tympanic membrane site with an infrared sensor provides a rapid temperature reading, it should be avoided in perioperative patients because the results are often inaccurate. To access the core temperature, the infrared probe must be able to reach deep into the aural canal, which it does not on current models. While the site may be used to screen for fever in pediatric patients and is more accurate in those patients to detect mild hypothermia, it needs to be followed up with a more accurate measuring probe to determine the true core temperature, as it often reads low.

144. C: If, during an operative procedure, a specimen containing a radioactive seed is excised, the location of the seed should be verified by a handheld radiation detection device and a radiograph. All seeds have to be accounted for, but handheld radiation detection devices cannot distinguish between seed locations unless they are at least 1.1 inches (2.8 cm) apart. Radiographs are generally taken intraoperatively to ensure that the seeds have been removed. All seeds should be accounted for before breakdown of the Mayo stand and instrument tables.

145. C: If reusable surgical attire is contaminated with blood or other body fluids, it must be bagged but not rinsed, sorted, or pretreated because this may expose the perioperative team member to infectious material. Surgical attire must remain at the workplace and cannot be taken home for laundering. If surgical attire has been penetrated by potentially infectious material, it should be changed as soon as possible to prevent infection. Any personal clothing (such as undergarments) that are contaminated with blood or other potentially infectious materials must be removed at the place of work and remain there for laundering.

146. B: Critical water should have a pH level in the range of 5–7. A pH of 7 is neutral, so a pH reading below 7 is acidic and one above 7 is basic (or alkaline). Utility water, on the other hand, has a pH level of 6–9. Utility water is most often used for decontamination and critical water for final rinsing. Disinfectants are affected by the pH of the water. For example, glutaraldehyde has improved antimicrobial action with increased pH, but hypochlorites have decreased antimicrobial action.

147. A: Developing headache, tachypnea, tachycardia, lightheadedness, decreasing oxygen saturation, and cyanosis 90 minutes after exposure to local anesthesia is consistent with methemoglobinemia. The medication the nurse should anticipate that the physician will order is methylene blue. The patient should receive high-flow oxygen and have an IV line inserted because methylene blue is administered intravenously. Laboratory testing typically includes arterial blood gases and complete blood count.

148. B: When using a brush in the decontamination area to clean soiled surgical instruments, it is necessary to brush under cool water. Brushing must be done under the water to avoid aerosolizing any chemicals or contaminants. Cool water is used because warm water denatures protein and coagulates blood, making them more difficult to remove. Lumens should be flushed and brushed the length of the lumen with the type, size, and material specified by the IFU.

149. B: With a hysteroscopy, the use of dextran, a high-viscosity fluid media, as an irrigating or distension media should be limited to a volume that does not exceed 500 mL. In fact, the recommended volume is 300 mL. Dextran (commonly 32% dextran 70) is a plasma expander and can lead to fluid overload, disseminated intravascular coagulation, overdose, pulmonary edema, increased bleeding time, and impaired platelet function. Because dextran does not mix with blood, bleeding is more easily seen.

150. A: When disposing of bodily waste with low levels of radioactivity, the appropriate method is to dilute and disperse, such as by emptying into the toilet and by double flushing into the sewer system. If bodily wastes have high levels of radiation, the delay and decay method (holding until radiation levels decrease) is used. A concentrate and contain method is rarely used because it is intended for wastes with very high levels of radiation. In this case, waste is contained and buried in an appropriate site. Some types of hazardous waste may be incinerated or returned to the vendor.

151. B: When reviewing a patient's history, the finding that should alert the nurse to a risk of the development of postoperative nausea and vomiting is a history of migraines. Other risk factors include female gender, history of being a nonsmoker, history of motion sickness, history of previous postoperative nausea and vomiting, dehydration, anxiety, and gastroparesis. Patients who receive opioids or nitric oxide also are at increased risk. Some surgical procedures also include risk, such as those involving the head (eyes, ears, nose, and throat), gastrointestinal (GI) tract procedures, gynecologic procedures, breast procedures, and laparoscopic procedures.

152. D: Before using a sterile pack, the nurse should always check the load control label because it typically lists the date of sterilization, expiration date, sterilizer used, and load control number. The load control number is an important factor in inventory control, ensuring that packs are rotated so that those with the earliest dates are used first before their expiration dates so that the instruments and materials in the packs do not need to be resterilized, which wastes time and increases energy costs.

153. A: The Richmond Agitation-Sedation Scale (RASS) assesses a patient's level of sedation. It is a 10-point scale ranging from +4 to –5. A score of 0 indicates that the patient is alert and calm.

Less Sedated	More Sedated
+4 combative	–5 unarousable
+3 very agitated	–4 deep sedation
+2 agitated	–3 moderate sedation
+1 restless	–2 light sedation
0 alert and calm	–1 drowsy

Steps to using the RASS begin with observing the patient, and they progress to asking the patient to state his or her name and open the eyes, and finally to physically stimulating the patient if there is no response to voice commands.

154. B: Visiting Nurse Association provides medical and personal care to patients who are homebound and unable to care for themselves. Public health departments offer vaccinations and various clinics. Nurses may visit people with communicable diseases, such as tuberculosis, but do not provide general medical or personal care. Social Services agencies have social workers who can evaluate a person's ability to remain independent, determine if abuse is occurring, and help provide financial support for the needy. Senior Citizens' organizations vary widely but usually offer social services, such as classes and activities.

155. C: The anatomical structures that pose the greatest risk of fire include the bowels and the trachea. The bowels may contain flammable gases, such as methane and hydrogen, and the anesthetic gases in the trachea are oxygen rich. In these areas, use of electrosurgical active electrodes should be avoided in favor of a scalpel or another method of creating an incision in order to minimize the risk of an ignition.

156. C: If a patient is to have open reduction and internal fixation surgery of a fracture of the femoral shaft, skin prep should extend from the umbilicus to below the knee. The prep should begin at the site of the fracture and extend outward from there. The prep should extend laterally to the operating room bed. During draping, a fluid-control drape, which contains a pouch to collect fluids, is recommended to prevent strike-through contamination of the sterile field from irrigant used during the procedure.

157. B: Screening is an important aspect of vertical perioperative decolonization. Vertical (or targeted) decolonization is focused on reducing a specific pathogen, such as *Staphylococcus aureus,* and it may include nasal and skin decolonization and contact precautions for a select group of patients. Horizontal perioperative decolonization, on the other hand, is focused on universal decolonization and typically includes nasal decolonization, chlorhexidine gluconate bathing, hand hygiene, and PPE. Blended perioperative decolonization uses some aspects of both.

158. D: Scribes document dictated patient information for only one healthcare provider at a time; they cannot document for multiple members of the surgical team. Scribes cannot participate in any procedures or patient care and cannot communicate dictated orders, which must be done directly by the healthcare provider. The scribe does not make independent notes. All documentation done by the scribe must be reviewed by the healthcare provider for accuracy because the healthcare provider is responsible for that documentation. Records must be signed by both the scribe and the healthcare provider.

159. A: Although remaining supportive and monitoring a parent's well-being are important, the primary role of the operating room nurse is to ensure that the parent is prepared to be in the operating room with the child. The parent must be properly attired and should be educated about what to expect in the operating room environment (e.g., its general setup and any special equipment) and about the induction process as well as what the parent's role is during that process and when the parent will exit. A staff member should be assigned to escort the parent in and out of the operating room.

160. D: A cost-benefit analysis uses average cost of an event and the cost of intervention to demonstrate savings. Cost-utility analysis (CUA) is essentially a subtype of cost-effective analysis, but it is more complex and the results are more difficult to quantify and use to justify expense because CUA measures benefit to society in general. An efficacy study may compare a series of cost-benefit analyses to determine the intervention with the best cost-benefit. A cost-effective analysis measures the effectiveness of an intervention rather than the monetary savings.

161. A: There are numerous handoff methods used to ensure that no important information is neglected during the transfer of patients from the operating room to the postanesthesia care unit or the ICU. One method is the five P handover:

- Patient: Demographic information, current condition, existence of a do-not-resuscitate order, reason for operative procedure, important medications, allergies.
- Plan: Goals of surgery and detailed postoperative care plan, pertinent past history, patient status, abnormalities.
- Purpose: Rationale for the plan of care.
- Problems: Problems or potential complications, risk factors, or concerns.
- Precautions: Fall risk, problems with IV access, isolation requirements.

162. C: The recommended temperature range for operating rooms is 68-75 °F (20-24 °C). In some cases, the temperature may be maintained at the lower end of the scale because the equipment used during the operative procedure may generate heat and the surgical staff may become overheated from their gowns if the temperature is too high. A temperature range of 70-75 °F (21-24 °C) is commonly used to prevent patient hypothermia.

163. A: Natural rubber latex gloves provide the best protection for glove punctures because they are more elastic. The bacterial passage through neoprene and nitrile is 10 times higher than through latex. Thermoplastic elastomer gloves are thinner and less resistant to mechanical damage. Powdered latex gloves are most likely to contribute to latex allergies, but the risk is lessened with low-protein latex gloves.

164. D: After steam sterilization and removal of the sterilization rack from the chamber, sterilized items can be removed when cooled to room temperature. The items should cool on the rack. The duration of time needed for the cooldown will vary depending on the initial temperature, the load, and the packing material. Warm or hot items should not be placed on cold surfaces. Before handling the sterilized items, the temperature should be checked with an infrared or similar thermometer.

165. C: The nasopharynx is one of several sites that provide reliable core temperatures before, during and after surgery. These sites include:

- Tympanic membrane: Accurate when measured by a thermocouple (not when by a standard thermometer which does not reach deep into the canal) and preferred for presurgical and postsurgical monitoring.
- Distal esophagus: Often used intraoperatively with probe in the distal portion of esophagus.
- Nasopharynx: Measured by thermistor probe inserted 10 to 20 cm into the nares.
- Pulmonary artery: The most accurate but most invasive.

Less reliable sites include axillary (wide variations due to operating room temperatures), bladder (close to core temperature but difficult to get during surgery), oral (close to core but does not detect malignant hyperthermia and inaccurate when the patient is intubated), rectal (close to core temperature but difficult to access), skin (wide variations), and temporal artery (unreliable).

166. D: If a formula-fed infant is scheduled for surgery, the minimal nothing-by-mouth (NPO) fasting guideline for infant formula is 6 hours. The stomach typically empties within 4–6 hours after ingestion, although this may vary somewhat. NPO status often starts at midnight before the scheduled procedure, although this length of time is not generally necessary.

Substance	Minimal Fasting (hours)
Clear liquids (water, apple juice, tea)	2
Breast milk	4
Milk (cow, goat, etc.)	6
Infant formula	6
Light meal	6

167. A: If using charting by exception, it is critically important to accurately record baseline data because subsequent charting is based on identifying deviations from the baseline. When deviations occur, they should be detailed in narrative form even though most documentation is through check marks/initials to indicate no deviation. Vital signs, even if they are stable, are typically documented. Charting by exception streamlines documentation and saves time by reducing duplication of information, but it does require training and development of protocols and standards.

168. C: An unexplained anaphylactic reaction while receiving treatment in the emergency department for flu should trigger an evaluation for latex allergy. Other triggers include a history of multiple surgeries or contact with healthcare institutions or workplaces in which recurrent exposure to latex may have occurred. Additionally, cross-reactivity allergic reactions may occur in those allergic to kiwi, bananas, avocadoes, pineapples, stone fruits, tomatoes, and raw potatoes.

169. D: If, during administration of local anesthesia, vasoconstrictor-induced ischemia occurs, the emergent treatment is phentolamine (1 mg/mL). This condition may occur with the "wide-awake, local anesthesia, no tourniquet technique" used for hand surgery. During this technique, a local anesthesia, such as lidocaine or bupivacaine, is used along with epinephrine for hemostasis. Phentolamine reverses the vasoconstrictive effects of the epinephrine.

170. B: When carrying out hand hygiene with soap and water, after wetting the hands and applying soap, the hands must be rubbed together vigorously for at least 15 seconds. All jewelry should be removed from the hands and wrist (including watches) before washing. After completing the soap scrub, the hands are rinsed with water and dried with a disposable towel. If using an alcohol-based rub, the hands should be rubbed together until the alcohol is completely dry.

171. D: When preparing a patient for surgery on the right hand, the nurse notes that there is no marking on the site even though this is required by protocol; the most appropriate response is to hold the procedure until the surgeon verifies the correct site. The site must be marked by the person who will carry out the surgery and must be done consistently for every surgical procedure to ensure safety. Marking the site is required by the Universal Protocol for Preventing Wrong Site, Wrong Procedure, Wrong Person Surgery.

172. B: Dysfunction of cranial nerves IX (glossopharyngeal) and X (vagus) can place the patient at increased risk for aspiration during anesthetic induction and extubation because these nerves control swallowing and the gag reflex. Additionally, cranial nerve X dysfunction can affect breathing patterns. Risk of corneal injury occurs with dysfunction of cranial nerve VII (facial). If cranial nerve V (trigeminal) is dysfunctional, this can impair the sensation in the face and may result in facial injuries with pain and palsy.

173. B: If the bispectral index system (BIS) is used with a patient to monitor the sedation level, the index level that is considered optimal anesthesia is 40-60. BIS measures the frequency of brain signals with a range of 0-100. Although the BIS monitors the hypnotic status of the brain, it provides less information about analgesia. The BIS allows anesthesia to be more accurately titrated to the needs of the individual patient.

174. B: The medication most commonly used for nasal decolonization is topical mupirocin 2%. Although protocols vary, application of mupirocin twice daily for 5 days is common. Nasal colonization is usually combined with preoperative bathing with soap or with an antiseptic such as chlorhexidine gluconate. The number of baths varies according to protocol, but the current recommendation is that the patient should bathe at least once the night before surgery or the morning of surgery. For procedures of the head or neck, patients should shampoo the hair.

175. D: Reservoirs of critical water used in the cleaning and reprocessing of instruments should be cleaned every 2 months because tanks that hold water may become contaminated and biofilms can form. Once a biofilm has developed, its removal can be difficult. The water quality should be checked frequently to ensure that the pH level is correct and has the appropriate mineral content.

176. B: If graduated compression stockings are applied to a patient and a reverse gradient occurs, this means that the proximal pressure is higher than the distal pressure, creating a tourniquet effect. To promote venous circulation, the distal pressure should be higher than the proximal pressure. If a reverse gradient occurs, this increases the risk of VTE. Improperly fitted or folded down compression stockings may result in a proximal indentation and a reverse gradient.

177. A: If a patient scheduled for moderate sedation has a history of sleep apnea, a necessary precaution is to prepare for possible noninvasive positive pressure ventilation during the procedure. Moderate sedation may cause the muscles of the throat to relax, resulting in complete or partial collapse of the airway. Continuous positive airway pressure or bilevel positive airway pressure may be necessary to prevent hypoxia. Opioids and other nonopioid analgesics must be carefully titrated because of their depressant effects on the respiratory system.

178. B: When the circulating nurse transfers a medication to the sterile field, the person receiving the medication must concurrently verify the name, strength, dosage, and expiration date. Only one medication can be transferred at a time, and medications should be transferred as close to the time of use as possible. Transfer devices should be used to place liquid medications into a secondary container on the sterile field in order to minimize splashing or spilling.

179. C: If, during the preoperative assessment, the patient reports taking routine morning medications before coming to the ambulatory surgery center, the medication that may be cause for concern is ibuprofen. NSAIDs should be discontinued 4 days before surgery, aspirin a week before surgery, and warfarin 3 days before surgery. It is common for patients to be advised to take one-quarter to one-half of the usual dosage of insulin the morning of surgery, but this may vary.

180. A: The AVPU scale is used to assess the level of consciousness at a point in time. Any point on the scale below A (i.e., V, P, or U) is considered abnormal. The AVPU scale does not quantify the level of consciousness because no score is assigned.

A	Alert and awake; oriented to person, place, time, and condition. Can follow commands, open eyes, track objects.	Yes	No
V	Responds to verbal stimuli; does not open eyes spontaneously.	Yes	No
P	Responds to painful stimuli but not to verbal stimuli.	Yes	No
U	Unconscious; does to respond to painful or verbal stimuli.	Yes	No

181. B: For patients with body piercings, the nurse should verify removal by checking the sites and documenting the sites of piercings as scar tissue may form and interfere with incisions. While procedures vary, in general, all jewelry, including that of body piercings, should be removed prior to surgery to avoid trauma or injury. All patients should be asked about body piercings as many, such as genital piercings, are not visible. With general anesthesia, all facial jewelry must be removed because it may interfere with intubation and oxygen masks.

182. D: Cushing's triad (i.e., bradycardia, hypertension with widened pulse pressure, and irregular respirations) is an indication of brain stem herniation, which is the result of increased intracranial pressure (ICP), usually from swelling or bleeding in the brain. Increased ICP can occur with subdural and epidural hematoma if bleeding is significant. The normal ICP level is 7–15 mmHg, and treatment to lower the ICP is usually initiated for ICP levels greater than 20–25 mmHg. With increasing ICP, the patient will lose all brain stem reflexes and eventually go into cardiac and respiratory arrest if the increased ICP is not immediately reduced.

183. C: If a solution is used to irrigate a surgical wound during an operative procedure, the maximum temperature of the solution should be no more than 104 °F (40 °C) (acceptable range: 91.4-104 °F [33-40 °C]) when used. Fluids should always be warmed before irrigation. If the irrigant is poured into a second container for use during surgery, some temperature loss occurs; therefore, if extensive irrigation is needed for a long procedure, then an irrigant warmer that keeps the fluid at a stable temperature should be used.

184. C: If, during the initial count, a standard 10-pack of surgical sponges is found to contain only 9 sponges, the correct response is to exclude the pack from the count and remove it from the field. Additionally, the pack should be isolated from countable items in the operating room and it should be labeled as to the discrepancy. If the patient has not yet entered the operating room, then the pack with the incorrect number of sponges can be removed from the room before the patient arrives.

185. D: The individual who has primary responsibility for initiating the counting process of surgical items before a surgical procedure is the circulating nurse. This individual should survey the room before the initial count to ensure that there are no items present from a previous procedure and initiate the counting process while viewing each item as it is counted. The count should be recorded in a visible location (e.g., on a whiteboard). The circulating nurse should check whether any items were dropped on the floor and conduct the closing count, reporting any discrepancies.

186. D: The dispersive electrode for an electrosurgical unit should be placed over a large perfused muscle mass. It should also be on the same side and as close as possible to the operative site so that the current has a short distance to travel before exiting the body. The dispersive electrode should not be placed over a bony prominence, scar tissue, skin folds, hairy areas, or distal to tourniquets, and it should not be placed over an implant containing metal.

187. D: Documentation regarding exposure incidents have to be maintained for the duration of the employee's employment and an additional 30 years. All exposures to blood, body fluids, or potentially infectious materials must be reported as soon as possible and documented. Documentation should include the route of exposure, description of the event, employee's name and social security number and vaccination status. If the source person's serological status is known, that should be documented as well. The results of all treatments should be recorded.

188. B: When preparing a 5-year-old child for a surgical procedure, the explanation to the child that is most appropriate is, "While you are sleeping, the doctor will make a small opening to remove that lump." Children are typically fearful of hospitals and procedures, and words such as "cut" and "pain" should be avoided. It is better to say that the child may be a little "sore" after the procedure because that is less frightening. Children need age-appropriate information and should not be told not to worry (which gives them no information) or that they will wake up and feel fine because this may not be true.

189. B: Although all of these nursing diagnoses (i.e., ineffective health maintenance, risk for injury, and risk for poisoning) may be appropriate for a patient with substance abuse, ineffective coping specifically addresses the issue of using drugs to relieve anxiety. This is a maladaptive coping mechanism. The nurse should respond with empathy and explore coping strategies (both positive and negative) that the patient has previously used in order to introduce healthy coping skills. The nurse should also help the patient identify the stressors that lead to ineffective coping.

190. C: 24%.

Rockall Risk Scoring System after Upper GI Tract Bleeding				
Risk factor	0	1	2	3
Age	<60	60–79	≥80	---
Shock	None	SBP >100, HR ≥100	SBP <100	
Comorbidities	None	---	Ischemic heart disease, cardiac failure, major disease	Renal/Liver failure Cancer metastasis
Endoscopic diagnosis	Mallory-Weiss tear, no recent bleeding	All other diagnoses	Upper GI tract malignancy	---
Evidence of bleeding	None	---	Blood in the upper GI tract, adherent clot, spurting blood vessel	---

Scores and approximate risk for rebleeding are as follows: 0 = 5%, 1 = 3.5%, 2 = 5.3%, 3 = 11%, 4 = 14%, 5 = 24%, 6 = 33%, and 7 = 44%.

191. C: If a large amount of blood has spilled on the floor, the first step is to apply an appropriate EPA-registered disinfectant (one that is effective against bloodborne pathogens) to decrease the risk of transmission. The next step is to use absorbent material (gel, lint-free towel) to confine the spill and then to clean and discard the material. Once the blood is removed, the surface must be thoroughly cleaned and disinfected. If an Environmental Protection Agency (EPA)-registered disinfectant is not available, a 1:100 dilution of sodium hypochlorite can be applied to small spills (<10 mL) and a 1:10 dilution to larger spills.

192. B: Heparin-induced thrombocytopenia is an immune-mediation adverse reaction to heparin that typically occurs 5–14 days after initiation of therapy, although it can occur within hours if the patient has previously been treated with heparin. Signs include the following:

- Thrombocytopenia: Drop by greater than 50% from base, although may still be within normal range in some patients
- Thrombosis: Deep vein thrombosis, pulmonary embolism, arterial thrombosis
- Skin reactions: Lesions at the injection site

Treatment includes discontinuation of heparin and administration of direct thrombin inhibitors, such as lepirudin and argatroban.

193. C: In an operating room, the vicinity of care extends 6 feet beyond the usual position of the operating bed and extends vertically above the bed at least 7.5 feet. This is the space intended for the care and treatment of a patient. Therefore, when disposing of flammable wet antiseptic materials after skin prep, the materials should be disposed of outside this vicinity of care to reduce the risk of fire. It is not necessary to remove these materials from the operating room.

194. D: Class 3B and class 4 lasers pose the greatest risk of materials burn hazard. Classes range from class 1, which poses few risks with exposure, to class 4, which poses the greatest risk. Classes are as follows:

- 1: No materials burn hazard
- 1M: Possible materials burn hazard under collecting optics such as microscopes
- 2: Laser is visible, but no materials burn hazard; eye protection is recommended
- 2M: Possible materials burn hazard under collecting optics
- 3R: Potential hazard if eyes are focused, though injury is minimal; no fire hazard
- 3B: Materials burn hazard if the beam is directed at close range for an extended period
- 4: Materials burn hazard when exposed to eyes or skin

Lightweight materials (paper, fabric) and dark materials burn most easily.

195. D: Risk factors for deep vein thrombosis (DVT) include age older than 50, a history of varicose veins, myocardial infarction, atrial fibrillation, cancer, ischemic stroke, previous DVT, diabetes, obesity, paralysis, and inhibitor deficiency state. A history of ovarian cysts does not increase the risk of DVT.

196. A: Coronary thrombosis. The five Ts of cardiac arrest are explained as follows:

Five Ts	Indications	Interventions
Cardiac tamponade	Tachycardia, narrow QRS, jugular venous distention, muffled heart sounds, absent pulse	Pericardiocentesis
Toxins	Prolonged QT interval	Specific to agent
Tension pneumothorax	Bradycardia, narrow QRS, tracheal deviation, asymmetric breathing, jugular venous distention	Needle decompression Chest tube insertion

Five Ts	Indications	Interventions
Pulmonary thrombosis	Tachycardia, dyspnea, narrow QRS, hypoxic, chest pain	Embolectomy, anticoagulation, fibrinolytic
Coronary thrombosis	ECG changes	Angioplasty, coronary artery bypass graft, stent

197. C: Nonoperative individuals in the operating room should avoid distracting the surgical team. In the case of a medical student who persists in making comments and asking questions during a surgical procedure, the nurse should advise the student of the importance of observing and remaining quiet but should encourage the student to make a list of questions and to hold the questions until after the surgical procedure has been completed. The nurse may also encourage the student to ask questions about the procedure beforehand.

198. B: Tissue vaporizes, producing surgical smoke when surgical energy devices (lasers, electrosurgical units, ultrasonic devices, and high-speed powered instruments) raise the intracellular temperature of the tissue to ≥212 °F (100 °C). Surgical smoke has a bad odor, is visible, and may contain toxic compounds (such as hydrogen cyanide and benzene), viruses, cancer cells, bacteria, dust particles, blood fragments, and water vapor.

199. A: Swallowing comprises three stages, but only the oral stage is voluntary. One or more stages may be impaired:

Stage	Description	Impairment
I—Oral	Preparatory phase: Food is held in the mouth, mixed with saliva, and chewed, forming a bolus. Propulsive phase: The bolus pushes against the hard palate and initiates the swallowing reflex.	Drooling, coughing or choking before swallowing. Unable to form a bolus.
II—Pharyngeal	The bolus enters the pharynx, the soft palate blocks the nasal passages, and the epiglottis covers the trachea.	Choking, coughing, delayed swallowing, gurgling, gagging.
III—Esophageal	The bolus moves from the esophagus to the stomach.	Bruxism, acidic breath, epigastric pain, regurgitation, vomiting.

200. B: If a cord is of insufficient length, the cord should be changed for a longer one. Extension cords should be avoided if possible because they increase the risk of falls and may cause overload of the electrical system or leakage of current. All cords in use should be safely secured with devices that can be cleaned or disposed of. Plugs should be hospital grade or have adequate strain relief. Electrical equipment, including cords and outlets, should be checked routinely and before each use and any damaged equipment repaired or replaced.

CNOR Practice Test #2

1. A patient with a traumatic crush injury to the lower leg is assessed for compartment syndrome. A fascial compartment pressure consistent with compartment syndrome is

a. 0-8 mmHg.
b. 10-12 mmHg.
c. 15-20 mmHg.
d. 30-40 mmHg.

2. Fatigue-reducing techniques should be used if the perioperative team member (not wearing a lead apron) stands in the same position continuously for more than:

a. 40 minutes
b. 60 minutes
c. 2 hours
d. 3 hours

3. The purpose of a neutral zone in surgery is to:

a. increase the speed of instrument transfer
b. decrease the risk of sharps injuries
c. facilitate transfer of instruments to the sterile field
d. facilitate communication among team members

4. Physician preference cards do which of the following?

a. list the physician's preferred sutures, dressings, special instruments, and equipment.
b. list the surgeon's phone number for questions.
c. list every instrument the surgeon may need.
d. list the physician's preferred staff.

5. Metoclopramide may be given as a preoperative medication in order to

a. relieve apprehension.
b. reduce risk of aspiration.
c. relieve discomfort.
d. to control secretions.

6. During invasive procedures, surgical gloves should be changed at least every:

a. 30–60 minutes
b. 60–90 minutes
c. 90–150 minutes
d. 120–180 minutes

7. Which of the following intraoperative positions most increases the risk of procedure-related VTE?

a. Excessive hip flexion
b. Trendelenburg position
c. Hyperextension of the elbow
d. Left lateral position

8. The Focused Assessment with Sonography for Trauma (FAST) is used primarily to assess

a. injury to solid organs.
b. retroperitoneal bleeding.
c. the source of bleeding.
d. internal bleeding or fluid accumulation.

9. During research, if staff members examine a testing instrument and agree that the instrument measures the intended concept, the instrument has

a. content validity.
b. face validity.
c. criterion-related validity.
d. construct validity.

10. Before transporting soiled instruments from the OR to the cleaning/decontamination area

a. soak in disinfecting solution.
b. rinse with cold water.
c. place in leak-proof container.
d. wipe with sponge saturated with normal saline.

11. All of the following should be placed in the sharps hazardous waste disposal container EXCEPT

a. needles.
b. saw blades.
c. partially empty medicine vial (rubber topped).
d. broken glass.

12. Bispectral index (BIS) is primarily used to monitor

a. anesthetic effects on consciousness.
b. cerebral ischemia.
c. head trauma.
d. hypothermia.

13. A patient scheduled for gastric bypass for obesity calls 2 days before surgery to ask if it is alright to get a tattoo on her arm. The best response is

a. "You are already at risk for infection because you are overweight, so you should wait."
b. "You absolutely should not get a tattoo!"
c. "A tattoo on the arm is all right because it won't interfere with surgery."
d. "Tattoos carry a risk of infection, so it's safer to wait until you've recovered from surgery."

14. With the Perioperative Nursing Data Set (PNDS), pain management is an element of

a. (D1) Safety.
b. (D2) Physiologic response to surgery.
c. (D3) Behavioral response to surgery.
d. (D4) Health system.

15. When the nurse asks a patient with advanced Parkinson's disease a question, the patient is very slow to respond, and the nurse wonders if the patient has understood. The best strategy is to

a. repeat the question slower and louder.
b. prompt the patient or suggest words.
c. wait patiently and give the person more time to respond.
d. ask the question in a different way.

16. The modified neutral zone may be indicated:

a. when the surgeon prefers it
b. when surgery is carried out under magnification
c. for procedures of duration longer than 1 hour
d. when the procedure requires many instruments

17. Following a coronary artery bypass graft procedure, the patient exhibits a tracheal deviation to the right with increased dyspnea, tachypnea, and tachycardia. Breath sounds are markedly decreased on the left. These signs and symptoms are consistent with

a. pleural effusion.
b. pneumothorax.
c. cardiac tamponade.
d. pulmonary embolism.

18. Under the American Society of Anesthesiologists (ASA) preoperative physical status classification, a status of P4 indicates

a. normal patient appears to be in good health.
b. systemic disease is present but mild.
c. systemic disease is severe and life-threatening.
d. patient is brain-dead.

19. Which of the following cleaning methods for operating rooms are the most environmentally friendly?

a. Chemical liquid disinfectants.
b. Steam cleaning methods.
c. Disposable wipes/mops.
d. Ultraviolet light disinfection.

20. If unsure how to properly clean a rigid sterilization container prior to use, the best recourse is to

a. ask another staff member.
b. clean it in the same manner as used for other containers.
c. refer to the manufacturer's instructions for use.
d. set it aside and use a different type of container.

21. If an organization has "deemed status," this means that:

a. it is exempt from some reporting requirements
b. it receives incentive payments for implementation of electronic health records
c. it can determine if a healthcare provider is in compliance with CMS regulations
d. it provides incentive payments for the implementation of electronic health records

22. A patient with a blunt chest injury is dyspneic and complains of pain in the upper abdomen, exacerbated by movement and deep breathing. There are decreased breath sounds on the left side with asymmetric chest movement, and bowel sounds are heard in the chest cavity. The nurse should suspect

a. pneumothorax.
b. pleural effusion.
c. diaphragmatic injury.
d. rib fractures.

23. Which model for performance improvement is easiest to apply when dealing with specific unit problems?

a. Plan-do-check-act.
b. Find-organize-clarify-uncover-start.
c. Six Sigma.
d. Lean Six Sigma.

24. Desflurane is contraindicated for induction for infants and children because of

a. increased risk of anesthesia-related hepatitis.
b. decreased cerebral metabolism.
c. decreased cardiac output.
d. upper airway complications.

25. A patient who experienced a motor vehicle accident complains of pain in the upper left abdomen radiating to the left shoulder (i.e., Kehr's sign) and dizziness. The patient exhibits hypotension; tachycardia; and cool, clammy skin. Kehr's sign is consistent with

a. pericardial effusion.
b. ruptured spleen.
c. aortic dissection.
d. diaphragmatic injury.

26. How close to the surgical site does the National Institute for Occupational Safety and Health recommend that smoke capture devices be located?

a. Within 5 cm (2 inches)
b. Within 10 cm (4 inches)
c. Within 15 cm (6 inches)
d. Within 20 cm (8 inches)

27. For a patient who has postoperative mechanical ventilation, in order to avoid toxicity, the fraction of inspired oxygen (FiO_2) should usually be maintained at

a. <30%.
b. <40%.
c. <50%.
d. <60%.

28. The purpose of separating sponges is

a. to ensure they are intact.
b. to make counting easier.
c. to facilitate use.
d. to promote better air circulation.

29. Which of the following is NOT true regarding discharge instructions?

a. Include the patient's medication instructions, dosage, schedule, diet, and physician's phone number.
b. Include the patient's wound care, signs of infection, and symptoms that require a call to a physician or a nurse practitioner.
c. Tell the patient when to make an appointment for follow-up care.
d. Remind the patient to call a physician or nurse practitioner if the wound itches or prickles.

30. When providing an interdisciplinary report about an adolescent patient who screamed at and threw an object at the nurse, the correct report is

a. the patient threw a screaming fit.
b. the patient screamed, "I hate shots," and threw a glass of water at the nurse.
c. the patient is obviously upset and angry.
d. the patient has been very uncooperative.

31. Following a total knee arthroplasty, which of the following side effects may indicate damage to the peroneal nerve?

a. Muscle cramps and tightness in the lower leg.
b. A burning, shooting pain down the lower leg.
c. Toe drag, slapping gait, and foot drop.
d. A continuous, dull, aching pain in the lower leg.

32. Which of the following roles is the perioperative nurse LEAST likely to assume?

a. Nurse anesthetist.
b. Scrub nurse.
c. RN First Assistant.
d. OR Manager.

33. The temperature in warming cabinets for blankets should not exceed

a. 98.6 °F (37 °C).
b. 110 °F (43.3 °C).
c. 130 °F (54 °C).
d. 150 °F (65.5 °C).

34. Which one of the following nerves is most commonly injured with a total hip arthroplasty?

a. Obturator nerve.
b. Femoral nerve.
c. Superior gluteal nerve.
d. Sciatic nerve.

35. To apply the 15-15 rule to treat mild to moderate hypoglycemia (54–70 mg/dL), a patient should be advised to consume 15 g of carbohydrate and then

a. repeat the carbohydrate dosage in 15 minutes.
b. repeat the carbohydrate dosage every 5 minutes for 15 minutes.
c. eat a small meal within 15 minutes.
d. recheck the blood glucose level in 15 minutes.

36. Which of the following is necessary when positioning a patient for bariatric surgery?

a. Padded footboard.
b. Padded headboard.
c. Side attachments.
d. Lift.

37. The initial medical treatment or drug of choice indicated for cardiac arrest related to pulseless electrical activity (PEA) or asystole (after initiating CPR) is

a. defibrillation.
b. epinephrine.
c. vasopressin.
d. atropine.

38. When documenting a subcutaneous injection, an acceptable abbreviation is

a. SC.
b. SQ.
c. Subcut.
d. sub q.

39. During the preoperative physical exam of a Hmong child, the nurse notes eight 2-inch reddened circles on the child's back. The nurse should

a. report the parents to Child Protective Services for abuse.
b. ask the parents if the child was treated with cupping.
c. immediately place the child on isolation.
d. take a skin culture.

40. The scope of practice of the perioperative nurse includes all of the following EXCEPT

a. admitting patients to the holding area.
b. assisting the physician during the surgical procedure.
c. providing critical care in the CCU after surgery.
d. providing postanesthesia care in the PACU.

41. The governmental agency responsible for bloodborne pathogens standard in medical institutions is

a. CDC.
b. OSHA.
c. EPA.
d. FDA.

42. When extending a patient's arm on an arm board, the arm should be placed in a supinated position (palm up) because this position:

a. decreases pressure on the median nerve
b. reduces risk to the brachial plexus
c. decreases pressure on the ulnar nerve
d. decreases pressure on the radial nerve

43. A patient suffered a severe blunt chest injury during an automobile accident and exhibits persistent hypotension despite no indication of ongoing blood loss as well as a drop of systolic pressure of 15 mmHg during inspiration. The patient should be assessed for

a. cardiac tamponade.
b. myocardial infarction.
c. aortic dissection.
d. tension pneumothorax.

44. Which of the following information points should be communicated to radiology when an MRI is scheduled for a patient?

a. Presence of orthopedic implants.
b. Allergy to seafood.
c. Small tattoo outside of area of scan.
d. Presence of tooth fillings.

45. If a patient is to undergo a nerve block and 10% dextrose is added to the anesthetic agent, this will result in a(n):

a. hypobaric block
b. hyperbaric block
c. isobaric block
d. neutral block

46. With Perioperative Nursing Data Set (PNDS) coding, the letter X is used to refer to

a. outcome.
b. intervention.
c. diagnosis.
d. domain.

47. When developing guidelines for evidence-based practice, the weakest justification for establishing a procedure is

a. evidence review.
b. staff preference.
c. policy considerations.
d. expert judgment.

48. The purpose of the Bowie-Dick test (chemical indicator, type 2) is to:

a. detect whether a package has been exposed to sterilization
b. monitor the temperature within the sterilization chamber
c. monitor the temperature and sterilant concentration
d. detect air leaks and adequate removal of air from the sterilization chamber

49. A patient with tuberculosis should be placed on

a. standard precautions.
b. airborne precautions.
c. contact precautions.
d. droplet precautions.

50. Following a lumbar laminectomy, the patient complains of tearing and discomfort of the right eye as well as sensitivity to light and blurred vision. The sclera is reddened. The most likely cause is

a. conjunctivitis.
b. dry eye syndrome.
c. allergic reaction.
d. corneal abrasion.

51. Dry heat sterilization is appropriate for all of the following EXCEPT

a. powders.
b. metal instruments.
c. glass syringes and needles.
d. rubber materials.

52. When performing a dressing change on an abdominal surgical wound because of a sudden increase in wound drainage, the nurse notes deep dehiscence of underlying fascia with beginning signs of evisceration. In addition to notifying the surgeon, what is the appropriate emergent response?

a. Cover the wound with a sterile saline dressing.
b. Cover the wound with a dry dressing.
c. Cover the wound with sterile plastic wrap.
d. Approximate the wound edges and apply adhesive strips.

53. For a patient with a history of alcoholism, how long after drinking cessation should the nurse anticipate that the individual may start to experience beginning withdrawal symptoms?

a. Within 4 hours.
b. Within 8 hours.
c. Within 24 hours.
d. Within 48 hours.

54. When carrying out a cost-benefit analysis for a desired new piece of surgical equipment, the analysis should consider cost of acquisition, maintenance costs, reimbursement, potential savings, and

a. training and implementation costs.
b. indirect environmental impact.
c. personal preferences.
d. unrelated and sunken costs.

55. The purpose of hemodilution is

a. to collect blood lost during surgery.
b. to decrease loss of red blood cells.
c. to increase hematopoiesis.
d. to prevent anemia.

56. The minimum number of air exchanges per hour in the OR in which general anesthesia is

a. 4.
b. 6.
c. 15.
d. 20.

57. If a surgeon is planning to use a new type of implant with technical support provided by a healthcare industry representative, what is the best method to ensure that the staff is knowledgeable about the implant?

a. Ask the surgeon to educate the staff.
b. Request literature about the implant.
c. Search for information on the internet.
d. Ask the healthcare industry representative to educate the staff.

58. In a natural disaster with multiple casualties, patients are triaged in the field by a physician. Upon arrival at the hospital, the patient should be

a. treated according to triage assignment.
b. retriaged.
c. treated according to triage assignment and then reassessed.
d. treated in order of arrival.

Refer to the following for questions 59 - 61:

> Some surgeries, especially orthopedic procedures on extremities, use pneumatic tourniquets to control intraoperative bleeding. Consider the following three questions in reference to the use of this device in the operating room.

59. Which of the following personnel determines the pressure setting on the tourniquet?

a. Surgeon.
b. Circulating RN.
c. Scrub RN.
d. Assistant.

60. Although pressure settings may be adjusted as needed, what is the normal recommended range for tourniquet pressure on upper extremities?

a. 30-70 mmHg below systolic blood pressure.
b. 30-70 mmHg below diastolic blood pressure.
c. 30-70 mmHg above systolic blood pressure.
d. 30-70 mmHg above diastolic blood pressure.

61. In order to prevent damage to a limb that is being constricted by a pneumatic tourniquet, it is vital to monitor the time the tourniquet has been inflated. After what amount of time should the tourniquet be briefly deflated and the limb be reevaluated?

a. 15 minutes.
b. 30 minutes.
c. 1 hour.
d. 2 hours.

62. A patient brings a list of medications. During the process of medication reconciliation, the nurse notices a problem in the medication list, shown here:

- Metformin 500 mg daily
- Benadryl 50 mg prn allergic reaction
- Cholecalciferol 2,000 units daily
- Calcium 1,000 mg per day
- Diphenhydramine 25 mg prn sleep

What is the potential problem?

a. One of the medications should not be taken with metformin.
b. One of the medications in inappropriately prescribed.
c. One of the medications should not be taken with cholecalciferol.
d. Two of the medications are duplicates.

63. The five rights of delegation include right task, circumstance, person, direction, and

a. authority.
b. responsibility.
c. time frame.
d. supervision.

64. When placing a patient in supine position, the patient's knees should be:

a. extended with the heels elevated
b. flexed 5–10 degrees
c. flexed 10–15 degrees
d. flexed 15–20 degrees

65. Noncritical items used during surgery of a patient with Creutzfeldt-Jakob disease may be disinfected with sodium chlorite solution of

a. 1:10 dilution.
b. 1:50 dilution.
c. 1:100 dilution.
d. 1:1000 dilution.

66. If the sponge count is incorrect, the person(s) responsible for searching the nonsterile field for the sponge is

a. the housekeeper.
b. both the scrub nurse and circulating nurse.
c. the scrub nurse.
d. the circulating nurse.

67. When administering or handling open containers of chemotherapeutic agents, the nurse should

a. wear double gloves and then remove the outer gloves upon completion.
b. wear single gloves and then change to new gloves upon completion.
c. wear single gloves and then use alcohol hand wash before changing to new gloves.
d. wear single gloves with no added precautions necessary.

68. The most appropriate nursing diagnosis for a surgical patient with neutropenia and absolute neutrophil count (ANC) of 900 is

a. risk of injury.
b. risk of aspiration.
c. risk of infection.
d. ineffective coping.

69. The nurse notes that a large part of the surgical department's budget goes to inventory but outdated products have resulted in unnecessary waste. Which approach is likely the most cost-effective?

a. Ordering when item numbers drop to a preestablished count.
b. Using just-in-time ordering.
c. Looking for less expensive supplies.
d. Educating staff members about avoiding waste.

70. When communicating with a patient with Wernicke's aphasia, it is important to

a. avoid verbal communication.
b. depend on gestures and signals.
c. prompt the patient and suggest words.
d. use multiple modes of communication.

71. The skin antiseptic with the most effective residual action is

a. alcohol.
b. povidone-iodine.
c. chlorhexidine gluconate.
d. parachlorometaxylenol (PCMX).

72. Long-term substance abuse is commonly suggested by all of the following physical assessment findings EXCEPT

a. nasal irritation and sniffing repeatedly.
b. needle tracks on arms.
c. burns on fingers and lips.
d. unequal pupils.

73. When transferring a patient that weighs less than 157 pounds (71 kg) in the supine position from a stretcher to an operating room bed, an appropriate method of transfer is:

a. mechanical lift with supine sling and three caregivers
b. mechanical lift with supine sling and two caregivers
c. lateral transfer device with at least two caregivers
d. lateral transfer device with at least four caregivers

74. A directive that promotes discussion regarding end-of-life decisions and the actions to take (as opposed to those actions to avoid) is

a. an allow-natural-death (AND) order.
b. a do-not-resuscitate (DNR) order.
c. a required reconsideration.
d. a durable power of attorney.

75. The safety precaution "As Low As Reasonably Achievable" or ALARA refers to

a. ventilation.
b. radiation dose.
c. electric current.
d. operation duration.

76. To prevent back strain for a patient in the lithotomy position

a. place a rolled towel under lower back.
b. avoid candy cane stirrups.
c. use stirrups that disperse support and pressure.
d. ensure the buttocks do not extend past the edge of the bed (torso section).

77. Considering the Standards of Perioperative Nursing, determining data collection priorities based on observations of patient's condition and needs is a measurement of

a. Standard 1: Assessment.
b. Standard 1: Diagnosis.
c. Standard 3: Outcome identification.
d. Standard 4: Planning.

78. In problem-oriented SOAP notes, which of the following is an example of subjective data?

a. Ativan 2 mg, instruction in relaxation and visualization.
b. Patient tearful, pacing about room, wringing hands.
c. Ineffective coping, anxiety.
d. "I can't stop crying!"

79. For a critically ill adult patient who is hospitalized and is at risk for an unstable glucose level, the patient's blood glucose level should generally be maintained at

a. 70–150 mg/dL.
b. 90–180 mg/dL.
c. 100–130 mg/dL.
d. 140–180 mg/dL.

80. Preoperative teaching by the CNOR must include all of the following EXCEPT

a. preoperative instructions.
b. an explanation of nothing by mouth (NPO) requirements.
c. postoperative pain management.
d. signing of consent for the procedure.

81. The responsibilities of the surgical team members who wear sterile attire are to

a. take directions from the surgeon.
b. set up non-sterile equipment.
c. assist the anesthetist during induction.
d. position the anesthetized patient.

82. The primary disadvantage of pasteurization is

a. lack of sporicidal activity.
b. time involved.
c. risk of splash burns.
d. cost.

83. An adult patient who underwent a craniotomy had a Glasgow Coma Scale score of 10–12 but now has a score of 8. What does this indicate?

a. The patient is showing improvement.
b. The patient is deteriorating.
c. The patient is near death.
d. The patient has a mild head injury.

84. The purpose of using chemical indicator tape to hold wrappers in place for surgical packs is to indicate

a. the pack has been exposed to sterilization.
b. the pack is completely sterilized and safe for use.
c. whether a pack has been opened.
d. the date of sterilization.

85. If a perioperative nurse is splashed in the face and eyes with blood, the first procedure is

a. flush the face and eyes at an eyewash station for 15 minutes.
b. report the exposure according to protocol.
c. wash the face with soap and water (or povidone-iodine) for 5 minutes and rinse the eyes with water.
d. wipe blood from face with alcohol swabs and rinse eyes for 15 minutes.

86. If a patient develops a gas embolism during insufflation for minimally invasive surgery, the emergent response includes discontinuation of insufflation and anesthesia and:

a. maintaining the supine position and increasing infusion of IV fluids
b. elevating the patient's head and decreasing infusion of IV fluids
c. placing the patient in the Trendelenburg or left lateral position and decreasing infusion of IV fluids
d. placing the patient in the Trendelenburg or left lateral position and increasing infusion of IV fluids

87. The AORN fire triangle consists of fuel, ignition source, and:

a. oxidizer (oxygen)
b. chemical reaction
c. air movement
d. time

88. If operating room turn-around time is slow because of an inadequate number of environmental services technicians, what kind of analysis should the nurse carry out to support the need for additional staff?

a. Cost allocation analysis.
b. Cost-effective analysis.
c. Cost–benefit analysis.
d. Cost–utility analysis.

89. According to the American Medical Association, informed consent must include all of the following EXCEPT

a. detailed cost analysis.
b. explanation of diagnosis.
c. risk and benefits.
d. alternative options.

90. For which procedure should a medical-surgical vacuum with an inline smoke evacuation filter be sufficient to evacuate surgical smoke?

a. Mastectomy
b. Transurethral resection of the prostate
c. Tonsillectomy
d. Arthroplasty

91. All of the following are steps to decrease turnover time EXCEPT

a. increase use of physician-specific instrument trays.
b. monitor instrument use and eliminate seldom-used instruments from sets.
c. use an integrated operative record.
d. do activities in tandem rather than sequentially.

92. When using the LEMON mnemonic to guide assessment of a difficult airway, the L stands for

a. landmark.
b. length of the uvula.
c. look externally.
d. likelihood of difficulty.

93. When setting patient-controlled analgesia (PCA) for pain management, the "Limit" setting refers to

a. the amount of medication received when the patient delivers a dose.
b. time required between administrations of boluses.
c. total amount of opioid that can be delivered in the preset time limit.
d. rate at which opioid is delivered per hour for continuous administration.

94. The equipment required by the perioperative nurse to monitor a patient receiving local anesthetic includes all of the following EXCEPT

a. blood pressure monitor and resuscitation equipment.
b. electrocardiograph.
c. anesthesia machine.
d. pulse oximeter.

95. When doing biologic testing for a steam sterilizer, the biological indicator (BI) should be placed

a. in an open container in the front, bottom section.
b. inside a pack in the front, bottom section.
c. in an open container in the back, top section.
d. inside a pack in the back, top section.

96. All of the following are factors necessary to achieve steam sterilization EXCEPT

a. time.
b. temperature.
c. cooling.
d. moisture.

97. To prevent transmission from a patient with *Clostridioides difficile* infection, which of the following precautions are indicated?

a. Standard precautions.
b. Airborne precautions.
c. Contact precautions.
d. Droplet precautions.

98. Which of the following would be a postoperative complication specific to below-the-knee amputations?

a. Postoperative bleeding.
b. Phantom limb syndrome.
c. Flexion contracture.
d. Poor stump care.

99. A patient's lab reports shows a slightly elevated total white blood cell count with equal elevations of all types of white blood cells, an elevated hemoglobin and hematocrit, normal creatinine but elevated blood urea nitrogen (BUN), increased urine specific gravity, and increased serum sodium. The most likely nursing diagnosis is

a. risk of infection.
b. deficient fluid volume.
c. excess fluid volume.
d. imbalanced nutrition.

100. The optimal operating room bed height is at the waist or elbow or:

a. 3 cm below the elbow
b. 3 cm above the elbow
c. 5 cm below the elbow
d. 5 cm above the elbow

101. If a patient with a patent foramen ovale is placed in the sitting position for surgery, the patient is at increased risk for:

a. venous air embolism
b. deep vein thrombosis
c. pulmonary embolism
d. myocardial infarction

102. If a fire in the operating room occurs with combustion of disposable drapes, what class of fire extinguisher is indicated?

a. Class A
b. Class B
c. Class C
d. Class K

103. The three components of a "fire triangle" include all of the following EXCEPT

a. oxygen.
b. heat.
c. fuel.
d. spark.

104. Patients who have developed cutaneous anthrax as a result of a terrorist attack require

a. standard precautions only.
b. contact precautions and high filtration masks.
c. standard and contact precautions
d. contact precautions and negative pressure rooms.

105. With the surgical smoke hierarchy of control, which one of the following interventions is the least effective?

a. Engineering controls
b. Substitution
c. PPE
d. Administrative controls

106. The most commonly injured intra-abdominal organ is the

a. spleen.
b. small intestine.
c. bladder.
d. liver.

107. All of the following are true about the Association for the Advancement of Medical Instrumentation (AAMI) standards EXCEPT

a. requirements should be based on performance.
b. one global standard should apply to each product, activity, or service.
c. current technology and consensus of opinion should be the basis of standards.
d. government should be the primary agent in establishing standards.

108. Knowles' characteristics of adult learners include all of the following characteristics EXCEPT

a. practical and goal-oriented.
b. motivated.
c. knowledgeable.
d. patient.

109. Which of the following medications is often given with intrathecal administration of morphine to prevent or control a common adverse effect?

a. Serotonin antagonist.
b. Antihistamine.
c. H_2 antagonist.
d. Corticosteroid.

110. When holding a sterile wrapped package, the correct procedure for opening the package is to begin with the:

a. farthest wrapper flap
b. right-sided wrapper flap
c. left-sided wrapper flap
d. closest wrapper flap

111. When using a manual retractor to retract laterally, the assistant should hold the retractor with:

a. the arm extended and palm facing downward
b. the arm flexed and palm facing downward
c. the arm extended and palm facing upward
d. the arm flexed and palm facing upward

112. The adoption of the electronic health record is a component of the:

a. Patient Safety and Quality Improvement Act (PSQIA)
b. American Recovery and Reinvestment Act (ARRA)
c. Healthcare Quality Improvement Act (HCQIA)
d. Health Insurance Portability and Accountability Act (HIPAA)

113. The purpose of pre-sterilization procedures is to

a. lower amount of bioburden.
b. speed sterilization process.
c. reduce cost of sterilization.
d. prevent cross-contamination.

114. In assessing for retroperitoneal trauma, in which retroperitoneal zone is the pancreas located?

a. Zone 1.
b. Zone 2.
c. Zone 3.
d. Zone 4.

115. When placing a patient in the lateral position, an axillary roll should be positioned at the level of the:

a. 5th to 6th ribs
b. 6th to 7th ribs
c. 7th to 9th ribs
d. 9th to 10th ribs

116. A do-not-resuscitate order (DNR) is most likely to be suspended and CPR performed if the patient experiences cardiac arrest in the preoperative period because of

a. acute myocardial infarction.
b. drug reaction.
c. advanced cancer.
d. sepsis.

117. When surgery requires the use of powered surgical instruments, the person responsible for removing blades and drill bit is

a. the physician.
b. the anesthesia provider.
c. the scrub nurse.
d. the circulating nurse.

118. Exposure to which of the following chemical sterilants is carcinogenic to humans?

a. Hydrogen peroxide gas plasma
b. Ethylene oxide
c. Vaporized hydrogen peroxide
d. Peracetic acid

119. If using the Munro Pressure Ulcer Risk Assessment Scale for Perioperative Patients to assess risks associated with positioning, a score of 12 indicates:

a. no risk
b. low risk
c. moderate risk
d. high risk

120. A perforation indicator system involves:

a. double gloving with a colored glove under a standard glove
b. wearing clear gloves to improve visualization of perforations
c. maintaining records of all perforations
d. single gloving with safety gloves

121. An adult Jehovah's Witness patient is hemorrhaging and might die without transfusions, but the patient refused any blood products prior to lapsing into unconsciousness. The correct procedure is

a. use volume replacement and fractionated blood cells only, as permitted by the religion.
b. contact family members and ask permission.
c. ask legal authorities to grant permission.
d. give transfusions, as the patient is not responsive.

122. Which of the following skin changes in older adults increases risk of pressure ulcers?

a. Thinning of the hypodermis.
b. Sweat glands decrease.
c. Epidermal-dermal junction flattens.
d. Langerhans cells decrease in number.

123. Elevating the surgical position above the level of the heart (such as with the sitting position)

a. decreases the danger of arterial air embolism.
b. increases the danger of arterial air embolism.
c. increases the danger of venous air embolism.
d. decreases the danger of venous air embolism.

124. The preferred method of checking effectiveness of sterilization is

a. chemical indicator.
b. mechanical monitoring.
c. physical monitoring.
d. biological indicator.

125. The most common cause of fires in the OR is

a. electrical outlets.
b. lasers.
c. electrosurgical units (ESU).
d. faulty wiring.

126. In the Pain Assessment in Advanced Dementia (PAINAD) scale, all of the following are common indicators of pain EXCEPT

a. compliant behavior.
b. hyperventilation.
c. grimacing.
d. combative behavior.

127. The best method to confirm a patient understands his discharge instructions is to

a. have the patient complete a competency quiz.
b. have the patient "teach back" the instructions.
c. ask the patient if he has any questions.
d. give the patient a postoperative instruction booklet.

128. If using the Scott Triggers tool to assess the risk of perioperative pressure ulcers, what laboratory test may be assessed?

a. Arterial blood gases
b. Serum albumin
c. Total protein
d. Hemoglobin and hematocrit

129. The positions that carry the greatest risk of eye injury include the:

a. prone and lateral
b. lateral and supine
c. Trendelenburg and prone
d. Trendelenburg and sitting

130. With the Continuous Quality Improvement (CQI) model, the focus of improvement is on

a. processes.
b. staff.
c. administrative personnel.
d. patients.

131. In a sterile processing area, the distance between the instrument washing sink and the area where the instruments are prepared for sterilization must be at least:

a. 3 feet
b. 4 feet
c. 5 feet
d. 6 feet

132. When educating a patient about wound care, the response that best indicates that the patient is engaged in the process is

a. the patient takes notes.
b. the patient states that the material is interesting.
c. the patient listens quietly.
d. the patient asks questions.

133. The typical duration of mechanical aeration of items sterilized with ethylene oxide at 50-55 °C is

a. 2-4 hours.
b. 4-8 hours.
c. 8-12 hours.
d. 12-16 hours.

134. A usually continent patient with functional urinary incontinence is often incontinent on the way to the bathroom because of impaired physical mobility. What is the best nursing intervention for this patient?

a. Schedule urination times.
b. Use incontinence pads.
c. Insert a Foley catheter.
d. Alert the staff to quickly answer the call bell.

135. Why should the surgical patient without a Foley catheter be encouraged to void in the preoperative area, if possible?

a. To check for pregnancy.
b. To run a stat urinalysis.
c. To prevent bladder distention.
d. To prevent urinary tract infection.

136. If a healthcare industry representative is going to be present during an operative procedure, then

a. the patient should be informed.
b. it is unnecessary to inform the patient.
c. the patient should be informed only if he or she inquires.
d. the patient must give consent.

137. The CDC's Standard Precautions should be applied in perioperative nursing when caring for

a. all patients.
b. patients with communicable infections.
c. patients with whom exposure to body fluids may occur.
d. intra- and postoperative patients.

138. The Mini-Cog test to assess for dementia includes

a. counting backward from 100 by 7s.
b. copying a picture of interlocking shapes.
c. following simple 3-part directions.
d. drawing the face of a clock with hands indicating a specified time.

139. When opening a pack of surgical instruments, the nurse notes that some instruments have been left in the closed or latched position, but the chemical indicators show adequate sterilization of the pack. The correct response is to

a. replace the entire surgical pack with a new one.
b. consider the instruments sterile and use them.
c. remove and replace the closed or latched instruments.
d. ensure that the instruments have no visible signs of debris.

140. A patient calls Ambulatory Surgery five days after a laparoscopic procedure with general anesthetic, complaining of a persistent cough. The best response is to

a. advise her to splint over the incision to eliminate pain when coughing.
b. ask if she has a fever.
c. advise her to call her physician's office.
d. ask if her cough is productive, and tell her how to achieve postural drainage.

141. Following treatment for an anaphylactic reaction, some patients experience a biphasic reaction with recurrence of symptoms, usually within

a. 30–60 minutes.
b. 5 hours.
c. 10 hours.
d. 24 hours.

142. With the Total Quality Management (TQM) model, the focus of improvement is on

a. improving processes.
b. meeting customer needs.
c. improving staff.
d. identifying inefficiency.

143. Which surgical attire is required in the semi-restricted perioperative zone?

a. Hospital-issued scrubs
b. A lab coat over street clothes
c. Hospital-issued scrubs and head coverings
d. Hospital-issued scrubs, head coverings, and shoe coverings

144. If a perioperative team member shouts angrily at another team member and this is the first instance of disruptive behavior, an appropriate response toward the disruptive person is to:

a. discuss the situation in an informal meeting
b. discuss the situation formally with the immediate supervisor
c. refer the issue to a department head
d. carry out disciplinary interventions

145. The biological indicator for what organism is used with steam sterilization and vaporized hydrogen peroxide sterilization for monitoring the effectiveness of sterilization?

a. *Geobacillus stearothermophilus* spores
b. *Bacillus atrophaeus* spores
c. *Paenibacillus spp. spores*
d. *Clostridioides difficile spores*

146. The label for radioactive waste must contain all of the following EXCEPT

a. name of radioisotope.
b. disposal date.
c. full name and contact information of authorized user.
d. type of patient protection used.

147. The purpose of the Joint Commission's "Do Not Use" List is to

a. promote standardization in documentation.
b. prevent errors.
c. promote cost-effectiveness.
d. comply with FDA regulations.

148. Following ventilator weaning, a patient has been maintained on oxygen with a nonrebreather mask. When weaning the patient from oxygen, the FiO_2 should be gradually reduced until the PaO_2 is at ________ on room air.

a. 70–100 mmHg
b. 50–70 mmHg
c. 40–60 mmHg
d. 30–40 mmHg

149. Open shelves used for storage of sterile packages require all of the following EXCEPT

a. lowest shelf 8-10 inches from floor.
b. highest shelf 8-10 inches from ceiling.
c. good ventilation with temperature and humidity control.
d. shelves 2 inches away from outside walls.

150. A PACU nurse is recovering a cesarean section patient in the PACU. If the patient received a regional anesthetic in the operating room, such as a spinal, which of the following would be the most important for the PACU nurse to monitor?

a. The patient's dermatome levels.
b. The patient's height and weight.
c. The patient's input and output.
d. The patient's level of consciousness.

151. If a patient suffers a gunshot injury to the abdomen with open wounds in the right abdomen and right back, the wounds should NOT be documented in terms of

a. entry and exit.
b. size, appearance, and location.
c. entry, exit, and trajectory.
d. entry, possible internal damage, and exit.

152. Under the National Pressure Injury Advisory Panel (NPIAP) staging system, a pressure ulcer that is superficial and appears as an abrasion or blistered area with partial thickness skin loss is

a. Stage I.
b. Stage II.
c. Stage III.
d. Stage IV.

153. In the event of a disaster, which initial strategy could be used to increase a hospital's surge capacity?

a. Identify clients who are safely eligible for early discharge.
b. Place extra beds in private rooms.
c. Recommend closing the emergency department to non-disaster-related clients.
d. Transfer clients so that open rooms are in close proximity.

154. A sharps injury log must contain the:

a. type and brand of device involved
b. name of the injured person
c. names of witnesses to the injury
d. treatment provided to the injured party

155. Core temperature of 30-32 °C (86-89.6 °F) is classified as

a. normothermia.
b. mild hypothermia.
c. moderate hypothermia.
d. severe hypothermia.

156. Which characteristics of support surfaces provide the best protection against positioning-related pressure injuries?

a. Shallow immersion, low envelopment
b. Shallow immersion, high envelopment
c. Deep immersion, low envelopment
d. Deep immersion, high envelopment

157. An absorbable suture material is

a. polyester.
b. catgut.
c. silk.
d. nylon.

158. If a metal plate is composed of stainless steel, the screws should be

a. stainless steel or cobalt-chromium.
b. stainless steel or titanium-vanadium aluminum.
c. stainless steel, cobalt-chromium, or titanium-vanadium aluminum.
d. stainless steel only.

159. The tasks delegated to the perioperative nurse in the role of the circulator are

a. coordinating care of the surgical patient.
b. patient advocacy during the preoperative period.
c. managing and implementing activities on the sterile field.
d. managing the transfer and care of the patient post-operatively through stabilization.

160. Which type of needle is indicated for suturing of fascia and muscle?

a. Cutting needle
b. Reverse cutting needle
c. Taper-point needle
d. Blunt-tip needle

161. Surgical staff in the presence of surgical smoke need

a. standard surgical masks.
b. high filtration surgical masks.
c. no special precautions.
d. smoke evacuation system only.

162. A patient with a newly implanted demand pacemaker exhibits the following cardiac monitor tracing:

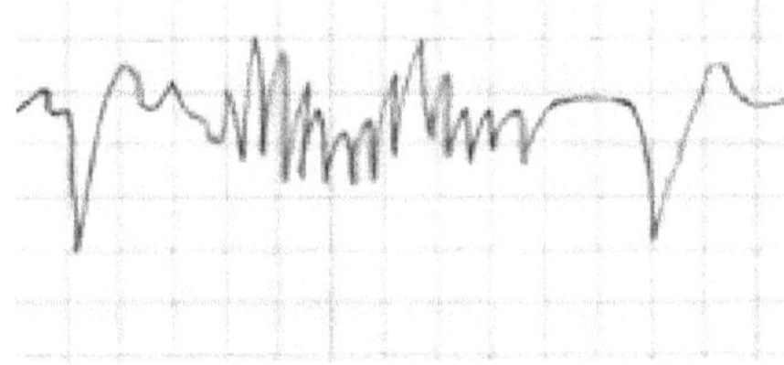

What does this indicate?

a. Undersensing.
b. Oversensing.
c. Noncapture.
d. Electrical interference.

163. After selecting a number of possible vendors for a complex upgrade of equipment and services, the next step is to develop a

a. business plan.
b. request for proposal.
c. request for quotation.
d. budget allowance.

164. Medication reconciliation should be completed

a. prior to admission.
b. during the admission assessment.
c. on discharge.
d. during all phases of care.

165. Midazolam is often combined with fentanyl for conscious sedation in order to

a. potentiate the effect of midazolam.
b. decrease pain associated with the procedure.
c. extend duration of the procedure.
d. decrease drug dosage.

166. For a patient with an IED in place, all of the following are true EXCEPT

a. the programming device and personnel to reprogram must be in the OR.
b. the active and dispersive electrodes should be placed as far from the IED and wires as possible.
c. environmental humidity should be between 50% and 60%.
d. monopolar electrosurgery should be used.

167. When documenting a medication, which of the following is an appropriate entry?

a. 4 ½ tsp Robitussin PO
b. 8 U regular insulin SQ left deltoid
c. Morphine sulfate 4 mg SQ right deltoid
d. Meperidine 50.0 mg IM right deltoid

168. Under the AABB (American Association of Blood Banks) standards, blood may be attached to a warmer for

a. ≤1 hour.
b. ≤2 hours.
c. ≤3 hours.
d. ≤4 hours.

169. If an afterloading modality, such as a MammoSite catheter, is used for insertion of radioactive seeds following a lumpectomy, the seeds are typically inserted:

a. immediately after insertion of the catheter
b. before insertion of the catheter
c. in the PACU
d. in a protected room outside of the operating room

170. The purpose of using neostigmine in surgical procedures is to

a. reverse effects of nondepolarizing neuromuscular blocking agents.
b. block effects of acetylcholine.
c. reverse activity of opioids.
d. potentiate intraoperative anesthetics.

171. The members of the surgery/procedure team who should participate in the "time out" as part of the Universal Protocol are

a. physician, anesthesia provider, and scrub nurse.
b. physician, scrub nurse, and circulating nurse.
c. physician, anesthesia provider, scrub nurse, and other assisting physicians.
d. all team members.

172. A preoperative RN is preparing to interview his patient for the preoperative assessment for her surgery. After washing his hands and introducing himself to her, what is the first thing the preoperative nurse should do?

a. Check that the patient's surgical consent is correct and complete.
b. Review the surgeon's history and physical for past surgeries that could affect his plan of care.
c. Properly identify the patient by name and date of birth.
d. Check for medication allergies.

173. The hand-off report to the PACU nurse must include all of the following EXCEPT

a. relevant preoperative information.
b. family request for information.
c. type and duration of anesthesia.
d. estimated fluid/blood loss.

174. Which type of tissue produces the most fine and ultrafine particulate matter in surgical smoke?

a. Lung
b. Renal cortex
c. Liver
d. Adipose

175. When developing quality improvement projects, the diagram that is used to help identify cause and effect and root causes is

a. Ishikawa diagram.
b. affinity diagram.
c. prioritization matrix.
d. Gantt chart.

176. A surgical gown is considered sterile from the:

a. neck to the level of the sterile field
b. chest to the level of the sterile field
c. neck to the waist
d. chest to the waist

177. In preparation for surgery, the scrub nurse sets up the back table according to

a. personal preference.
b. surgeon preference.
c. circulating nurse preference.
d. standardized procedure.

178. During administration of intravenous methylene blue dye, the expected effect on pulse oximetry is

a. slight increase.
b. no effect.
c. decrease to 65% for 1-2 minutes.
d. slight decrease to 90-94% for 1-2 minutes.

179. Intraoperative blood salvage is contraindicated in

a. orthopedic surgery.
b. transplant surgery.
c. vascular surgery.
d. cancer surgery.

180. All of the following are factors that the nurse manager considers when making scrub assignments for the following day's surgeries EXCEPT

a. necessary expertise.
b. staffing skill mix.
c. seniority.
d. availability.

181. When monitoring the intracranial pressure (ICP) of an adult following a craniotomy, a pressure greater than ______ is considered pathological.

a. 10 mmHg
b. 15 mmHg
c. 20 mmHg
d. 30 mmHg

182. Chemical solutions used specifically to disinfect body parts are called

a. antiseptics.
b. disinfectants.
c. germicides.
d. sporicides.

183. Alcohols are effective disinfectants for

a. instruments contaminated with blood.
b. lensed instruments.
c. plastic tubing.
d. rubber stoppers on medication vials.

184. During surgical procedures, it is recommended that double gloving be used by:

a. all perioperative team members
b. surgeons and first assistants
c. scrubbed team members
d. scrub persons

185. Isotonic crystalloid solutions are used to

a. replace water and electrolytes.
b. treat hyponatremia.
c. treat severe hypovolemic shock.
d. replace water.

186. The purpose of diluting ethylene oxide with inert gases (such as CO_2) and hydrochlorofluorocarbon (HCFC) is to

a. reduce flammability.
b. destroy spores.
c. increase bactericidal activity.
d. decrease carcinogenicity.

187. The person responsible for documenting sponge, sharp, and instrument counts is

a. the physician.
b. the scrub nurse.
c. the circulating nurse.
d. the scrub nurse and circulating nurse.

188. All of the following conditions are contraindications to ambulatory or outpatient surgery EXCEPT

a. controlled diabetes.
b. untreated obstructive sleep apnea.
c. history of poorly controlled epileptic seizures.
d. current alcoholism.

189. The following demonstrates proper body mechanics

a. squatting down with knees bent to retrieve an item on the floor.
b. bending at the waist to retrieve to lift an item.
c. pushing a full box of materials with the arms.
d. stretching to reach an item on a high shelf.

190. Low-pressure/high-volume adult endotracheal tubes (ETTs) increase risk of all of the following EXCEPT

a. sore throat.
b. aspiration.
c. spontaneous extubation.
d. mucosal trauma.

191. Breastfeeding infants scheduled for surgery must not breastfeed or receive breast milk for

a. 8 hours before surgery.
b. 6 hours before surgery.
c. 4 hours before surgery.
d. 2 hours before surgery.

192. According to the ANA Code of Ethics for Nurses, the nurse's primary commitment is to

a. the provision of care.
b. the institution.
c. the patient.
d. the self.

193. The isolation technique should be used during surgeries that involve the:

a. respiratory system
b. bowel and metastatic tumors
c. GU system
d. respiratory system and tumors >6 cm

194. Which pediatric assessment tool was developed specifically for the perioperative pediatric patient?

a. Braden Q scale
b. Braden Q+P scale
c. Glamorgan scale
d. Neonatal Skin Risk Assessment scale

195. A preanesthesia evaluation and assessment may not be required for

a. minor surgical procedures.
b. patients with recent history of anesthesia.
c. patients receiving local anesthesia.
d. outpatient surgery procedures.

196. Which of the following is an example of resistive warming?

a. Heated water circulating through blankets that do not contain heating elements.
b. A blanket warmed in a warming cabinet.
c. A covering reduces the loss of body heat.
d. The air is heated.

197. Personal protective equipment (PPE) includes all of the following EXCEPT

a. gloves.
b. face shields.
c. uniform.
d. gown.

198. During a preoperative assessment, the patient tells the preoperative nurse she takes ginkgo biloba to help with her memory. What should the nurse do?

a. Nothing, this is an herbal and has no effect on the surgery.
b. Cancel the surgery because this medication has severe adverse reactions with the anesthetic agents.
c. Be sure this medication is added to her home medication list, and verify that the surgeon and anesthesia care provider are aware she takes it.
d. Ask the physician for a stat electrocardiogram (EKG), because this herbal can cause cardiac arrhythmias.

199. Hazardous waste that is contaminated by chemotherapeutic agents must be disposed of in a waste container that is:

a. red
b. yellow
c. green
d. brown

200. The airborne concentration of a chemical substance that workers can be exposed to repeatedly without it adversely affecting their health is the:

a. ceiling limit
b. short-term exposure limit
c. threshold limit value
d. time-weighted average

Answer Key and Explanations for Test #2

1. D: Normal fascial compartment pressure varies (0-8 or higher) with 30-40 mmHg consistent with compartment syndrome. Compartment syndrome occurs when myofascial compartment size decreases because of constriction (casts, splints, dressings, excessive traction, premature fascia closure) or contents of a compartment increase (swelling, hemorrhage, infiltrated IV). The increased compartment pressure reduces capillary perfusion below the level necessary for tissue viability and damages nerves. Symptoms include the 6 P's: paresthesia, pain (deep, throbbing, relentless pain, and positive Homans sign for lower extremities), pressure, pallor, paralysis, and pulselessness (peripheral pulses), although pulselessness may indicate arterial occlusion rather than compartment syndrome.

2. C: Fatigue-reducing techniques should be used if the perioperative team member (not wearing a lead apron) stands in the same position continuously for more than 2 hours or more than 30% of the workday. Fatigue-reducing techniques include antifatigue mats, sit-stand stools, supportive footwear, and adjusting the height of the operating room bed. If the procedure requires that the team member wear a lead apron, then fatigue-reducing techniques should be used after 1 hour.

3. B: The purpose of a neutral zone in surgery is to decrease the risk of sharps injuries. A neutral zone is a hands-free technique in which the surgeon and the scrub person do not touch a sharp instrument at the same time. The scrub person places the sharp in the neutral zone (a magnetic pad, container, or specified area) for transfer, and the surgeon then takes the instrument from the zone and vice versa. Using a neutral or hands-free technique reduces sharps injuries markedly.

4. A: The physician's preference cards include the preferred sutures, special instruments or equipment, and types of dressing. The surgeon's phone number is not included. The physician's preference card does not contain each and every instrument the surgeon would use, since most specialties have pre-arranged trays that include common instruments. The surgeon does not decide on the staff; that is the prerogative of the nurse manager.

5. B: Metoclopramide is often given as a preoperative medication in order to speed emptying of the stomach and prevent nausea and vomiting to reduce the risk of aspiration. An antacid or H_2 receptor blocker (such as famotidine) may be given to reduce production of gastric acids or decrease acidity. Midazolam is given to relieve anxiety and apprehension prior to surgery as well as to provide amnesia. Anticholinergics (atropine, glycopyrrolate) are given to control secretions, resulting in the "dry mouth" associated with surgery.

6. C: During invasive procedures, surgical gloves should be changed at least every 90 to 150 minutes. In addition, gloves should be changed after each patient procedure, if there is a visible defect or perforation, after contact with methyl methacrylate (bone cement), after touching optics eyepieces or a fluoroscopy machine, after touching a surgical helmet system, and when contamination is suspected. Gloves may be changed after completing draping and after handling heavy or sharp instruments or rough bones and before handling implants.

7. A: The intraoperative position that most increases the risk of procedure-related VTE is excessive hip flexion. Other positions that increase risk are hyperextension of the knee and the reverse Trendelenburg position. Other risk factors include general anesthesia for longer than 90 minutes or longer than 60 minutes if the operative procedure involves a lower extremity or the pelvic area. Almost all major surgeries increase the risk of VTE; therefore, careful monitoring of patients, early ambulation, and prophylaxis as indicated are essential preventive measures.

8. D: The focused assessment with sonography for trauma (FAST) is used primarily to assess trauma patients for signs of internal bleeding or fluid accumulation; however, it is not sensitive enough to determine the source of bleeding, injury to solid organs, or retroperitoneal bleeding. Areas of the body assessed include the following:

- Pericardial area: Pericardial effusion, cardiac tamponade
- Abdomen: Right upper quadrant for fluid between the liver and right kidney; left upper quadrant to assess fluid between the spleen and the kidney
- Pelvis: To assess the rectovesical pouch or rectouterine pouch for signs of pelvic bleeding

9. B: Face validity is the weakest form of validity because it depends on subjective opinions rather than objective evaluation and empirical evidence. However, assessing for face validity may be helpful during preliminary steps of research. Content validity occurs when the instrument effectively measures the intended concept. Criterion-related validity measures how well the instrument correlates with the results found in another instrument and how well it can predict an outcome. Construct validity evaluates whether the instrument represents the concept being measured.

10. C: Soiled instruments should be transported from the OR to the cleaning/decontamination area in leak-proof containers or in trays placed inside a leak-proof sealed plastic bag and labeled as a biohazard. Instruments should not be placed in soaking solution before transport because of the danger of spills. Instruments should be wiped after use during surgery but with water rather than normal saline, which may result in pitting. Rinsing of the instruments with cold water is done in the cleaning/decontamination area. Instruments may also be soaked in water with enzymes to dissolve protein and blood.

11. C: A partially empty medicine vial should not be placed in the sharps hazardous waste disposal container, which is intended for those materials that could puncture or cut the skin of someone handling them. Sharps include needles, saws, pins, nails, broken glass, and syringes. A partially empty medicine vial is classified as a pharmaceutical, and disposal should be conducted according to protocol. Disposing of materials correctly is especially important because some materials are incinerated and others disposed of in different manners.

12. A: Modified EEG, such as bispectral index (BIS), measures anesthetic effects on consciousness to avoid anesthesia awareness by applying an algorithm to EEG activity and showing the results as a single number rather than a tracing. Scores:

$40 - 60$ = Optimal scores for a generally healthy individual undergoing surgery
> 60 = Indicates inability to respond to verbal commands
$65 - 85$ = Indicates sedation
> 70 = Indicates likelihood of awareness
100 = Indicates awake state

However, the numbers may not be accurate with head trauma, and EEG changes caused by conditions such as hypothermia can affect BIS scores.

13. D: Tattoos carry a risk of infection because they involve repeated small punctures of the skin and injection of dye. Additionally, they itch during the healing, so this will add to the patient's discomfort. The nurse should always give a reason when advising a patient about an action and should always try to avoid giving orders. While it is true an obese patient is at increased risk of infection, focusing on the problem with the procedure rather than with the patient is more supportive and likely to cause less anxiety.

14. C: Pain management is an element of (D3) patient/family behavioral responses to surgery in the Perioperative Nursing Data Set (PNDS), which promotes standardized documentation. Other behavioral responses include comfort level and anxiety, as well as ethnic, cultural, and religious or spiritual issues. Patient safety (D1) includes positioning, chemical burns, radiation exposure, fires, and falls or other injuries. Patient physiologic responses (D2) include infection, hypothermia, hyperthermia, and tissue perfusion. Health system (D4) includes benchmarking and other types of data.

15. C: Patients with advanced Parkinson's disease may respond slowly; therefore, if the nurse asks a question, the nurse should give the patient two to three times longer to answer compared to a patient with normal speech production. Parkinson's disease can result in impaired muscle control of the muscles essential for speech, and the bradykinesia that is characteristic of Parkinson's disease makes speech production slow. Additionally, Parkinson's disease can cause dysarthria, resulting in slurred and mumbled speech; also, patients have decreased speech volume and variations in pitch.

16. B: The modified neutral zone may be indicated when surgery is carried out under magnification during which time the surgeon is unable to look away from the surgical field. With the modified neutral zone, the scrub person hands an instrument to the surgeon, but the surgeon returns the instrument to the neutral zone. By doing it this way, an instrument that is contaminated is handled by only one person rather than two. The modified neutral zone may also be used during critical parts of surgery in which the surgeon's attention must remain focused on the surgical site.

17. B: Pneumothorax (i.e., air in the pleural space) can occur as a complication of surgical procedures, such as thoracic, cardiothoracic, and laparoscopic procedures. Pneumothorax is characterized by a sudden onset of chest pain, dyspnea, tachypnea, and tachycardia. Tracheal deviation toward the unaffected side and decreased expansion of the chest on the affected side may be evident as well as markedly decreased or absent breath sounds in the affected lung. Emergent treatment includes needle decompression and chest tube insertion to expand the lung.

18. C: P4 in the ASA preoperative classification system indicates that the patient has systemic disease that is life-threatening. There are 6 categories for physical status:

- P1 – Normal patient appears to be in good health.
- P2 – Systemic disease is present but is mild.
- P3 – Systemic disease is severe but not incapacitating.
- P4 – Systemic disease is life-threatening.
- P5 – Moribund patient will likely not survive without surgical intervention.
- P6 – Brain-dead patient whose surgery is for the purpose of harvesting organs.

19. D: Although ultraviolet disinfection requires some energy consumption, and the manufacturing and disposal processes may have some environmental impact, ultraviolet cleaning is the most environmentally friendly option. It reduces the uses of chemical disinfectants, which may contain substances that contribute to pollution and require water. Ultraviolet light disinfection systems are generally energy efficient, do not require water (unlike steam cleaning), leave no residue that must be rinsed off, and reduce the overall use of chemical disinfectants. Disposable wipes and mops contribute to waste.

20. C: If unsure how to clean a rigid sterilization container or any other type of container or device, the nurse should refer to the manufacturer's instructions for use (IFU). The IFU contains information about the product description and indications for use, storage, maintenance, disposal, and cleaning and will list cleaning agents that can be used with the device. The IFU provides guidance regarding compliance with regulatory standards. IFUs should be maintained electronically or in a central storage place for easy access.

21. C: If an organization has deemed status, this means that it can determine if a healthcare provider is in compliance with CMS regulations to receive payment from CMS. National accrediting agencies, such as The Joint Commission and the American Association for Accreditation of Ambulatory Surgery Facilities, have deeming authority in six different areas: (1) quality insurance, (2) antidiscrimination, (3) access to service, (4) confidentiality and accuracy of records, (5) advance directives, and (6) provider participation rules.

22. C: Although dyspnea, pain, decreased breath sounds, and asymmetric chest movements may be found with different types of injuries and conditions, bowel sounds heard in the chest cavity are strong predictors of diaphragmatic injury because this occurs when the abdominal contents herniate into the thoracic cavity. The displaced organs result in decreased or even absent breath sounds on the side affected by the injury. Diaphragmatic injuries on the left are the most common because the liver provides a cushion on the right side, protecting the diaphragm.

23. A: Plan-do-check-act is a simple method of continuous quality improvement to apply when dealing with specific unit problems, but it is less well suited for organization-wide problems. Note that "check" may be replaced with "study":

P	Plan	Identify, analyze, define the problem and set goals, brainstorm.
D	Do	Generate solutions and choose one on a trial basis.
C/S	Check/Study	Gather and analyze data regarding effectiveness. If ineffective, return to "do" and select another option.
A	Act	Identify modifications needed for implementation, and monitor the results.

24. D: Desflurane is used for induction and maintenance of anesthesia in adults but is contraindicated for induction in infants and children because of upper airway complications (coughing, apnea, laryngospasm), although it can be used for maintenance. Halothane is associated with many adverse effects, so other anesthetic agents are often used. Halothane effects include increased risk of anesthesia-related hepatitis in those with liver dysfunction and 50% reduction in BP and cardiac output. Cerebral blood flow and ICP are moderately increased, but cerebral metabolism is decreased and autoregulation is impaired.

25. B: Kehr's sign (i.e., pain radiating from the upper left abdomen to the left shoulder) is consistent with a ruptured spleen. Kehr's sign occurs because blood from the ruptured spleen pools and irritates the diaphragm. Other signs of a ruptured spleen include indications of shock including dizziness; altered mental status; hypotension; tachycardia; and cool, clammy skin. A ruptured spleen is often associated with fractures of ribs 9–12, and it most often results from blunt trauma rather than penetrating trauma with most traumatic injuries resulting from motor vehicle accidents.

26. A: The National Institute for Occupational Safety and Health recommends that smoke capture devices be located within 5 cm (2 in.) of the surgical site. Vacuum pressure should be no greater than 150 mmHg, and the minimum capture velocity should be 100-150 feet per minute. The smoke evacuation system should eliminate odor, so if an odor is detectable, the device should be examined to make sure it is functioning properly and has an unexpired charcoal filter in place.

27. B: Postoperative ventilator settings generally include the following:

- Fraction of inspired oxygen (FiO_2, i.e., the percentage of oxygen in the inspired air) ranging from 21% to 100% but usually maintained at <40% to avoid toxicity

Toxicity can occur if the FiO_2 setting is significantly higher than the normal atmospheric level of 21% because this high level can cause oxidative stress, which can result in the release of proinflammatory cytokines and can damage the alveolar-capillary barrier, increasing permeability and leading to pulmonary edema. High levels can also disrupt the production and function of surfactants, and this can lead to atelectasis. Over time, high levels of oxygen can lead to pulmonary fibrosis.

28. B: Sponges should be separated and counted out loud during the initial count to ensure the count is accurate and that each package contains the correct number of sponges. The circulating nurse and one other person should participate in the count. Used sponges should also be kept separated for counting. If a package holds an incorrect number, the entire package should be removed, bagged, labeled, and isolated from the sterile field. The same sequence of counting (large to small, small to large, proximal to distal) should be used during every count as an established routine minimizes errors.

29. D: Discharge instructions include: Medication directions; pain management; wound care; signs and symptoms of infection and other complications; the surgeon's phone number; date to schedule a follow-up appointment; and any education specific to the surgery (e.g., a dialysis overview for a graft recipient). Itching and prickly sensations around the incision site are common during the healing process.

30. B: Nurses should use objective descriptions (threw a glass of water at the nurse) that describe an action rather than judging it, including direct quotations ("I hate shots" when describing patient behavior) and should avoid the use of subjective terms (especially those that are negative), such as "upset," "angry," and "uncooperative," or "screaming fit," as the use of these terms may be used to establish bias in the event of legal action. Verbal and written reports should always remain neutral and objective.

31. C: With a total knee arthroplasty, damage can occur to the saphenous nerve or the peroneal nerve, although the peroneal nerve is most at risk of injury. Peroneal nerve damage is characterized by toe drag, slapping gait, and foot drop, resulting in weakness of the foot and ankle and difficulty ambulating. Muscle mass may be lost because of the lack of enervation to the muscles; the patient may also experience a reduction in sensation and numbness and tingling in the foot and lower leg.

32. A: In order to practice as a nurse anesthetist, the registered nurse must obtain an advanced degree (masters or doctorate) in nurse anesthesia. This is not within the scope and definition of a perioperative nurse. The perioperative nurse's scope includes the following roles: scrub nurse, circulating nurse, RN First Assistant (an expanded role in which the perioperative nurse assists the surgeon), and OR Nurse Manager (in which an experienced perioperative nurse takes on the administrative duties of managing the daily operations of an OR).

33. C: The temperature in warming cabinets for blankets should not exceed 130 °F (54 °C) because patients are at risk for thermal burns because sedation or unconsciousness renders them insensitive to the high temperatures. Solution cabinets are maintained at a lower temperature because fluids used for intracorporeal irrigation or IV fluids should not exceed normal body temperature (98.6 °F [37 °C]). Temperatures should be maintained according to fluid manufacturers' guidelines, and all solutions should be labeled with the date they are placed inside the warming cabinet and disposed of if they exceed maximum length of time for warming.

34. D: About 9 out of 10 nerve injuries associated with total hip arthroplasty involve the sciatic nerve, although the incidence is still low. Injury may result from compression on the nerve, stretching, inadequate perfusion, and/or transection. Compression also often causes direct nerve damage and inadequate perfusion at the same time. Signs and symptoms can include pain, numbness, weakness, tingling, foot drop, and reduced knee and ankle reflexes. Femoral nerve injury can occur with the anterior approach; superior gluteal nerve injury can occur with the lateral approach. Obturator injury causes the fewest adverse effects and is the least common.

35. D: For mild/moderate hypoglycemia (54–70 mg/dL), patients should ingest 15 g carbohydrate, wait 15 minutes, and recheck the blood glucose level. If the level remains <70, then the patient should repeat the process until the blood glucose stays ≥70. Once stable, the patient should eat a small meal. If the patient's blood glucose drops to <54 but there is no mental impairment, the patient should use the same process but increase the dosage of carbohydrates to 30 g. If any confusion or mental impairment occurs, regardless of the blood glucose level, this is a medical emergency that requires immediate medical attention.

36. A: Because patients are placed in reverse Trendelenburg position, padded footboards are necessary to prevent the patient from sliding. The patient's feet should be secured to the footboard in neutral position. Two straps secure the legs at the thighs and lower legs. Side attachments may be necessary for some patients. Arms are usually placed on an extended armboard, although some procedures may require arms at the sides (duodenal switch). Sequential compression devices or arterial venous compression boots should be in place.

37. B: PEA and asystole do not respond to defibrillation. CPR with supplementary oxygen is begun immediately:

16. CPR up to 2 minutes and then epinephrine 1 mg (drug of choice) every 3 to 5 minutes or replace first or second dose of epinephrine with vasopressin 40 units. Atropine 1 mg may be given every 3 to 5 minutes (≤ 3 doses).
17. If asystole continues, step 1 is repeated.
18. If shockable rhythm begins, a shock is given and CPR resumed. At this point, the procedure follows that for ventricular fibrillation or ventricular tachycardia.
19. If normal (non-shockable) rhythm begins, postresuscitation care is begun.

38. C: An acceptable abbreviation for a subcutaneous injection is "subcut" or "subcutaneous" because shorter abbreviations may be misinterpreted. "S" may be read as 5, SC may be misread as SL, and the "q" may be understood as "every." Many traditional abbreviations, such as BID, TID, QID, and QHS can be easily misinterpreted, especially if they are not written clearly, so these abbreviations should no longer be used. For example, HS may be interpreted as half-strength or hour of sleep. Nurses should always refer to institutional lists of accepted abbreviations.

39. B: The nurse should ask the parents if the child was treated with cupping, a traditional healing procedure used in many Asian cultures. Round cups, usually now made of glass, are flamed with alcohol to reduce inside pressure and then they are applied to the skin, where suction forms as the glasses cool. The combination of heat and suction causes skin discoloration or bruising that can be mistaken for abuse, but the discolorations are usually very regular in size and parallel to the spine if done on the back.

40. C: Critical care is outside the scope of practice of the perioperative nurse. Preoperative care may include preadmission assessment and teaching as well as admission, evaluation, and assessment in the holding area before surgery. Intraoperative care includes working as a circulating nurse outside the sterile field and/or as a scrub nurse within the sterile field, supervising, and transferring patients to the PACU. Postoperative care includes assessment and treatment within the PACU and transfer of patients to other units.

41. B: OSHA, under the Department of Labor, is responsible for bloodborne pathogens standards, as well as other workplace standards, and inspection of workplaces to ensure safety standards are met. The CDC provides treatment guidelines and recommendations and monitors public health, compiling statistics regarding reportable disease. The EPA is not a statutory agency but provides information about the environment to other governmental agencies. The FDA is a consumer protection agency ensuring safety of medications, biological products, medical devices, and food.

42. C: When extending a patient's arm on an arm board, the arm should be placed in a supinated position (palm up) because this position decreases pressure on the ulnar nerve. Padding the arm board also decreases the risk of injury. Compression of the ulnar nerve is one of the most frequently implicated causes of perioperative neuropathy. Compression injuries may take up to 6 weeks to heal. Severe injury may result in permanent disability.

43. A: Cardiac tamponade is characterized by persistent hypotension despite there being no indication of ongoing blood loss and a drop of systolic pressure of greater than 10 mmHg with inspiration. Beck's triad (i.e., hypotension, muffled heart sounds, and jugular venous distention) is only present in approximately one-third of patients presenting with cardiac tamponade. Kussmaul's sign (i.e., decreased jugular venous distention with inspiration) may not be evident in the presence of hypovolemia. FAST is used to quickly assess the pericardial area for fluid in the pericardial sac.

44. A: For an MRI, the presence of orthopedic implants should be communicated, although those in place for more than 6 weeks should be imbedded and pose no problem. However, they should be evaluated individually as they may cause artifacts and some older implants are more ferromagnetic. Allergy to seafood, which precludes use of some contrast material for x-rays and CT scans, does not apply to MRIs as the contrast material contains gadolinium, a paramagnetic metal ion. Large tattoos may heat during MRI but small tattoos outside the area pose no problem. Fillings pose no risk but may distort facial images.

45. B: If a patient is to undergo a nerve block, adding 10% dextrose to the anesthetic agent will result in a hyperbaric block because it is heavier than the cerebrospinal fluid. Because of this, it will gravitate accordingly. If, for example, the patient is in the sitting position, it will flow downward. A hypobaric block with sterile water added is lighter than the cerebrospinal fluid, so the anesthetic rises. With an isobaric block, the anesthetic tends to stay localized. After a nerve block is administered, the patient may be placed in a temporary position until the anesthetic takes effect.

46. C: In the Perioperative Nursing Data Set (PNDS), X refers to diagnosis. PNDS is a specialized nursing language for use in perioperative care to ensure that care is documented and reported accurately and consistently. PNDS is based on the 4 domains of the Perioperative Patient Focused Model: (D1) safety, (D2) physiologic response to surgery, (D3) behavioral responses to surgery, and (D4) the health system. Each of these domains is associated with nursing diagnosis (X), interventions (I), and outcomes (O). The PNDS focuses on patient outcomes and methods to achieve those outcomes. Nursing diagnoses are linked to outcomes and expected interventions.

47. B: Staff preference is subjective and is the weakest justification for establishing a procedure. Evidence review includes review of literature, critical analysis of studies, and summarizing of results, including pooled meta-analysis. Expert judgment, recommendations based on personal experience from a number of experts, may be utilized, especially if there is inadequate evidence based on review, but this subjective evidence should be explicitly acknowledged. Policy considerations include cost-effectiveness, access to care, insurance coverage, availability of qualified staff, and legal implications.

48. D: The purpose of the Bowie-Dick test is to detect air leaks and adequate removal of air from the sterilization chamber. The Bowie-Dick test is a type 2 chemical indicator. Adequate removal of air is essential for sterilization because the air in a sterilization chamber (non-condensable gas) does not condense if it comes into contact with a cold item and can create a barrier between the item being sterilized and the steam. If some air remains, the items may not be completely sterilized.

49. B: A patient with tuberculosis should be placed on airborne precautions because transmission is per particles ≤ 5 micrometer, which can be widely dispersed through the air and inhaled by others. Airborne precautions are used in addition to standard precautions and include use of private negative-pressure rooms. Staff should use respiratory precautions (N95 respirators are required for TB), and patients should wear masks if they must leave their rooms. Persons who are susceptible to the disease or immunocompromised in any way should not enter the room.

50. D: Corneal abrasion is the most common ophthalmic disorder associated with nonophthalmic operative procedures, especially when the patient is placed in positions in which the eyes may be subjected to pressure, such as when the patient is placed in the prone position for spinal surgeries. Other positions for which there is risk for corneal injury include the lateral decubitus position, the Trendelenburg position, and the lithotomy position. To decrease risk, it is essential that eye protection, such as lubricating ointments and eye shields, be used and that patients be positioned carefully to prevent pressure on their eyes.

51. D: Rubber materials are not sterilized by dry heat because the high temperature (usually 160 °C for 2 hours or 170 °C for 1 hour) may result in deterioration of the materials. Dry heat can be used with anything that is not altered by high heat, such as instruments, glassware, needles, powders, grease, and anhydrous oils. Dry heat sterilizers include gravity convection sterilizers with the heating element at the bottom of the oven and the mechanical convection sterilizer with the healing element in a separate chamber from the oven.

52. A: If evisceration is occurring, this is a surgical emergency, and the patient must be surgically repaired. The emergent response should be to cover the wound with a sterile saline dressing to prevent eviscerating organs from drying out and to reduce the risk of infection. Risk factors for dehiscence and evisceration include infection, inadequate perfusion, inadequate nutrition, diabetes mellitus, and obesity. Dehiscence most commonly occurs 5–8 days postoperatively. If only dehiscence is present but no evisceration, then an abdominal binder may be used to reduce traction on the incision.

53. B: Alcohol withdrawal stages are described as follows:

- Beginning withdrawal: Within 8 hours—Characterized by tremors, abdominal cramping, anorexia, general weakness, nausea and vomiting, excessive sweating, irritability, mood swings, and depression.

- Withdrawal: Within 24 hours—As above plus increased anxiety and mood swings. The person may have increased BP and respiratory rate and may exhibit urinary and fecal incontinence, muscle rigidity, and clenching of the teeth.
- Severe withdrawal: Up to 3–4 or even up to 14 days after cessation but can also occur within 12 hours—Characterized by extreme confusion with hallucinations and severe agitation, possible seizures.

54. A: A cost–benefit analysis compares the average cost of an event and the cost of intervention to the benefits of the event to demonstrate savings. In the case of a new piece of equipment for the surgical department, costs can include such things as the cost of acquisition; maintenance costs; depreciation; and costs of additional staff, training, and implementation. Offsets for costs (benefits) can include such things as increased reimbursement for procedures, faster patient turnaround, decreased need for other equipment and supplies, and decreased staffing requirements.

55. B: Hemodilution is used to decrease the loss of red blood cells during surgery. One or more units of blood are removed immediately before surgery for transfusion back to the patient intraoperatively or postoperatively. After the blood is withdrawn, the patient is immediately given IV fluids to compensate for the volume of blood lost. Since this procedure dilutes the number of red blood cells in the person's circulatory system, fewer red blood cells will be lost from bleeding during the operation. The patient's blood is reinfused after the surgery. This causes a temporary anemia that the patient must be able to tolerate.

56. D: Because the OR environment and air are contaminated by dust, respiratory droplets, and surgical smoke, air exchanges should be done at a minimum of 20 per hour per AORN guidelines. In ORs where only local or topical anesthesia is being administered, a minimum of 15 air exchanges are recommended. The PACU should have 6 air exchanges and sterile storage area 4 air exchanges. Air exchanges must be monitored and airflow patterns uninterrupted. OR doors should remain closed with the pressure gradient inside the OR positive to the outer corridor.

57. D: One of the responsibilities of a healthcare industry representative is to educate healthcare personnel, including physicians, nurses, and technicians, about medical devices. The healthcare industry representative is generally better prepared to educate the staff than physicians, who may also be learning from the representative or who may have little extra time. Additionally, the healthcare industry representative typically has access to models that the staff can examine and they can provide educational materials, such as videos and literature, as well as answer questions.

58. B: Patients should be retriaged by an experienced trauma surgeon on arrival at the hospital because conditions may have changed in route to the hospital and field conditions sometimes are chaotic and may lead to error. Ideally, the trauma surgeon in charge of triage should not also be operating on the patients but should remain free to assess patient needs and to contact other surgeons and specialists, as they are needed to care for the patients. Patients are particularly at risk for hypothermia, metabolic acidosis, and coagulopathy. Immediate care includes controlling hemorrhage, decontaminating wounds, and applying temporary closure to open wounds.

59. A: The surgeon and/or the anesthesia care provider are the healthcare professionals who should determine the appropriate setting of pressure when using a pneumatic tourniquet due to the potential harm to the patient.

60. C: The pressure setting for upper extremities is usually 30-70 mmHg above the patient's systolic pressure. This has been found to be acceptable to control blood loss but limit damage to the occluded tissues.

61. C: In order to reduce damage to the limb, after each hour of surgery the limb should be evaluated. The tourniquet may be deflated briefly to restore blood flow to the limb as needed during these one-hour evaluations. This is especially important during very lengthy surgeries, because the tissue will die without proper blood circulation.

62. D: Two of the medications are duplicates: Benadryl is the brand name for diphenhydramine. Benadryl/diphenhydramine can be taken both to relieve an allergic reaction and to promote sleep with temporary insomnia. The Benadryl is prescribed at a 50 mg dosage and the diphenhydramine at 25 mg. There is a risk that the patient may take both drugs at the same time because the patient is unaware that they are the same medication, which could result in adverse effects.

63. D: Supervision. The five rights of delegation include the following:

- Right task: An appropriate task to delegate for a specific individual
- Right circumstance: Considering the setting, resources, time factors, safety factors, and all other relevant factors to determine appropriateness
- Right person: By virtue of education/skills to perform a task for the right individual
- Right direction: Clear description of the task, the purpose, any limits, and expected outcomes
- Right supervision: Able to supervise, intervene as needed, and evaluate performance of the task

64. B: When placing a patient in the supine position, the patient's knees should be flexed 5–10 degrees in order to prevent compression of the popliteal vein and reduce the risk of developing deep vein thrombosis. Extension of the knees with elevated heels is unsafe because it increases sacral pressure and can result in hyperextension of the knees and pressure on the popliteal vein. Patients with BMI >25 are especially at risk for compression of the popliteal vein and deep venous thrombosis.

65. A: When used for noncritical items associated with care of a patient with Creutzfeldt-Jakob disease (CJD), sodium chlorite solution should be at 1:10 dilution. A solution of 1:50 is usually able to provide high-level disinfection, but the CDC recommends routine use of 1:10 dilution. With CJD, environmental surfaces should be covered with disposable, impermeable material, which can be removed and incinerated. After removal, the surfaces must be further decontaminated with sodium hypochlorite 1:10 solution. Critical and semi critical items are cleaned with germicide and then autoclaved or immersed in 1N NaOH and then steam sterilized.

66. D: If a sponge count is incorrect, the circulating nurse searches the nonsterile field. Both the scrub nurse and the circulating nurse search the entire sterile field (scrub nurse manually and circulating nurse visually), and the surgeon does a manual search of the wound. If the sponge is found within the sterile field, it is placed with other sponges for counting. If it is found outside the sterile field, it is shown to the scrub nurse by the circulating nurse and isolated for later counting. If the sponge is not found, an x-ray should be taken before final wound closure.

67. A: When administering or handling open containers of chemotherapeutic agents, the nurse should wear double gloves and then remove the outer gloves upon completion. These agents should be transported in warning-labeled, leak-proof, break-resistant containers, and staff should wear PPE as indicated by the type of possible exposure. A gown impervious to chemotherapeutic agents should be worn if the agent may come in contact with arms or torso, and face shields should be used if a danger of splashing or splattering is present. Manufacturer's guidelines should be followed regarding handling and discarding hazardous chemotherapeutic agents.

68. C: Surgical patients with neutropenia are at risk for both exogenous and endogenous infection. Total ANC should be 1,800-2,000/mm^3 or higher. Risk of infection is significant if the level falls to 1,000 and severe at 500. ANC is calculated indirectly from the total white blood cell count (WBC) and the percentages of neutrophils and bands:

- ANC = Total WBC x (% neutrophils + % bands)/100

If, for example, the WBC is 5,300 with 11% neutrophils and 2% bands, neutropenia is evident despite the normal WBC:

- ANC = 5,300 X 13/100 = 689

69. B: The most cost-effective method of inventory is just-in-time ordering, in which new supplies are ordered when the stock is almost depleted so that less money is tied up in inventory. This method is most effective with automatic reordering, which is more efficient with computerized inventories to ensure that an adequate supply of materials is always on hand. If there may be delays in deliveries or if manual reordering is required, then reordering when items drop to a preestablished count may be preferable.

70. D: Wernicke's aphasia is characterized by impaired language comprehension. Often, the patient's spoken language is the most affected, so the patient speaks, but the content is often confused, and the patient may be unaware of this and believe that the communication is clear. Multiple strategies must be used, such as using gestures to provide clues and writing down key words or providing drawings to help the patient understand. The patient may have slowed comprehension, so speaking slowly and clearly is important.

71. C: Chlorhexidine gluconate is the skin antiseptic with the most residual action and has excellent effectiveness against gram-positive bacteria and good effectiveness against gram-negative bacteria and viruses. Alcohol has no residual action but has excellent effectiveness against gram-positive and gram-negative bacteria and good effectiveness against viruses. Povidone-iodine has minimal residual action and excellent effectiveness against gram-positive bacteria and good effectiveness against gram-negative bacteria and viruses. PCMX has moderate residual action and good effectiveness against gram-positive bacteria and fair effectiveness against gram-negative bacteria and viruses.

72. D: While pupils may be abnormally dilated or constricted and watery because of drug use, they are usually equal in size. Physical signs of drug use include:

- Needle tracks on arms or legs.
- Burns on fingers or lips.
- Slurring, slow speech.
- Lack of coordination, unstable gait.
- Tremors.
- Sniffing repeatedly, nasal irritation.
- Persistent cough.
- Weight loss.
- Dysrhythmias.
- Facial pallor, puffiness.

Other signs include:

- Odor of alcohol/marijuana on clothing or breath.
- Labile emotions, including mood swings, agitation, and anger.
- Inappropriate, impulsive, and/or risky behavior.
- Lying.
- Missing appointments.
- Difficulty concentrating/short-term memory loss, disoriented/confused.
- Blackouts.
- Insomnia or excessive sleeping.
- Lack of personal hygiene.

73. D: When transferring a patient that weighs less than 157 pounds (71 kg) in the supine position from a stretcher to an operating room bed, an appropriate method of transfer is a lateral transfer device with a minimum of four caregivers—one at the head, one at the foot, one on the receiving side, and one on the transferring side. Lateral transfer devices may include friction-reducing sheets or air-assisted transfer devices. Using draw sheets should be avoided.

74. A: An allow-natural-death order is a directive that promotes discussion regarding end-of-life decisions and the actions to take rather than to avoid, thus outlining the intent of care. A do-not-resuscitate order directs that CPR or other life-extending measures not be performed in the event of cardiac arrest. Required reconsideration is those events that allow discussion and participation of the patient/surrogate regarding the use of procedures and interventions during the perioperative period. A durable power of attorney empowers a specific person to make decisions on behalf of the patient.

75. B: ALARA refers to reducing radiation dose because a lower dose to the patient results in lower risk of exposure to health care personnel. Staff should stay ≥ 6 feet from the source of radiation or remain behind leaded shielding if ionizing radiation is in use. Health care providers who are nonessential should leave the OR, and those on the sterile scrub team should wear protective equipment. Radiation sources that pose a hazard include portable x-ray and fluoroscopy (ionizing) equipment and lasers (nonionizing).

76. D: To prevent back strain from the lithotomy position, the patient should be positioned so that the buttocks do not extend past the edge of the bed (torso section). Rolled towels should not be used as support. Stirrups that disperse support and pressure are used to prevent pressure injuries to the knees, ankles, and feet. Candy cane stirrups should be avoided if possible as a measure to prevent hip dislocations or fractures and muscle and nerve injuries.

77. A: Standard 1: Assessment includes a systemic, ongoing method of data collection from the patient and his or her condition and needs, as well as other support persons and health care providers. Assessment includes reviewing diagnostic studies and documenting data that are relevant in the correct format. Standard 2: Diagnosis utilizes the assessment data for development of a nursing diagnosis. Standard 3: Outcome Identification includes developing expected outcomes that are culturally and age appropriate, measurable, and retrievable. Standard 4: Planning includes developing a plan to achieve the expected outcomes.

78. D: Problem-oriented SOAP notes begin with subjective data:

- Subjective: "I can't stop crying."
- Objective: Patient tearful, pacing about room, wringing hands.

- Assessment: Ineffective coping, anxiety.
- Plan: Ativan 2 mg, instruction in relaxation and visualization.

With SOAP notes, each individual problem is numbered and the SOAP format used for each problem. With some charting systems, an extended version (SOAPIER) is used and includes Intervention, Evaluation, and Revision. This form of charting is time-consuming and may be repetitive if problems overlap.

79. D: Because the patient is at risk for an unstable glucose level, it is generally important to maintain the blood glucose level at 140–180 mg/dL because this level balances the risk of hyperglycemia against the greater risk of hypoglycemia, which can occur if the blood glucose level is maintained at a lower level. Patients may have individual factors that influence the target range, but if the glucose levels are more stringently controlled, the patient must be very closely monitored.

80. D: The CNOR is not responsible for obtaining consent for a procedure. This must be done by the surgeon performing the procedure (and also separately for anesthesia if anesthesia is being used). The CNOR may only act as a witness and an advocate for the patient in the consent process. Topics to cover by the CNOR in preoperative education should include all preoperative instructions (such as any preparations needed), NPO requirements, procedures, routine care, premedications, postoperative pain management, as well as possible complications (such as nausea) and management. Family members should be included in the preoperative teaching when appropriate. Preoperative teaching should include discussions of personal issues, such as anxiety or fears regarding surgery.

81. A: The sterile surgical team takes direction from the surgeon. The non-sterile team set up the non-sterile equipment, assist the anesthetist, and position the anesthetized patient.

82. A: The primary disadvantage of pasteurization is the lack of sporicidal activity, so it provides only high to intermediate levels of disinfection but not sterilization. Pasteurization requires submersion in hot water at temperature range of 65.5-76.6 °C (150-170 °F) for 30 minutes. Pasteurization may be used for semi critical items after initial cleaning to reduce the bioburden. The risk of splash burns is also a problem with pasteurization, so safety procedures must be followed carefully.

83. B: The patient is deteriorating: Mild = 13–15, moderate = 9–12, severe = ≤8, and comatose = 3–7.

Eye opening	4: Spontaneous. 3: To verbal stimuli. 2: To pain (not of the face). 1: No response.
Verbal	5: Oriented. 4: Conversation is confused, but can answer questions. 3: Uses inappropriate words. 2: Speech is incomprehensible. 1: No response.

Motor	6: Moves on command. 5: Moves purposefully in response to pain. 4: Withdraws in response to pain. 3: Decorticate posturing (flexion) in response to pain. 2: Decerebrate posturing (extension) in response to pain. 1: No response.

84. A: Chemical indicator tape on the outside of surgical packs indicates only that the pack has been exposed to the sterilization process but it does not guarantee that the inside of the pack is sterile; interior chemical or biological indicators must be checked to ensure the effectiveness of sterilization. The chemical indicator tape should be torn first when opening the pack to ensure the pack is not resealed and should be removed from reusable wrappers.

85. A: If splashed in the face with blood or body fluids, the perioperative nurse should immediately flush the area and the eyes with copious amounts of water for approximately 15 minutes and then report the exposure, according to established protocol. In some cases, the nurse may require postexposure prophylaxis for HIV or HCV. Needle sticks require that the person express blood from the wound and then wash the area thoroughly with soap and water (or povidone-iodine). Alcohol inactivates in the presence of organic material and is not useful for cleansing skin of blood.

86. D: If a patient develops a gas embolism during insufflation for minimally invasive surgery, the emergent response includes discontinuation of insufflation and anesthesia, placing the patient in the Trendelenburg or left lateral position, and increasing infusion of IV fluids as well as ventilation with 100% oxygen and hyperventilation. The hyperventilation, oxygen, and IV fluids are intended to reduce hypoxemia and push the gas into the lungs so it can be exhaled.

87. A: The AORN fire triangle consists of:

- Fuel: Any type of flammable/combustible material/gas. In the surgical area, this can include surgical drapes, tissue, and gas.
- Ignition source: A heat source sufficient to ignite a flammable or combustible material/gas.
- Oxidizer (oxygen): Air typically contains 21% oxygen, and fires require only 16% oxygen to burn, so the surgical environment, with oxygen in use, provides the ideal circumstances for fire.

88. C: The nurse should carry out a cost–benefit analysis to try to demonstrate that the expenditure involved in hiring additional staff will be offset by faster operating room turnaround time. Decisions about hiring are often based on monetary considerations as the cost of providing healthcare has escalated, and there is often considerable competition in a healthcare organization for limited funds. Cost–utility analysis measures benefits to society. Cost allocation analysis measures direct and indirect costs. Cost-effective analysis measures effectiveness rather than monetary savings.

89. A: A detailed cost analysis is not required as part of informed consent according to American Medical Association (AMA) guidelines, but options must be presented regardless of cost or insurance coverage. Providing informed consent is a requirement of all states. AMA guidelines for informed consent include:

- Explanation of diagnosis.
- Nature of, and reason for, treatment or procedure.
- Risks and benefits.
- Alternative options.
- Risks and benefits of alternative options.
- Risks and benefits of not having a treatment or procedure.

90. C: A medical-surgical vacuum with an inline smoke evacuation filter is sufficient to evacuate surgical smoke produced during a tonsillectomy because the smoke produced is in small amounts. Other procedures that generally produce small amounts of surgical smoke include hand surgery, craniotomy, breast biopsy, Mohs procedures, and oral surgery. Mastectomy, transurethral resection of the prostate, and arthroplasty produce large amounts of surgical smoke and require a smoke evacuation and filtration device to evacuate smoke effectively.

91. A: The use of physician-specific instrument trays requires extra setup time and should be replaced with standard trays as much as possible. Turnover time is the time between one patient leaving an OR and another entering. Ideally, turnover time should be ≤30 minutes. Turnover time may be decreased by simplifying instrument sets, eliminating seldom-used instruments, and using an integrated operative record. Doing activities in tandem rather than sequentially can also improve turnover time.

92. C: The LEMON mnemonic is used to assess a difficult airway and is described as follows:

L	Look externally	Facial trauma, large incisors, beard, mustache, obesity, abnormalities.
E	Evaluate the 3-3-2 rule	Can the patient open the mouth three finger widths, is the mandible length three finger widths from the chin to the hyoid bone, and is the thyromental distance from the thyroid notch to the mentum at least two finger widths?
M	Mallampati score	I–IV. Higher scores indicate a more difficult airway.
O	Obstruction	Stridor, hoarseness, masses are evident.
N	Neck mobility	Limited extension or flexion may cause difficult intubation.

93. C: The Patient-controlled analgesia (PCA) device is filled with opioid and must be programmed correctly and checked regularly to ensure that it is functioning properly and that controls are set. The most commonly administered medications include morphine, meperidine, fentanyl, and sufentanil.

- Limit (usually set at 4 hours): Total amount of opioid that can be delivered in the preset time limit.
- Bolus: Determines the amount of medication received when the patient delivers a dose.
- Lockout interval: Time required between administrations of boluses.
- Continuous infusion: Rate at which opioid is delivered per hour for continuous analgesia.

94. C: The perioperative nurse monitors blood pressure, EKG, and oxygen saturation for the patient who receives local anesthetic. The nurse also ensures the crash cart (resuscitation equipment) stands ready nearby. The anesthesia machine is managed by the anesthetist; therefore, it is not the responsibility of the perioperative nurse to monitor.

95. B: The biological indicator (BI) should be placed inside a pack (on end) in the front bottom section of a steam sterilizer for biologic testing because this area is most likely to be deficient. After sterilization is completed, the BI is removed and incubated to determine if any spores remain viable. A negative report for spores indicates that the sterilization process is sufficient. Testing should be completed at least weekly with daily checking during the first sterilization of the day preferable. Results of biologic testing should be documented.

96. C: Cooling is not one of the factors necessary to achieve steam sterilization. Time and temperature are the two interrelated factors as time may decrease with increased temperature, and both affect the production of steam from moisture. The time may vary according to the type and size of packaging. Each type of sterilizer has specific use guidelines that should be consulted. Common time and temperatures include:

- Gravity displacement: 121-123 °C for 15-30 minutes or 132-136 °C for 10-25 minutes.
- Prevacuum: 132-135 °C for 3-4 minutes.
- Steam flush/pressure pulse: 121-123 °C for 20 minutes or 132-135 °C for 3-4 minutes.

97. C: Contact precautions are indicated to prevent transmission of *Clostridioides difficile*, which is a spore-forming, gram-positive anaerobic bacterium that produces virulent toxins. *C. difficile* infections usually develop when antibiotic use kills off normal flora in the bowel, allowing *C. difficile* to multiply rapidly in the colon, resulting in severe diarrhea, colitis, and toxic megacolon. Patients may become severely dehydrated and the bowel may perforate, resulting in severe peritonitis and death. Spores are resistant to drying, heat, and many disinfectants, and can survive for 5 months in the environment.

98. C: All the answers could be possible complications of all amputations, but flexion contractures are specific to below-the-knee amputations. As a result, many surgeons may choose to splint the operative leg postoperatively and order special exercises to prevent this.

99. B: These laboratory findings are consistent with deficient fluid volume. An increased WBC indicating infection results from 1 or 2 cell types, but if all cell types show equal elevations, this results from concentration of the blood. Both hemoglobin and hematocrit increase as the blood volume decreases. An elevation of both BUN and creatinine indicates kidney disease, but elevated BUN alone may indicate dehydration. Serum sodium increases with dehydration. The most common cause of increased urine specific gravity is dehydration.

100. D: The optimal operating room bed height is at the waist or elbow or 5 cm above the elbow. If the operating room bed height is too high or too low, this can result in low back pain to the caregiver. When team members are at different heights, adjusting the operating room bed for the comfort of all can be difficult and the height is most often adjusted to the comfort of the lead surgeon. Standing stools can be used to help relieve discomfort.

101. A: If a patient with a patent foramen ovale is placed in the sitting position for surgery, the patient is at increased risk for venous air embolism. Venous air embolism occurs when venous blood entraps gas from the operative site, and the venous blood mixes with arterial blood and enters into the general circulation. If a large volume of gas circulates, it can have devastating effects, such as a CVA and symptoms such as pulmonary embolism. Patients undergoing neurosurgical procedures in the sitting position are especially at risk.

102. A: If a fire in the operating room occurs with combustion of disposable drapes, the class of fire extinguisher indicated is class A. The most common classes of fire extinguishers include:

- Class A: Used for wood, cloth, paper, common combustibles
- Class B: Flammable liquids, alcohol, grease, gasoline, oil
- Class C: Electrical appliances
- Class K: Cooking oils, grease

Type A (water mist) and type B (carbon dioxide) are the two types of fire extinguishers that are generally recommended for operating rooms. Carbon dioxide extinguishers are classed as types A and C, so they can be used for electrical fires.

103. D: Spark is not one of the components of the "fire triangle." The most common site for fires is the patient's airway where oxygen pools. Heat, oxygen, and fuel combine to create combustion:

- Oxygen: Leakage from about connections and pooled oxygen in drapes and body cavities. Oxygen-enriched atmosphere (OEA) is associated with about three-quarters of OR fires.
- Heat: Electrosurgical units (ESUs), lasers, and fiberoptic equipment,
- Fuel: Ointments, solutions, dressing supplies, electrical equipment, and body and facial hair.

The RACE procedure for fires includes rescuing the patients, activating the fire alarm, confining the fire, and extinguishing/evacuating.

104. C: Anthrax requires both standard and contact precautions and avoidance of direct touching of wound or drainage. After exposure, symptoms begin within a day. The patient complains of itching at site of skin contact with spores or bacilli and develops a papular lesion that becomes vesicular with development of black eschar within about 1 week to 10 days. Cultures should be taken immediately before treatment with antibiotics. Cutaneous anthrax does not spread through the air so negative pressure rooms and high filtration masks are not necessary.

105. C: With the surgical smoke hierarchy of control, the intervention that is the least effective is the use of PPE. The hierarchy from least to most effective is as follows:

- PPE: Provides secondary protection.
- Administrative controls: Provide safety education and policies.
- Engineering controls: Evacuate surgical smoke to prevent exposure.
- Substitution: Evaluate the use of alternate surgical devices.
- Elimination: Stop producing surgical smoke.

106. D: The liver is the most commonly injured intra-abdominal organ because of its size and vulnerable position in the abdomen. Most hepatic injuries are penetrating (such as gunshot and knife wounds); however, blunt hepatic injury carries a higher mortality rate. Injuries to the left hemiliver are usually more severe than those to the right hemiliver because the left hemiliver is less contained. If the patient is hemodynamically stable, conservative treatment is usually indicated to give the liver time to heal; however, with hemodynamic instability and evidence of an enlarging lesion, immediate laparotomy or angiographic intervention is required.

107. D: AAMI standards should include participation of government, but the government should not be the primary agent in establishing standards unless there are compelling safety concerns. The AAMI is a nonprofit agency whose mission is to educate people about medical instrumentation and develop standards and recommended practices for medical device users. AAMI members include medical institutions, research facilities, governmental agencies, manufacturers of medical instrumentation, testing facilities, unions, and individuals in health care. Standards should be performance based, with one global standard, so international organizations should be involved to avoid duplication of effort. Current technology and consensus of opinion should be the basis of standards.

108. D: Patience is not necessarily a characteristic of adult learners.

Knowles' characteristics of adult learners

Practical and goal-oriented	Provide overviews or summaries and examples. Use collaborative discussions with problem-solving exercises. Remain organized with the goal in mind.
Self-directed	Provide active involvement, asking for input. Allow different options toward achieving the goal. Give them responsibilities.
Knowledgeable	Show respect for their life experiences/education. Validate their knowledge and ask for feedback. Relate new material to information with which they are familiar.
Relevancy-oriented	Explain how information will be applied. Clearly identify objectives.
Motivated	Provide certificates of achievement or some type of recognition for achievement.

109. B: An antihistamine may be given with intrathecal administration of morphine to prevent or control pruritus, a common adverse effect that occurs in approximately 40% of patients. Intrathecal (subarachnoid/spinal) administration of opioids is used for patients whose pain is not controlled with other methods (such as oral, IM, IV drugs). Intrathecal narcotics (commonly morphine, fentanyl, or a combination) are frequently administered during surgical procedures employing a spinal anesthesia or as an adjunct to general anesthesia to control postoperative pain.

110. A: When holding a sterile wrapped package, the correct procedure for opening the package is to begin with the farthest wrapper flap, folding it back and securing it with the hand holding the package. Next, open one side flap and then the other, again securing with the hand holding the package. The last flap to open is the one closest to the body. The wrapper should be carefully inspected to ensure that there are no holes, punctures, tears, or signs of moisture before transferring the items to the sterile field.

111. D: When using a manual retractor to retract laterally, the assistant should hold the retractor with the arm flexed and the palm facing upward. If retracting toward the assistant's body, the arm should be flexed but with the palm facing downward. Using retractors in either direction can result in muscle strain to the neck and shoulders, especially if the retractors are held for an extended period of time without relief. Additionally, gripping the retractor too tightly can result in strain in the hands, arms, shoulders, and back.

112. B: The adoption of the electronic health record is a component of the American Recovery and Reinvestment Act (ARRA) (2009), which includes the Health Information Technology and Economic and Clinical Health Act. ARRA provided Medicare and Medicaid incentives to healthcare providers to adopt electronic health records. By 2019, 88% of healthcare providers had instituted the use of electronic health records. Electronic health records are often completed at the point of care, increasing synchronous documentation and reducing errors.

113. A: The purpose of presterilization procedures is to lower the bioburden as much as possible in order to facilitate sterilization. Contaminated instruments and equipment should be cleaned manually or by machine. Mechanical cleaning reduces the risk to staff. Mechanical cleaners include washers that sterilize, decontaminate, and disinfect. Other cleaners include ultrasonic cleaners, cart washers, and utensil washers. Staff involved in presterilization procedures should wear PPE as well as waterproof gown, waterproof foot coverings, and face and eye protection.

114. A: Zone 1. For assessment purposes, the retroperitoneal area is divided into three zones:

- The central retroperitoneal zone includes the abdominal aorta, inferior vena cava, celiac axis, superior and inferior mesenteric arteries, pancreas, esophagus, and duodenum.
- The right and left lateral peritoneal zones include the ascending and descending colon, kidneys, proximal ureters, and adrenal glands.
- The pelvic retroperitoneal zone includes the iliofemoral vessels, bladder, and extraperitoneal rectum.

If retroperitoneal bleeding occurs, zones 1 and 3 require immediate surgical exploration, and if the bleeding is ongoing, zone 2 right and left should be explored. Exploration of zone 3 with blunt pelvic trauma may worsen bleeding.

115. C: When placing a patient in the lateral position, an axillary roll (which is not actually placed in the axilla) should be positioned at the level of the 7th to 9th ribs. The roll reduces pressure on the dependent humerus head and prevents compression of axillary nerves. The arms should be on parallel arm boards, maintaining abduction of less than 90 degrees. The lower forearm and wrist should be in a neutral position with the palm up on the same plane as the operating bed. The upper arm, on the same plane as the shoulder, should be positioned similarly but with the palm down.

116. B: The DNR order is most likely to be suspended and CPR performed if a cardiac arrest is medically induced or directly relates to treatment, such as a drug reaction, rather than to a physical disorder, such as an acute MI, or the progress of a disease, such as advanced cancer or sepsis. Surgery in itself is an effort to improve health, so reasonable steps to ensure a positive outcome are usually undertaken. Medications and anesthetic agents may be the cause of cardiac arrest that would not otherwise occur; however, this is a complex ethical issue.

117. C: The scrub nurse is responsible for removing blades and drill bits from powered surgical instruments the end of the operative procedure. The equipment should be thoroughly cleaned and decontaminated, using care to remove all organic debris, such as blood and tissue. Equipment must be cleaned according to manufacturer's guidelines for detergents and germicides. Powered instruments should not be immersed or placed in ultrasonic cleaners or washer disinfectors/sterilizers except when manufacturer's guidelines specify. Air hoses should be attached to pneumatic hand pieces prior to cleaning.

118. B: Exposure to ethylene oxide is carcinogenic to humans and poses a reproductive hazard. Inhalation of ethylene oxide may cause nausea and vomiting as well as neurological disorders. In solution, it its irritating to the eyes, skin, and the lungs and can damage the kidneys and liver. Ethylene oxide cannot be mixed with other gases, and the sterilizer must not be opened until the aeration process is completed. Perioperative team members with potential exposure to ethylene oxide should wear ethylene oxide monitoring badges.

119. C: If using the Munro Pressure Ulcer Risk Assessment Scale for Perioperative Patients to assess risks associated with positioning, a score of 12 indicates moderate risk. The tool assesses mobility, nutritional status, BMI, recent weight loss, age, and comorbidities on a scale of 1 to 3. The higher the total score, the greater the risk:

- Low risk: 5–6
- Moderate risk: 7–14
- High risk: 15 or higher

120. A: A perforation indicator system involves double-gloving with a colored glove under a standard glove. The underglove is a bright color, such as blue, and the overglove is a neutral, straw color. When the overglove is punctured and fluid flows through the puncture site, this causes light to pass through and reveal the color of the underglove so that the puncture is rapidly evident. Commercial double gloving indicator systems are available.

121. A: Volume replacement and fractionated blood cells should be used because this is permitted for Jehovah's Witnesses. Adults have the right to refuse treatment even if this refusal may result in death, and health care providers do not have the right to override or ignore the patient's wishes. In the case of minors, legal authorities may grant permission to override the wishes of parents or legal guardians.

Basic blood standards for Jehovah's Witnesses	
Not acceptable	Whole blood: red cells, white cells, platelets, plasma
Acceptable	Fractions from red cells, white cells, platelets, and plasma

122. A: The thinning of the hypodermis in older adults can lead to increased risk of pressure sores. The sweat glands, vascularity, and subcutaneous fat all decrease, interfering with thermoregulation and contributing to dryness and irritation of the skin. The epidermal-dermal junction flattens, resulting in skin prone to tearing. Langerhans cells decrease in number, making the skin more prone to cancer, and the inflammatory reactions decrease. Age is an important consideration when evaluating the skin because the characteristics of the skin change as people age.

123. C: Elevating the surgical position above the level of the heart increases the danger of venous air embolism, which may cause dysrhythmias, arterial oxygen desaturation, pulmonary hypertension, and cardiac arrest. The sitting position may be used for surgical procedures involving the posterior fossa, cervical spine, shoulder, and breast. In the sitting position, the head must be supported in neutral position; excessive flexion, which can impair blood flow, must be avoided. There should be at least 2 finger widths between the chin and sternum if the head is flexed.

124. D: The preferred, and most accurate, method of checking the effectiveness of sterilization is with a biological indicator (BI). BIs commonly contain *Geobacillus stearothermophilus*, a spore-forming, nonpathogenic microorganism that is highly heat resistant. In some cases, spores are applied to a carrier, such as a disk or paper strips. Products to be sterilized may also be inoculated with a spore suspension. Self-contained BIs are also available. These include a growth medium. In some cases, more than 1 species of microorganism is present in a BI.

125. C: Electrosurgical units (ESUs) cause 68% of fires and lasers 13%. Most fires occur because oxygen pools in drapes around the face and neck or inside the throat. This oxygen-enriched atmosphere (OEA) sparks easily. Precautions include:

- Dry prepping solutions for 2-3 minutes before drapes are applied around the head and neck and then place drapes carefully to avoid creating pockets for oxygen to pool.
- Apply wet packing and keep it wet.

- Keep all dressing materials away from heat sources.
- Apply water-soluble jelly to facial hair.
- Use medical air (<30% oxygen) to decrease risk.
- Keep sterile water or normal saline on the back table.

126. A: Patients with dementia and pain do not usually react with compliance. PAINAD indicators include:

- Respirations: Rapid and labored breathing as pain increases, with short periods of hyperventilation or Cheyne-Stokes respirations.
- Vocalization: Negative or quiet and reluctant. As pain increases, patients may call out, moan or groan loudly, or cry.
- Facial expression: Sad or frightened, frowning or grimacing, especially on activities that increase pain.
- Body language: Tense, fidgeting, pacing. As pain increases, patients may become increasingly combative, rigid, fists clenched, or lie in fetal position.
- Consolability: Less distractible or consolable with increased pain.

127. B: When the patient has to *"teach back"* (explain the instructions back to the educator), it allows the nurse to evaluate his/her understanding of the discharge instructions. Correct any areas of misunderstanding. A written instruction booklet supports the verbal information provided.

128. B: If using the Scott Triggers tool to assess the risk of perioperative pressure ulcers, the laboratory test that may be assessed is serum albumin. The tool assesses four parameters, and two or more "yeses" or the presence of a finding indicates a high-risk surgical patient. Triggers include the following:

- Age: 62 or older
- Serum albumin or BMI: Albumin <3.5 g/L or BMI <19 or >40
- ASA score: 3 or greater
- Estimated surgery time in minutes: >180 minutes (3 hours)

129. A: The positions that carry the greatest risk of eye injury include the prone and lateral positions. Patients in these positions should be assessed and monitored carefully after positioning and during the procedure. Patients' bodies may shift slightly during procedures, and this can result in pressure on an eye in the dependent position. Horseshoe-shaped head positioners should be avoided because they increase the risk of eye injuries such as corneal abrasion.

130. A: CQI emphasizes the organization, systems, and processes within that organization rather than individuals. It recognizes internal customers (staff) and external customers (patients) and utilizes data to improve processes, recognizing that most processes can be improved. CQI uses the scientific method of experimentation to meet needs and improve services and utilizes various tools, such as brainstorming, multivoting, various charts and diagrams, storyboarding, and meetings. Core concepts include:

- Quality and success are meeting or exceeding internal and external customer's needs and expectations.
- Problems relate to processes, and variations in process lead to variations in results.
- Change can be incremental.

131. B: In a sterile processing area, the distance between the instrument washing sink and the area where the instruments are prepared for sterilization must be at least 4 feet. Cleaning and decontamination spaces must also be separated by a wall with a door or pass-through and a partial wall/partition that is at least 4 feet high. Separate sinks must be available for washing instruments and for hand washing, and there must be storage space for PPE and cleaning supplies in the decontamination area.

132. D: If a patient is learning a new process, such as wound care, the response that best indicates that the patient is engaged in the process is if the patient asks questions. Taking notes or referring to notes can be distracting, especially when the patient must learn to do a task, so the nurse should print out directions for the patient to read. These directions may be provided prior to actual instruction by the nurse or after instruction and demonstration. The patient should be encouraged to ask questions throughout the process and should carry out and talk through a return demonstration.

133. C: EO-sterilized items must be aerated before handling, as EO is a carcinogen. The typical duration of mechanical aeration of EO-sterilized items at 50-55 °C is 8-12 hours. With a temperature of 38 °C, aeration time extends to 12-16 hours. Carts carrying EO-sterilized items from the sterilizer to the mechanical aerator should be pulled so that the staff person is not walking behind the cart and breathing the air that passes over it. Both the sterilizer and aerator should be in a room well ventilated to the outside atmosphere to reduce danger of explosion.

134. A: Functional incontinence occurs when a continent patient is unable to reach the toilet in time, resulting in unintentional incontinence. The best intervention is to assess the patient's usual frequency of urination and then to schedule urination on a routine basis, typically every 2–3 hours, so that a nurse assists the patient to the bathroom before the patient's need to urinate becomes acute. In some cases, a bedside commode may be needed, especially if the toilet is at a distance.

135. C: Although urine may be needed to perform lab work prior to surgery, the main reason patients without a Foley catheter already in place are encouraged to void is to prevent bladder distention and incontinence, because an anesthetized patient cannot feel the urge to urinate. This is very important in abdominal surgeries, because an enlarged bladder could be damaged during surgery. The pooled fluid from an incontinent patient could also cause skin damage.

136. D: Patients should give consent for a healthcare industry representative to be present during an operative procedure. There is no federal law that specifically addresses this issue; however, some state laws require consent for any nonmedical personnel in the operating room. Additionally, it is a matter of informed consent and protection of the privacy and confidentiality of the patient. Patients have the right to autonomy in making decisions regarding their care and should be made aware of all aspects of their care, ensuring transparency in the healthcare process.

137. A: The CDC's Standard Precautions should be applied when caring for all patients from first contact to last. The precautions apply toward body fluids and excretions (except sweat), blood, mucous membranes, and nonintact skin, and include hand hygiene (soap and water or alcohol rub), gloves (clean, nonsterile), masks and other face protection (such as face shield), gowns (clean, nonsterile), sharps, patient care equipment (single-use and reusable), linens, environmental controls (procedures for cleaning), and patient placement (private, nonprivate, cohorting, and airflow considerations).

138. D: The Mini-Cog test to assess for dementia has 2 components:

- Drawing the face of a clock with all 12 numbers and the hands indicating the time specified by the examiner.
- Remembering and later repeating the names of 3 common objects.

The Mini-Mental State Exam includes:

- Remembering and later repeating the names of 3 common objects.
- Counting backward from 100 by 7s or spelling "world" backward.
- Naming items.
- Providing the address and location of the exam.
- Repeating common phrases.
- Copying a picture of interlocking shapes.
- Following simple 3-part instructions.

139. A: If surgical instruments are left in the closed or latched position, it is possible that sterilant cannot reach all of the surfaces, so the instruments should be considered unsterile, and any unsterile item in a surgical pack renders the entire pack unsterile. Therefore, the correct response is to replace the entire surgical pack with a new one. Devices such as racks, stringers, and V-shaped pouches are available to ensure that instruments stay in their open or unlatched position during sterilization.

140. C: Any postoperative patient who received general anesthetic could develop a persistent cough. The *best* advice is for the patient to inform her physician. The conversation may include questions regarding her temperature, and instructions for splinting and postural drainage. However, the patient needs to inform the physician in case she needs further treatment, such as chest physiotherapy, or prescriptions, such as antibiotics.

141. C: Up to 20% of patients who are treated for anaphylaxis develop a sudden biphasic reaction in which their symptoms recur. Although this reaction can occur within 1–72 hours, it most commonly occurs within 10 hours. The cause of biphasic reactions is not clear but is likely related to a prolonged immune response. The biphasic reaction can be similar to the first reaction, or it may be more or less severe; therefore, it is important that patients are carefully monitored for several hours after the initial treatment, and patients should be provided with an epinephrine autoinjector (such as the EpiPen) if discharged.

142. B: TQM focuses on meeting the needs of the customers at all levels within an organization, promoting both continuous improvement and dedication to quality. Outcomes should include increased customer satisfaction, productivity, and profits through efficiency and reduction in costs. In order to provide TQM, an organization must seek the following:

- Information regarding customer's needs and opinions.
- Involvement of staff at all levels in decision making, goal setting, and problem solving.
- Commitment of management to empowering staff and being accountable through active leadership and participation.
- Institution of teamwork with incentives and rewards for accomplishments.

143. C: Semi-restricted perioperative zones require the donning of hospital-issued scrubs and head coverings. Perioperative zones are broken down as follows:

- Non-restricted: Street clothes. Labs coats are recommended if entering from a restricted or semi-restricted zone and there is a plan to return to those zones.
- Semi-restricted: Hospital-issued scrubs and head coverings. Religious head coverings that cover only part of the scalp may be worn under surgical head coverings.
- Restricted: Hospital-issued scrubs, head coverings, and shoe coverings or clean dedicated shoes. All jewelry must be removed prior to scrubbing.

144. A: An appropriate response toward a disruptive team member is to discuss the situation in an informal meeting by saying, "I could see that you were very upset earlier, and I'd like to talk about that with you." If the first disruption was egregious or if, in fact, it was an example of a pattern of behavior, then the situation should be discussed formally with the immediate supervisor. If the behavior persists after this, the matter should be referred to the department head, and, if that doesn't resolve the problem, then disciplinary action may be indicated.

145. A: The biological indicator that is used with steam sterilization and vaporized hydrogen peroxide sterilization for monitoring the effectiveness of sterilization is assessing for the presence of *Geobacillus stearothermophilus* spores because they are highly resistant to these types of sterilization. *Bacillus atrophaeus* spores are used as biological indicators for dry heat and ethylene oxide. Biological indicators contain lot numbers, the name of the organism that is tested for, the organism's population, and the expiration date. Usually, biological and chemical indicators are used during sterilization.

146. D: The label for radioactive waste does not require the type of patient protection used, although this information must be documented on the patient's operative record as well as assessment of patient's skin, including any indications of injury, such as redness, blistering, swelling, or abrasions. Radioactive waste must be placed in special containers and labeled as radioactive waste with the name of the radioisotope, activity, disposal date, and full name and contact information of the authorized user.

147. B: The purpose of the Joint Commission's "Do Not Use" List is to prevent errors and protect patient safety by eliminating abbreviations, acronyms, and symbols that can be easily mistaken or misconstrued. In many cases, abbreviations have been eliminated in favor of words (QD is replaced with daily and QID with 4 times daily). With numbers, trailing zeroes are eliminated (7.0 mg is replaced with 7 mg), although a leading zero (.7 mg replaced with 0.7 mg) is required. Many symbols (e.g., @, <, >, µg) are replaced with words. Acronyms (e.g., SOB) are replaced with words.

148. A: When a patient is ready for oxygen weaning based on oxygen saturation and blood gas levels, the FiO_2 is gradually reduced to the lowest level at which the patient's respiratory rate, oxygen saturation, and PaO_2 are adequate for the patient: 90%–92% for oxygen saturation and PaO_2 at 70–100 mmHg on room air. Once the patient is stabilized at this level, then trial periods on room air without oxygen are carried out, with the trial periods gradually being lengthened until oxygen is discontinued. The patient should be closely monitored during the weaning process and after oxygen is discontinued.

149. B: When open shelving is used to store sterile packages, the highest shelf should be 18 inches from the ceiling to ensure adequate air circulation. The lowest shelf must be 8-10 inches from floor to prevent contamination from the floor. The shelving unit should be at least 2 inches away from outside walls to promote circulation of air as well. All surgical storage equipment, including cabinets and shelving, should have good ventilation with temperature and humidity control.

150. A: Although all of these answers are recorded for a surgical patient, only the dermatome levels are specific to regional anesthetic patients. This is to determine the level of the anesthetic as it wears off postoperatively.

151. A: When describing gunshot wounds, they should not be described in terms of entry and exit because this is a forensic determination and it is not always possible to immediately differentiate the entry wound from the exit wound. The wounds should be documented with a detailed description of their size, appearance, and location. Examining the location of the two wounds can help determine the trajectory, which is important in assessing possible damage to internal organs.

152. B: Stage II. NPIAP Staging:

- Stage I: Red or purple discoloration of defined area of intact skin, which may exhibit change in temperature (warm or cool), consistency (firm or soft), or sensation (itching, pain).
- Stage II: Superficial ulcer may appear as an abrasion or blistered area or slightly depressed. Skin loss is partial-thickness and involves the epidermis and/or dermis.
- Stage III: Deep full-thickness ulceration of skin with damaged or necrotic subcutaneous tissue. Ulceration may extend to the fascia, and there may be tunneling of adjacent tissue.
- Stage IV: Deep full-thickness ulceration of skin with extensive damage, and necrosis of tissue extending to muscle, bone, tendons, or joints.

153. A: In the event of a disaster, increasing surge capacity allows for admission of large numbers of injured clients. The initial strategy is to identify clients who are safely eligible for early discharge. This may also include canceling scheduled procedures, such as elective surgeries. Extra beds can be placed in outpatient areas and in hallways because this is more time-effective than attempting to transfer existing patients to different rooms and cleaning and preparing the rooms. In some cases, non-disaster-related patients may be diverted to other hospitals; however, in many cases, other facilities will also be impacted by the disaster.

154. A: A sharps injury log must contain the type and brand of the device involved in the injury, a description of the area in which the injury occurred, and a description of the how injury occurred, such as the engineering controls and work practices in use, the PPE in use, and the type of procedure being carried out. The sharps injury log is an OSHA requirement. The log must protect the confidentiality of the person who incurred the injury.

155. C: Moderate hypothermia: Core temperature of 30-32 °C (86-89.6 °F) with or without shivering, requires forced-air warming device, warm blankets, and warmed IV fluids. Normothermia: Core temperature more than 36 °C (96.8 °F). Mild hypothermia: Core temperature of 32-36 °C (89.6-96.8 °F) with skin pale or gray and cool to touch, requires rewarming with warm blankets, fluids, lights, or warm ambient environmental temperature. Severe hypothermia: Core temperature less than 30 °C (86 °F) with patient comatose and near death, requiring cardiopulmonary bypass to warm core first.

156. D: The characteristics of support surfaces that provide the best protection against positioning-related pressure injuries are deep immersion and high envelopment. Immersion is the depth to which the body part sinks into the surface of the support surface. The deeper the immersion, the more pressure is distributed rather than localized. Envelopment is the ability of the support surface to adjust to irregularities, such as wrinkles in the bedding, without markedly increasing pressure on the skin.

157. B: Catgut is an absorbable suture material but it has less tensile strength and greater tissue reactivity than other absorbable sutures (such as polyglactin 910, polyglycolic acid, poliglecaprone), and the absorption rate is more unpredictable (about 12 weeks). Polyester has good tensile strength and minimal tissue reactivity. It is easily seen and does not absorb fluids. Silk has excellent tensile strength but loses strength if wet and loses strength in about a year in tissue. Nylon has good tensile strength and little tissue reactivity but poor knot security, requiring multiple knots. Nylon can be manufactured in very fine sizes.

158. D: All implants should have the same metal composition, so only stainless-steel screws should be used with a stainless-steel metal plate; otherwise, galvanic corrosion may occur and damage the device. Implants are devices intended to replace a biological body part (such as the hip), support injured parts (such as plates and screws), or enhance a body part (such as breast implants). Implants can include plates, screws, intramedullary nails, rods, hip prosthesis, external fixators, and pins.

159. A: The circulating nurse coordinates care of the surgical patient. They are the patient's advocate, who coordinates intraoperative (rather than preoperative) patient care. The circulating nurse manages and implements activities outside the sterile field. The goal of the circulating nurse is to achieve desirable patient outcomes, but they do not manage the transfer and care of the patient through stabilization. This PACU nurse cares for the post-operative patient through stabilization.

160. D: The type of needle that is indicated for suturing of fascia and muscle as well as for perineal lacerations and episiotomy repair is the blunt-tip needle. Studies indicate that the use of blunt-tip needles reduces the incidence of glove perforation risk by more than 50%. Blunt-tip needles do not appear to affect wound morbidity, although some studies show that surgeons are less satisfied with blunt-tip needles. Blunt-tip needles dissect the tissue instead of cutting it.

161. B: Staff need high filtration surgical masks (filtering particulate matter ≥ 0.1 micrometer in size), along with a smoke evacuation system to prevent exposure to surgical smoke produced by lasers and other electrosurgical devices; the plume is hazardous and may contain toxic gases, aerosolized biological material (such as blood fragments and bacteria), and viruses. The National Institute for Occupational Safety and Health (NIOSH) recommends that the suction device for the smoke evacuation system be as close as possible to the source of surgical smoke.

162. B: For a patient with a demand pacemaker, this cardiac monitor tracing indicates oversensing. The sensitivity setting is too high, so the pacemaker is misinterpreting artifacts, such as muscle contractions and nondepolarization events, as contractions and therefore fails to trigger a contraction. This results in decreased cardiac output. Oversensing can also occur as the result of damage to the pacemaker or disconnection of a lead.

163. B: After selecting a number of possible vendors for a complex upgrade of equipment and services, the next step is to develop a request for proposal. With the request for proposal, there may be considerable differences among the different vendors related to the types of equipment and the costs of services. A request for quotation, on the other hand, is usually submitted for products or services that are essentially the same or very similar with cost being just one of the deciding factors.

164. D: Medication reconciliation should be an ongoing process during all phases of care. Medication reconciliation includes making a list of all current medications (dose and frequency), including herbs and nonprescription drugs and vitamins, as well as drug allergies or intolerances. This list should be posted prominently in the patient's chart so physicians can check the list whenever ordering medications. The patient must receive a new/revised list on discharge with thorough explanation of any changes and access to drug information and the advice of a pharmacist.

165. B: The fentanyl/midazolam combination provides both sedation and pain control. Conscious sedation uses a combination of analgesia and sedation so that patients can remain responsive and follow verbal cues but have a brief amnesia that prevents recall of the procedures. The patient must be monitored carefully, including pulse oximetry, during this type of sedation.

- Midazolam (Versed): Short-acting, water-soluble sedative, with onset of 1-5 minutes, peaking in 30, and duration usually about 1 hour (but may last up to 6 hours).
- Fentanyl: Short-acting opioid with immediate onset, peaking in 10-15 minutes and with duration of about 20-45 minutes.

166. D: Bipolar (not monopolar) electrosurgery should be used if at all possible. Before the procedure begins, the programming device and personnel to reprogram must be in the OR in case electrosurgery reprograms the device. The active and dispersive electrodes should be placed as far from the IED and wires as possible and the current path should not pass through the area of the IED or the electrodes. Temperature should be maintained at 68-76 °F (20-24 °C) and humidity at 50%-60% to reduce production of static electricity.

167. C: When documenting a medication, an appropriate entry is "morphine sulfate 4 mg SQ right deltoid." Fractions (such as 4 ½) should be replaced with decimals (4.5). Abbreviations that should be avoided include the use of U or u for units and IU for international units; QD or QOD (and variations); MS, MSO_4, and $MgSO_4$ for morphine or magnesium sulfate. Trailing zeros (50.0) should not be used with medication orders, although they may be used in laboratory reports.

168. D: AABB standards require that blood be attached to a warmer for no more than 4 hours. Overheating of blood (>42 °C) may cause hemolysis, so blood warmers must have temperature controls with a visible thermometer and online monitor that includes an audible alarm system. Blood warmers warm blood to approximately 32-38 °C: Indications for blood warmers include:

- Prevention of or increase in hypothermia.
- Blood flow rate > 100 mL/min (adult) or >15 mL/kg/hr (children).
- Patient evidence of significant cold agglutinins.
- Rapid infusion using central lines.

169. D: If an afterloading modality, such as a MammoSite catheter, is used for insertion of radioactive seeds following a lumpectomy, the seeds are typically inserted in a protected room outside of the operating room. Only low-dose radioactive materials are placed in the operating room, although, increasingly, afterloading modalities (catheters, needles, hollow tubing) are placed during surgery. The actual radiotherapy is then administered later in the day or the next day. Afterloading decreases exposure to personnel, improves accuracy, and simplifies the surgical procedure.

170. A: Neostigmine is a cholinesterase inhibitor used as a reversing agent after administration of nondepolarizing neuromuscular blocking agent. Neostigmine binds to acetylcholinesterase and makes the molecule lipid soluble so that it cannot penetrate the blood-brain barrier. It is usually given either with an anticholinergic in separate syringes or immediately after the anticholinergic.

Glycopyrrolate is recommended as an anticholinergic because its onset and duration are similar to neostigmine and it is less likely to cause tachycardia than atropine.

171. D: All team members should participate in the "time out" as part of the Universal Protocol established by the Joint Commission to avoid wrong site, wrong procedure, and wrong person surgery. One person on the team should be responsible for initiating the time out and ensuring that adequate time is taken for a final review of the verification process and operative site marking. The procedure should be delayed until the time out is completed and all concerns resolved.

172. C: All of these items should be addressed in a preoperative assessment, but first the nurse should make sure to have the right patient. The nurse cannot just do this by asking the patient's name because there are often patients with the same or similar names. Hence, a demographic piece of information, such as date of birth, should also be verified. This information should be compared with the patient's armband, and the correct spelling is verified. If the patient cannot verbally answer, then staff or visitors accompanying the patient to the preoperative area should do this verification.

173. B: While family request for information is important, the focus of transfer from OR to the PACU is on the patient, and PACUs should have established protocols for providing information to families. The hand-off report, both written and oral, includes all relevant preoperative information (conditions, allergies, laboratory findings, substance abuse, sensory limitations, age, and mobility), surgical information (type of operation, anesthetic agent, duration of anesthesia, drains, and complications), preoperative emotional status, estimated fluid/blood loss, treatments provided, and pain management plans.

174. C: The liver contains the type of tissue that produces the most fine and ultrafine particulate matter in surgical smoke at a rate that is three times higher than the next tissue, muscle. The renal cortex and renal pelvis are next. Lung and adipose tissue produce relatively lower amounts of particulate matter. For surgical smoke-generating procedures involving the liver, perioperative team members may wear N95 filtering facepiece respirators in addition to the use of smoke evacuation and filtration devices.

175. A: The Ishikawa "fishbone" diagram, resembling the head and bones of a fish, is an analysis tool to determine causes and effects. In performance improvement, it is used to help identify root causes. An affinity diagram is used to brainstorm and organize large numbers of ideas, items, or issues (>15) into major categories. A prioritization matrix is used to prioritize items or select one from a number of alternatives based on preselected criteria, such as benefit and cost. A Gantt chart is used to manage schedules and estimate time needed to complete tasks.

176. B: A surgical gown is considered sterile from the chest to the level of the sterile field. The areas of the gown that tend to be the most contaminated are above the chest and below the operating room bed. The neckline, shoulder areas, and axillary regions are generally considered unsterile, as well as the back of the gown. The arms of the gown are considered sterile from the cuff seam to two inches above the elbow. Sterile gloves should completely cover the cuff seams.

177. D: The back table(s) and Mayo stand should be set up according to standardized procedures rather than the preference of surgeon or nurses so that if the scrub nurse is relieved during the procedure, the incoming staff will be familiar with the setup. The most frequently used instruments are placed on the Mayo stand, which is usually positioned across the patient's legs. All medications and solutions must be carefully and clearly labeled. The scrub nurse must be familiar with setups for different procedures and surgeon preferences for instruments, prepping, and draping.

178. C: Intravenous methylene blue dye may cause the pulse oximetry reading to drop to 65% for 1-2 minutes. Indigo carmine and indocyanine green cause slight decrease. Pulse oximetry utilizes an external oximeter that attaches to the patient's finger or earlobe to measure arterial oxygen saturation (SpO_2), the percentage of hemoglobin that is saturated with oxygen. The oximeter uses light waves to determine oxygen saturation (SpO_2). Oxygen saturation should be maintained at more than 95%, although some patients with chronic respiratory disorders, such as COPD, may have lower SpO_2.

179. D: Intraoperative blood salvage is contraindicated in cancer surgery. Blood collection is used for surgical procedures, such as cardiac, vascular, orthopedic, urologic, trauma, gynecologic, and transplant surgery, where the anticipated blood loss is ≥ 20% and there is no expected contamination from bacteria or cancer cells. Machines can collect up to 4 L/min, depending on the unit. Care must be taken to suction from pooled blood rather than skimming blood off of the top because this may result in suctioning of air.

180. C: The nurse manager assigns scrub personnel based on their expertise. The staffing skill mix must be appropriate to the procedure and hospital policy. Staff availability must also be considered. Seniority does not equate with expertise.

181. C: The normal intracranial pressure (ICP) level ranges from 7 to 15 mmHg; values greater than 20 mmHg are considered pathological and should trigger ICP-lowering interventions. The Monro-Kellie hypothesis states that there are three compartments in the brain: brain tissue, cerebrospinal fluid, and blood. Because of limitations in the size of the skull, the total volume needs to remain constant, so an increase in one volume requires compensatory changes in the volumes in the other compartments. When there is an expanding volume in the brain (such as from bleeding), the brain is unable to compensate, and the ICP can begin to dangerously increase.

182. A: Antiseptics, such as alcohols, hydrogen peroxide, chlorhexidine gluconate, and povidone-iodine, are chemical solutions specifically used to disinfect body parts. Disinfectants, such as glutaraldehyde, sodium hypochlorite, phenolics, and quaternary ammonium compounds, are used to disinfect inanimate objects. Germicide is a general term for solutions that destroy microorganisms, including both antiseptics and disinfectants. Sporicides, such as glutaraldehyde, sodium hypochlorite, and stabilized hydrogen peroxide 6%, are disinfectants that also destroy bacterial spores. Disinfectants may be used alone or in combination with other products to achieve maximal disinfection.

183. D: Alcohols (70% or 90% isopropyl) are effective disinfectants for the rubber stops on medication vials, but alcohols are inactivated by blood and other protein material, so they cannot be used for instruments contaminated with blood. They may impair the coating on lenses instruments and cause hardening of some rubber and plastic materials. Alcohols are bacteriocidal against vegetative forms of bacteria but do not kill spores or hydrophilic viruses. Alcohols evaporate rapidly and may be used to speed drying of flexible endoscope channels.

184. C: During surgical procedures, it is recommended that double gloving be used by scrubbed team members, such as the scrub person, surgeon, and first assistant. These individuals have the greatest risk of sharps injuries. Double gloving reduces the risk of injury by about 71%. Exceptions may be made by surgeons for some situations, such as delicate neurosurgical procedures in which the sense of touch is essential.

185. A: Isotonic crystalloids: Replacement solutions for loss of water and electrolytes. Isotonic crystalloids, such as normal saline (0.9%), lactated Ringer's (contains potassium), and Plasma-Lyte (contains potassium), are most commonly used. Different solutions contain different electrolytes (sodium, chloride, potassium calcium, lactate, and magnesium), so monitoring electrolytes is essential. Hypotonic: Maintenance solutions used to replace water loss. Dextrose in water (D5W) is commonly used with water deficit and for those with sodium restriction. Hypertonic: Used for hyponatremia (3% saline) and severe hypovolemic shock (3-7.5% saline).

186. A: Ethylene oxide (EO) is highly flammable and may lead to explosions, so it is diluted with inert gases (such as CO_2) and hydrochlorofluorocarbon (HCFC) to reduce flammability. EO can be used for items that are heat labile and moisture sensitive, such as some microinstruments, electrical instruments, and large pieces of equipment. EO sterilization typically takes 105-300 minutes at temperatures of 37-63 °C, humidity 45-75%, and gas concentration of 450-1,200 mg/L. Duration is inversely proportional to concentration of the gas.

187. C: The circulating nurse is responsible for documenting sponge, sharp, and instrument counts. Documentation includes types of counts, numbers of counts, identification of those performing counts, results, and physician notification. If instruments or sponges (used for packing, for example) are left with the patient, the circulating nurse should explain the reason and the number of each. If the count is incorrect, this information must be documented, as well as actions taken to account for missing items and the results of those actions.

188. A: Controlled diabetes is not a contraindication to ambulatory or outpatient surgery, although uncontrolled diabetes is because it puts the patient at increased risk. Contraindications include conditions that prevent the patient from adequately managing care or pain in the postoperative period, including active substance or alcohol abuse, unstable condition, infections requiring isolation, surgery that may result in the need for parenteral analgesia, and dementia or other condition that prevents self-care unless assistance (such as a caregiver) is available.

189. A: Squatting down with knees bent to retrieve an item on the floor demonstrates proper body mechanics. Bending at the waist to retrieve or lift an item can cause back strain. The nurse should avoid stretching overhead but should use a step stool or grip tool with an extension to retrieve items out of reach. Pushing or pulling with the arms may result in muscle strains in the arms and back, so the person should use the whole body to push or pull. The nurse should avoid reaching, bending, or twisting while lifting.

190. D: Low-pressure/high-volume ETTs, used more frequently than high-pressure/low-volume, cause less mucosal trauma and ischemia but increase risk of sore throat, aspiration, and spontaneous extubation. ETTs are usually made of radiopaque polyvinyl chloride plastic that is pliable and able to mold to the shape of the airway. ETTs are sized according to internal diameter. A large size increases airflow but can cause more trauma than smaller sizes. Adult ETTs usually have an inflatable cuff to affect a tracheal seal, which allows positive-pressure ventilation and prevents aspiration.

191. C: While NPO guidelines may vary somewhat from one institution to another, generally breastfeeding infants must not breastfeed or receive breast milk for 4 hours before surgery. Infants usually may not be fed formula for 6 hours before surgery. Many institutions no longer require the traditional NPO after midnight but may restrict foods and fluids for 6 or 8 hours prior to scheduled surgery. In some cases, clear fluids may be allowed 6 to 3 (or even 2) hours preoperatively, depending on risk factors for aspiration.

192. C: According to the ANA Code of Ethics for Nurses: Provision 2, the nurse's primary commitment is to the patient. Issues of concern with provision 2 include avoiding conflict of interest (such as financial concerns), collaborating with other individuals and groups to meet the patient's needs and to plan and provide care, and establishing professional boundaries. The Code of Ethics contains 9 provisions with a number of subcategories for each provision that outline the goal, values, and obligations of nurses.

193. B: The isolation technique should be used during surgeries that involve the bowel and metastatic tumors. The isolation technique is used to prevent the spread of bacteria or other microorganisms or cancer cells from one area to another. The sterile field should be organized to minimize the risk of contamination. The isolation technique should begin immediately before resection and end when resection is complete. Instruments used for the resection are removed from the sterile field, gloves and soiled gowns are changed, new sterile drapes are applied over existing ones, and new instruments are used for closing the wound.

194. B: The pediatric assessment tool that was developed specifically for the perioperative pediatric patient is the Braden Q+P scale. It is a more comprehensive assessment than the Braden Q scale and includes assessment of height and weight, ASA score, surgical position, procedure length, devices used, underlying condition, sensory perception, moisture, mobility, nutrition, friction and shear, and tissue perfusion. Items are scored yes or no to indicate presence or absence. The higher the score, the greater the risk.

195. C: Preanesthesia evaluation and assessment should be done by the anesthesiologist or nurse anesthetist prior to administration of anesthesia in all cases except for local anesthesia to determine the degree of anesthesia required. In some cases, even those receiving local anesthesia should be evaluated, particularly those with risk factors, such as obesity or diabetes. The evaluation and assessment should include history (including previous response to anesthesia), physical assessment, and a review of laboratory studies. The anesthesia plan is developed as part of the evaluation and assessment.

196. A: Heated water circulating through blankets or pads that do not contain heating elements is an example of resistive warming. The heat is generated conductively, that is, by electricity passing through a conductor. With convective warming, a device warms the air that surrounds the patient. With passive insulation, a device such as an insulating garment or warmed blanket prevents hypothermia. Active warming involves direct application of heat and may be either convective or conductive.

197. C: The uniform is not PPE. PPE must be supplied without cost to employees and includes gowns and gloves. The face is particularly vulnerable to splashing and splattering of blood and body fluids. Goggles should be nonvented or indirectly vented with an anti-fog coating and solid side shields and should allow for direct and peripheral vision. They should be large enough to cover eyeglasses if necessary and still fit snugly to provide protection. Face shields provide protection to the eyes and face. The shields should have both crown and chin protection and extend around the face to the ears.

198. C: Many herbal medications can cause interactions with intraoperative medications and should be noted. Ginkgo biloba can increase bleeding, not cardiac arrhythmias. It is usually not substantial enough to delay or cancel surgery, but the physicians caring for the patient should be made aware that she is taking ginkgo biloba, so they may plan accordingly.

199. B: Hazardous waste that is contaminated by chemotherapeutic agents must be disposed of in a yellow waste container. This may include PPE, IV bags used to administer chemotherapeutic agents, empty vials syringes, or ampules. Contaminated empty devices are placed in the yellow containers, but if they are not empty, they are placed in black containers. Special red containers are used for sharps (not associated with chemotherapeutic agents), and red biohazard containers are used for blood, body fluids, and items contaminated with blood or body fluids (IV bags, blood-saturated materials).

200. C: The airborne concentration of a chemical substance that workers can be exposed to repeatedly without it adversely affecting their health is the threshold limit value (TLV), which serves as a guide to the control of health hazards. The time-weighted average (TWA) is the average concentration that a worker can safely be exposed to over the typical work week (8 hours daily times 5 days). The short-term exposure limit is what the worker can be continuously exposed for a short period (without exceeding the TLV-TWA) without developing adverse effects, such as irritation and tissue damage. The TLV ceiling limit (TLV-C) is the highest degree of concentration that the person should be exposed to at any time.

CNOR Practice Test #3

To take this additional CNOR practice test, visit our bonus page:
mometrix.com/bonus948/cnor

How to Overcome Test Anxiety

Just the thought of taking a test is enough to make most people a little nervous. A test is an important event that can have a long-term impact on your future, so it's important to take it seriously and it's natural to feel anxious about performing well. But just because anxiety is normal, that doesn't mean that it's helpful in test taking, or that you should simply accept it as part of your life. Anxiety can have a variety of effects. These effects can be mild, like making you feel slightly nervous, or severe, like blocking your ability to focus or remember even a simple detail.

If you experience test anxiety—whether severe or mild—it's important to know how to beat it. To discover this, first you need to understand what causes test anxiety.

Causes of Test Anxiety

While we often think of anxiety as an uncontrollable emotional state, it can actually be caused by simple, practical things. One of the most common causes of test anxiety is that a person does not feel adequately prepared for their test. This feeling can be the result of many different issues such as poor study habits or lack of organization, but the most common culprit is time management. Starting to study too late, failing to organize your study time to cover all of the material, or being distracted while you study will mean that you're not well prepared for the test. This may lead to cramming the night before, which will cause you to be physically and mentally exhausted for the test. Poor time management also contributes to feelings of stress, fear, and hopelessness as you realize you are not well prepared but don't know what to do about it.

Other times, test anxiety is not related to your preparation for the test but comes from unresolved fear. This may be a past failure on a test, or poor performance on tests in general. It may come from comparing yourself to others who seem to be performing better or from the stress of living up to expectations. Anxiety may be driven by fears of the future—how failure on this test would affect your educational and career goals. These fears are often completely irrational, but they can still negatively impact your test performance.

Elements of Test Anxiety

As mentioned earlier, test anxiety is considered to be an emotional state, but it has physical and mental components as well. Sometimes you may not even realize that you are suffering from test anxiety until you notice the physical symptoms. These can include trembling hands, rapid heartbeat, sweating, nausea, and tense muscles. Extreme anxiety may lead to fainting or vomiting. Obviously, any of these symptoms can have a negative impact on testing. It is important to recognize them as soon as they begin to occur so that you can address the problem before it damages your performance.

The mental components of test anxiety include trouble focusing and inability to remember learned information. During a test, your mind is on high alert, which can help you recall information and stay focused for an extended period of time. However, anxiety interferes with your mind's natural processes, causing you to blank out, even on the questions you know well. The strain of testing during anxiety makes it difficult to stay focused, especially on a test that may take several hours. Extreme anxiety can take a huge mental toll, making it difficult not only to recall test information but even to understand the test questions or pull your thoughts together.

Effects of Test Anxiety

Test anxiety is like a disease—if left untreated, it will get progressively worse. Anxiety leads to poor performance, and this reinforces the feelings of fear and failure, which in turn lead to poor performances on subsequent tests. It can grow from a mild nervousness to a crippling condition. If allowed to progress, test anxiety can have a big impact on your schooling, and consequently on your future.

Test anxiety can spread to other parts of your life. Anxiety on tests can become anxiety in any stressful situation, and blanking on a test can turn into panicking in a job situation. But fortunately, you don't have to let anxiety rule your testing and determine your grades. There are a number of relatively simple steps you can take to move past anxiety and function normally on a test and in the rest of life.

Physical Steps for Beating Test Anxiety

While test anxiety is a serious problem, the good news is that it can be overcome. It doesn't have to control your ability to think and remember information. While it may take time, you can begin taking steps today to beat anxiety.

Just as your first hint that you may be struggling with anxiety comes from the physical symptoms, the first step to treating it is also physical. Rest is crucial for having a clear, strong mind. If you are tired, it is much easier to give in to anxiety. But if you establish good sleep habits, your body and mind will be ready to perform optimally, without the strain of exhaustion. Additionally, sleeping well helps you to retain information better, so you're more likely to recall the answers when you see the test questions.

Getting good sleep means more than going to bed on time. It's important to allow your brain time to relax. Take study breaks from time to time so it doesn't get overworked, and don't study right before bed. Take time to rest your mind before trying to rest your body, or you may find it difficult to fall asleep.

Along with sleep, other aspects of physical health are important in preparing for a test. Good nutrition is vital for good brain function. Sugary foods and drinks may give a burst of energy but this burst is followed by a crash, both physically and emotionally. Instead, fuel your body with protein and vitamin-rich foods.

Also, drink plenty of water. Dehydration can lead to headaches and exhaustion, especially if your brain is already under stress from the rigors of the test. Particularly if your test is a long one, drink water during the breaks. And if possible, take an energy-boosting snack to eat between sections.

Along with sleep and diet, a third important part of physical health is exercise. Maintaining a steady workout schedule is helpful, but even taking 5-minute study breaks to walk can help get your blood pumping faster and clear your head. Exercise also releases endorphins, which contribute to a positive feeling and can help combat test anxiety.

When you nurture your physical health, you are also contributing to your mental health. If your body is healthy, your mind is much more likely to be healthy as well. So take time to rest, nourish your body with healthy food and water, and get moving as much as possible. Taking these physical steps will make you stronger and more able to take the mental steps necessary to overcome test anxiety.

Mental Steps for Beating Test Anxiety

Working on the mental side of test anxiety can be more challenging, but as with the physical side, there are clear steps you can take to overcome it. As mentioned earlier, test anxiety often stems from lack of preparation, so the obvious solution is to prepare for the test. Effective studying may be the most important weapon you have for beating test anxiety, but you can and should employ several other mental tools to combat fear.

First, boost your confidence by reminding yourself of past success—tests or projects that you aced. If you're putting as much effort into preparing for this test as you did for those, there's no reason you should expect to fail here. Work hard to prepare; then trust your preparation.

Second, surround yourself with encouraging people. It can be helpful to find a study group, but be sure that the people you're around will encourage a positive attitude. If you spend time with others who are anxious or cynical, this will only contribute to your own anxiety. Look for others who are motivated to study hard from a desire to succeed, not from a fear of failure.

Third, reward yourself. A test is physically and mentally tiring, even without anxiety, and it can be helpful to have something to look forward to. Plan an activity following the test, regardless of the outcome, such as going to a movie or getting ice cream.

When you are taking the test, if you find yourself beginning to feel anxious, remind yourself that you know the material. Visualize successfully completing the test. Then take a few deep, relaxing breaths and return to it. Work through the questions carefully but with confidence, knowing that you are capable of succeeding.

Developing a healthy mental approach to test taking will also aid in other areas of life. Test anxiety affects more than just the actual test—it can be damaging to your mental health and even contribute to depression. It's important to beat test anxiety before it becomes a problem for more than testing.

Study Strategy

Being prepared for the test is necessary to combat anxiety, but what does being prepared look like? You may study for hours on end and still not feel prepared. What you need is a strategy for test prep. The next few pages outline our recommended steps to help you plan out and conquer the challenge of preparation.

Step 1: Scope Out the Test

Learn everything you can about the format (multiple choice, essay, etc.) and what will be on the test. Gather any study materials, course outlines, or sample exams that may be available. Not only will this help you to prepare, but knowing what to expect can help to alleviate test anxiety.

Step 2: Map Out the Material

Look through the textbook or study guide and make note of how many chapters or sections it has. Then divide these over the time you have. For example, if a book has 15 chapters and you have five days to study, you need to cover three chapters each day. Even better, if you have the time, leave an extra day at the end for overall review after you have gone through the material in depth.

If time is limited, you may need to prioritize the material. Look through it and make note of which sections you think you already have a good grasp on, and which need review. While you are studying, skim quickly through the familiar sections and take more time on the challenging parts.

Write out your plan so you don't get lost as you go. Having a written plan also helps you feel more in control of the study, so anxiety is less likely to arise from feeling overwhelmed at the amount to cover.

Step 3: Gather Your Tools

Decide what study method works best for you. Do you prefer to highlight in the book as you study and then go back over the highlighted portions? Or do you type out notes of the important information? Or is it helpful to make flashcards that you can carry with you? Assemble the pens, index cards, highlighters, post-it notes, and any other materials you may need so you won't be distracted by getting up to find things while you study.

If you're having a hard time retaining the information or organizing your notes, experiment with different methods. For example, try color-coding by subject with colored pens, highlighters, or post-it notes. If you learn better by hearing, try recording yourself reading your notes so you can listen while in the car, working out, or simply sitting at your desk. Ask a friend to quiz you from your flashcards, or try teaching someone the material to solidify it in your mind.

Step 4: Create Your Environment

It's important to avoid distractions while you study. This includes both the obvious distractions like visitors and the subtle distractions like an uncomfortable chair (or a too-comfortable couch that makes you want to fall asleep). Set up the best study environment possible: good lighting and a comfortable work area. If background music helps you focus, you may want to turn it on, but otherwise keep the room quiet. If you are using a computer to take notes, be sure you don't have any other windows open, especially applications like social media, games, or anything else that could distract you. Silence your phone and turn off notifications. Be sure to keep water close by so you stay hydrated while you study (but avoid unhealthy drinks and snacks).

Also, take into account the best time of day to study. Are you freshest first thing in the morning? Try to set aside some time then to work through the material. Is your mind clearer in the afternoon or evening? Schedule your study session then. Another method is to study at the same time of day that you will take the test, so that your brain gets used to working on the material at that time and will be ready to focus at test time.

Step 5: Study!

Once you have done all the study preparation, it's time to settle into the actual studying. Sit down, take a few moments to settle your mind so you can focus, and begin to follow your study plan. Don't give in to distractions or let yourself procrastinate. This is your time to prepare so you'll be ready to fearlessly approach the test. Make the most of the time and stay focused.

Of course, you don't want to burn out. If you study too long you may find that you're not retaining the information very well. Take regular study breaks. For example, taking five minutes out of every hour to walk briskly, breathing deeply and swinging your arms, can help your mind stay fresh.

As you get to the end of each chapter or section, it's a good idea to do a quick review. Remind yourself of what you learned and work on any difficult parts. When you feel that you've mastered the material, move on to the next part. At the end of your study session, briefly skim through your notes again.

But while review is helpful, cramming last minute is NOT. If at all possible, work ahead so that you won't need to fit all your study into the last day. Cramming overloads your brain with more information than it can process and retain, and your tired mind may struggle to recall even previously learned information when it is overwhelmed with last-minute study. Also, the urgent nature of cramming and the stress placed on your brain contribute to anxiety. You'll be more likely to go to the test feeling unprepared and having trouble thinking clearly.

So don't cram, and don't stay up late before the test, even just to review your notes at a leisurely pace. Your brain needs rest more than it needs to go over the information again. In fact, plan to finish your studies by noon or early afternoon the day before the test. Give your brain the rest of the day to relax or focus on other things, and get a good night's sleep. Then you will be fresh for the test and better able to recall what you've studied.

Step 6: Take a Practice Test

Many courses offer sample tests, either online or in the study materials. This is an excellent resource to check whether you have mastered the material, as well as to prepare for the test format and environment.

Check the test format ahead of time: the number of questions, the type (multiple choice, free response, etc.), and the time limit. Then create a plan for working through them. For example, if you have 30 minutes to take a 60-question test, your limit is 30 seconds per question. Spend less time on the questions you know well so that you can take more time on the difficult ones.

If you have time to take several practice tests, take the first one open book, with no time limit. Work through the questions at your own pace and make sure you fully understand them. Gradually work up to taking a test under test conditions: sit at a desk with all study materials put away and set a timer. Pace yourself to make sure you finish the test with time to spare and go back to check your answers if you have time.

After each test, check your answers. On the questions you missed, be sure you understand why you missed them. Did you misread the question (tests can use tricky wording)? Did you forget the information? Or was it something you hadn't learned? Go back and study any shaky areas that the practice tests reveal.

Taking these tests not only helps with your grade, but also aids in combating test anxiety. If you're already used to the test conditions, you're less likely to worry about it, and working through tests until you're scoring well gives you a confidence boost. Go through the practice tests until you feel comfortable, and then you can go into the test knowing that you're ready for it.

Test Tips

On test day, you should be confident, knowing that you've prepared well and are ready to answer the questions. But aside from preparation, there are several test day strategies you can employ to maximize your performance.

First, as stated before, get a good night's sleep the night before the test (and for several nights before that, if possible). Go into the test with a fresh, alert mind rather than staying up late to study.

Try not to change too much about your normal routine on the day of the test. It's important to eat a nutritious breakfast, but if you normally don't eat breakfast at all, consider eating just a protein bar. If you're a coffee drinker, go ahead and have your normal coffee. Just make sure you time it so that the caffeine doesn't wear off right in the middle of your test. Avoid sugary beverages, and drink enough water to stay hydrated but not so much that you need a restroom break 10 minutes into the test. If your test isn't first thing in the morning, consider going for a walk or doing a light workout before the test to get your blood flowing.

Allow yourself enough time to get ready, and leave for the test with plenty of time to spare so you won't have the anxiety of scrambling to arrive in time. Another reason to be early is to select a good seat. It's helpful to sit away from doors and windows, which can be distracting. Find a good seat, get out your supplies, and settle your mind before the test begins.

When the test begins, start by going over the instructions carefully, even if you already know what to expect. Make sure you avoid any careless mistakes by following the directions.

Then begin working through the questions, pacing yourself as you've practiced. If you're not sure on an answer, don't spend too much time on it, and don't let it shake your confidence. Either skip it and come back later, or eliminate as many wrong answers as possible and guess among the remaining ones. Don't dwell on these questions as you continue—put them out of your mind and focus on what lies ahead.

Be sure to read all of the answer choices, even if you're sure the first one is the right answer. Sometimes you'll find a better one if you keep reading. But don't second-guess yourself if you do immediately know the answer. Your gut instinct is usually right. Don't let test anxiety rob you of the information you know.

If you have time at the end of the test (and if the test format allows), go back and review your answers. Be cautious about changing any, since your first instinct tends to be correct, but make sure you didn't misread any of the questions or accidentally mark the wrong answer choice. Look over any you skipped and make an educated guess.

At the end, leave the test feeling confident. You've done your best, so don't waste time worrying about your performance or wishing you could change anything. Instead, celebrate the successful completion of this test. And finally, use this test to learn how to deal with anxiety even better next time.

Review Video: Test Anxiety
Visit mometrix.com/academy and enter code: 100340

Important Qualification

Not all anxiety is created equal. If your test anxiety is causing major issues in your life beyond the classroom or testing center, or if you are experiencing troubling physical symptoms related to your anxiety, it may be a sign of a serious physiological or psychological condition. If this sounds like your situation, we strongly encourage you to seek professional help.

Additional Bonus Material

Due to our efforts to try to keep this book to a manageable length, we've created a link that will give you access to all of your additional bonus material:

mometrix.com/bonus948/cnor

www.ingramcontent.com/pod-product-compliance
Lightning Source LLC
LaVergne TN
LVHW081527100826
845153LV00003B/220